Crafts and Creative Media in Therapy

Fourth Edition

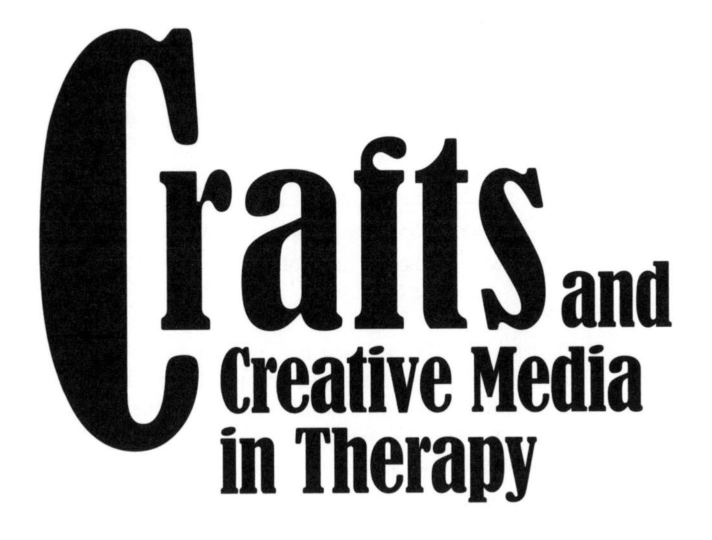

Fourth Edition

Carol Crellin Tubbs, MA, OTR/L
University of Mississippi Medical Center
Jackson, Mississippi

Margaret Drake, PhD, OTR/L, ATR-BC, LPAT, FAOTA
Retired Professor
University of Mississippi Medical Center
Jackson, Mississippi

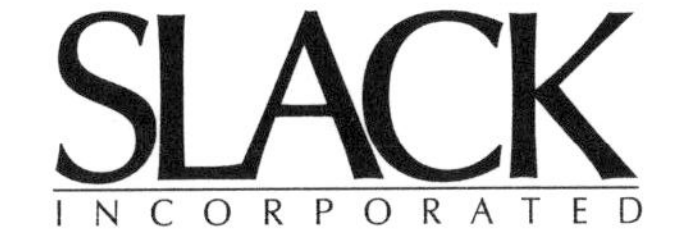

www.slackbooks.com

ISBN: 978-1-55642-976-7

Carol Crellin Tubbs and Margaret Drake have no financial or proprietary interest in the materials presented herein.

Crafts and Creative Media in Therapy, Fourth Edition includes ancillary materials specifically available for faculty use. Included are lesson plans, discussion questions, and activity ideas. Please visit www.efacultylounge.com to obtain access.

The procedures and practices described in this publication should be implemented in a manner consistent with the professional standards set for the circumstances that apply in each specific situation. Every effort has been made to confirm the accuracy of the information presented and to correctly relate generally accepted practices. The authors, editors, and publisher cannot accept responsibility for errors or exclusions or for the outcome of the material presented herein. There is no expressed or implied warranty of this book or information imparted by it. Care has been taken to ensure that drug selection and dosages are in accordance with currently accepted/recommended practice. Off-label uses of drugs may be discussed. Due to continuing research, changes in government policy and regulations, and various effects of drug reactions and interactions, it is recommended that the reader carefully review all materials and literature provided for each drug, especially those that are new or not frequently used. Some drugs or devices in this publication have clearance for use in a restricted research setting by the Food and Drug and Administration or FDA. Each professional should determine the FDA status of any drug or device prior to use in their practice.

Any review or mention of specific companies or products is not intended as an endorsement by the author or publisher.

SLACK Incorporated uses a review process to evaluate submitted material. Prior to publication, educators or clinicians provide important feedback on the content that we publish. We welcome feedback on this work.

Published by: SLACK Incorporated
6900 Grove Road
Thorofare, NJ 08086 USA
Telephone: 856-848-1000
Fax: 856-848-6091
www.slackbooks.com

Contact SLACK Incorporated for more information about other books in this field or about the availability of our books from distributors outside the United States.

Library of Congress Cataloging-in-Publication Data

Tubbs, Carol, 1959-
Crafts and creative media in therapy / Carol Tubbs, Magaret Drake. -- 4th ed.
p. ; cm.
Includes bibliographical references and index.
ISBN 978-1-55642-976-7 (alk. paper)
I. Drake, Margaret, 1940- II. Title.
[DNLM: 1. Occupational Therapy--methods. 2. Art Therapy--methods. WB 555]
LC classification not assigned
615.8'515--dc23

2011045464

Printed in the United States of America.

Last digit is print number: 10 9 8 7 6 5 4 3 2

Contents

Crafts and Creative Media in Therapy, Fourth Edition includes ancillary materials specifically available for faculty use. Included are lesson plans, discussion questions, and activity ideas. Please visit www.efacultylounge.com to obtain access.

Acknowledgements

With the completion of this *Fourth Edition*, I want to once again thank Dr. Margaret Drake for entrusting this project to me in the first place, and for being the inspiration that she is to everyone she meets. Thank you to therapists Stacey Dupre and Pauline du Plessis for sharing their testimonials on the benefits of crafting, and for keeping them alive in the clinic. I would also like to extend my sincere appreciation to friends and coworkers: Drs. Lorraine Street and Tonia Taylor—for their daily encouragement and willingness to be frequent sounding boards, and for loaning me some of their books; Dr. Dona Lee Andrew—especially for her help with class during the final stages of manuscript completion; Joyce Titus and Jeff Foster—for their helpful ideas, valuable feedback about the use of this text, and advocacy of crafts in the OT curriculum; Dr. Christy Morgan, my department chair, and Bette Groat, my former department chair—for their support of this project and their confidence in my ability to do it; and Kayla Abraham, Robin Davis, and Peter Giroux—for their patience, support, and sympathetic ears throughout this process (and I probably borrowed some of their books too!).

An extra thank you to Sandy Lowman, our administrative assistant, for her ready smile and willingness to help, even in the midst of her own deadlines. Thank you to students Lori Swords, Christa Anderson, Megan Wood, Monica Bane, and Anna Deen—crafters all—for being photographic models in the book and sharing neat craft ideas with me. And a special thank you to Megan Wood for her insight and keen observation skills, and her willingness to share them with the readers of this book.

I am eternally grateful to all the rest of my students, past and present, for being such an inspiration and the reason I enjoy going to work every day. Most especially the last few groups of craft lovers—classes of 2010, 2011, 2012, 2013—you know who you are. Thank you to my mom, the youngest "older adult" I've ever known, who never doubts that I can do anything; and lastly to my husband, for his patience, his humor, and his affirmation of my efforts every step of the way.

—Carol Crellin Tubbs

About the Authors

Carol Crellin Tubbs, MA, OTR/L has been a practicing occupational therapist for 25 years. A graduate of the Louisiana State University (Baton Rouge, Louisiana) Occupational Therapy program, she is currently an associate professor and assistant chair at the University of Mississippi Medical Center (Jackson, Mississippi) in the School of Health Related Professions. she has served as an Item Writer for NBCOT and practices on an as-needed basis in an outpatient clinic. She is involved with a community homeless program, and along with her students and other faculty, enjoys working with the population there on crafts and other productive activities. She is a lifetime crafter and believes in the healing and skill-building power of creative involvement.

Margaret Drake, PhD, OTR/L, ATR-BC, LPAT, FAOTA splits her time between writing historical novels, typing family documents (e.g., her mother's 1912 diary) to preserve them for future generations, volunteering for civic groups, and most recently, returning to professional work in long-term care on an "on-call" basis after a 5-year hiatus from practice following retirement from the University of Mississippi Medical Center.

Preface

A group of occupational therapy students at the University of Mississippi Medical Center recently completed a survey regarding the prevailing use of crafts and other creative media in the profession. Not surprisingly, they found that many therapists do not use them at all, or use them only seldom in daily practice. The primary reasons cited were cost, lack of time, inability to explain their benefits to patients, and insecurity about documenting the use of these activities for reimbursement. The *Fourth Edition* of this text was written with these barriers in mind. The first section of the book provides justification for and examples of the successful use of creative media in therapeutic programs; the second section contains practical tips for the implementation of crafts/creative activities; and the third section contains basic information about the crafts themselves. More ideas have been added to assist the student and practicing therapist in planning appropriate activities and providing rationale, such as tips for activity preparation, approximate cost and time required, ways to vary and grade the project, and suggestions for ways to document the session. The text resources have been updated, and this edition also contains more Internet resources and ways of thinking about crafts far beyond the traditional state hospital tile mosaic ashtray. Occupational therapists can and should capitalize on the current media attention on the "do-it-yourselfer" and the online market for handcrafted goods. An instructor's manual for the *Fourth Edition* is also available at www.efacultylounge.com; it provides suggestions for structuring classes around craft activities and also contains additional resources.

While crafts are assuredly not appropriate for *every* patient, they are appropriate and preferable for some. Crafts are uniquely suited to address the whole person and certainly have a stronger relationship to occupation than do physical agent modalities or rote exercise. Since the thoughtful, skilled application of crafts and other creative activities in rehabilitation seems to be one of the last areas of which OT seems to have sole possession, it is important that students and practitioners realize that the judicious use of crafts can be done without excessive cost or time, can be reimbursed as readily as other modalities, and can sometimes motivate a patient to participate in therapy like no other therapeutic approach.

Section I

Why Use Crafts?

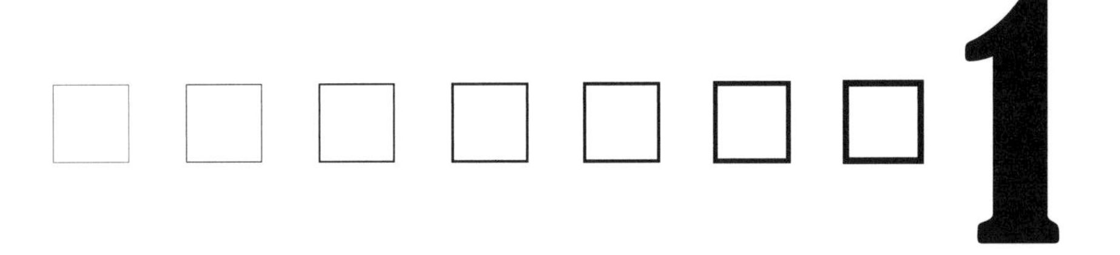

Introduction
Crafts in Perspective

Objectives

The student should be able to:

- Describe the historical roots of craftwork and its cultural significance
- Give examples from the past of the use of crafts in healing
- Describe trends in craft use in occupational therapy since the founding of the profession
- Explain the benefits of crafts and other creative activities as therapeutic tools
- Describe how crafts promote integrated brain function and are consistent with the holistic philosophy of occupational therapy

[1]*Craft (kraft)*: an occupation or trade requiring manual dexterity or artistic skill
[2]*Craft:* to make or produce with care, skill, or ingenuity

—*Merriam Webster's Collegiate Dictionary* (1994)

Add "–craft" to any production process and it seems to take on a more noble connotation (e.g., compare woodwork to woodcraft, or cooking to culinary craft). Many of the occupations we consider crafts were once work, partially accounting for their significance in early occupational therapy. Prior to the development of mass production methods, needed articles such as furniture had to be crafted by hand. Our earliest ancestors used animal hides to make shelters and clothing, and clay vessels to hold food and water. As civilization progressed, other crafted creations, such as mosaics and jewelry, had a more aesthetic purpose and held importance in religious, ritualistic, and cultural realms. Both productive and creative processes, in one form or another, have always been—and will probably always be—part of human existence. They also embody the holistic approach of occupational therapy: both utilitarian and beautiful, of both manual and spiritual origin.

Over the centuries, certain crafts were connected with a particular culture/ethnicity, socioeconomic status, or gender. Pottery and weaving were associated with goddess worship, suggesting that these crafts were invented by women (Eisler, 1987). Women originated other crafts as well, probably to assist them in their primary role as mother and nurturer. They made cradles and cradleboards from wood and leather to carry babies on their backs while they gathered food or tended animals. In hunter-gatherer cultures, men killed and brought home game, but women prepared the hides (Boserup, 1970; Danday, 1981; Morgan, 1972; Rich, 1976) and sewed them together for clothes, shelter, and food containers. With the development of metal,

Tubbs, C., & Drake, M. *Crafts and Creative Media in Therapy, Fourth Edition (pp. 3-10).*

men began crafting weapons and tools. As patriarchy prevailed, men took over many prestigious crafts such as woodworking and pottery. When the industrial revolution rendered many handicrafts obsolete, those that remained (e.g., needlework and china painting) again became the province of women (Boserup, 1970; Danday, 1981; Morgan, 1972; Rich, 1976; Sochen, 1974; Whyte, 1978). Men continued to dominate woodworking, leather craft, and pottery in western culture; the decline in status for some other crafts may have related to their continued identification with women. It is interesting to note that, regardless of region or environment, skills were developed universally for certain kinds of crafts, such as pottery, basketry, and fabric-making (Breines, 1995).

Documentation of arts and crafts in the treatment of illness is scarce until the late 18th century; however, music as treatment is commonly mentioned among the ancients (Willard & Spackman, 1947). Since early crafts were undoubtedly a necessity for daily function—even survival—they may not have been recognized as having the healing properties that we attribute to crafts today. Although Rich (1976) perceived early arts such as weaving and pottery as having magical qualities, rituals and taboos have been given more credit for cures among primitive peoples than have crafts (Achternecht, 1971).

Galen, the Greek physician who adopted Rome as his home, recommended exercise (MacKenzie, 1979) and thought patients were healed by being occupied (Willard & Spackman, 1954); however, he did not specify crafts. The Arabs adopted portions of Greek and Roman medicine; Ibn Jazlah, an Arabic physician in the Middle Ages (500 to 1500 AD), recommended physical treatments such as baths and exercise (Granziani, 1980). Some tribes of Native Americans, such as the Navajo and Cheyenne, have traditionally used painting and sand painting in healing and medicine (Achternecht, 1971).

Beginning around the Middle Ages and for centuries thereafter, these compassionate forms of healing treatment were abandoned. Then, at the beginning of the 19th century, Phillipe Pinel persuaded tradesmen in Paris to give craftwork to his asylum patients in Aisle de Bicetre; throughout Europe, similar developments in more humane treatment followed (Pinel, 1806). At about the same time, Dr. Benjamin Rush, a signer of the Declaration of Independence and father of American psychiatry, used work therapy—and some crafts—with his clients at Pennsylvania Hospital in Philadelphia, founded in 1751 as the nation's first hospital (Haworth & MacDonald, 1946; Willard & Spackman, 1954). By mid-century, patients' craftwork was being advertised for sale in London (Haworth & MacDonald 1946). "Activity" became synonymous with "craft" and crafts were often used with upper and middle class patients as an alternative to manual labor (Holder, 2001). Throughout the rest of the 1800's, many mental hospitals developed programs that included occupations, amusements, and crafts.

One of the first professional writings about crafts in occupational therapy is *Studies in Invalid Occupations* (Tracy, 1910). The author, Susan Tracy, espoused utilizing activities that were motivating and engaging, as she reasoned these elements were essential for recovery (Kielhofner, 2004). She was the first to utilize and promote specific crafts for specific physical or psychological needs. Tracy described the various contents and scheduling of the "occupation room" and emphasized the importance of a skilled leader (Tracy in Kielhofner, 2004). From that time on, publications in occupational therapy began to include instructions on how to use crafts to treat clients. A 2005 issue of *Occupational Therapy in Health Care* reprised the work of Dr. Herbert J. Hall, another pioneer in the use of crafts as a rehabilitation tool and influential force in early occupational therapy practice (Anthony, 2005). In the late 1930s, craftwork was the chief method of occupational therapy in the British Isles and practitioners related them to capacities and health conditions (Hocking, 2007). In the United States, craft use was prevalent in every treatment setting, including general medicine; surgery; tuberculosis sanitariums; and across practice specialties such as pediatrics, orthopedics, and psychiatry (Breines, 2008). A 1943 *New Yorker* magazine article described the use of crafts in a military hospital: "Most of the boys make leather lanyards for their identification tags or ashtrays for their girls...Some have bits of plastic from the turrets of planes and turn them into heart-shaped trinkets." Convalescing soldiers also made belts, clay objects, scarves, toys, and dioramas (Hamburger, 1943).

A look at the indices and tables of contents of the profession's textbooks over the years gives some insight into how crafts were viewed. A 1945 text, *Prescribing Occupational Therapy* (Dunton), had a 10-page section entitled "Suggestions of the Use of Crafts in Functional Restoration," plus a guide for selection that emphasized craft quality and usefulness.

The very first edition of *Principles of Occupational Therapy*, by Willard and Spackman (1947), lists seven crafts under activities in the index. The word "handicrafts" was used to define another 18 items. All but one of the 15 photographs shows a craft in progress. The second edition, *Principles of Occupational Therapy* (1954), does not use the word crafts in the index, but under activities, lists 14 separate crafts. One section of the chapter "Activities in Occupational Therapy" is titled "Handicrafts."

Most of the "Activities Suggested to Provide Treatment" in the third edition (Willard & Spackman, 1963) are crafts; however, a glance through the table of contents and index gives almost no hint that crafts are a major activity or occupation. Growing concern over the image of occupational therapy regarding the use of crafts is evident in the Eleanor Clark Slagle lecture given by Mary Reilly in the early 1960s. Reilly eloquently states, "The wide and gaping chasm which exists between the complexity of illness and the commonplaceness of our treatment tools, is, and always will be, both the pride and the anguish of our profession" (1962, p. 87). As the diversional use of crafts became the public's perception of the domain of occupational therapy, practitioners became increasingly uncomfortable with their use and began to distance themselves from them (Holder, 2001).

The fourth edition of Willard and Spackman's *Occupational Therapy* (1971) continues to list crafts under "Activities for Restoration of Function," but by the fifth edition (Hopkins & Smith, 1978), one must search to find any allusion to crafts. More generic terms such as functional activities or avocational activities are used instead. This trend continued, and the seventh edition (Hopkins & Smith, 1988) has listings for computers over crafts at eleven to one. In the eighth edition (Hopkins & Smith, 1993), crafts are only named as components of assessments, and photographs show formal assessments that have taken pieces of crafts and isolated them as evaluation tools. The ninth edition (Neistadt & Crepeau, 1997) has photographs of expressive activities such as art, dance, and related crafts, while the eleventh edition places greater emphasis on play, and recreational and social activities in terms of leisure (Crepeau, Cohn, & Schell, 2009).

In 1991, a new comprehensive occupational therapy textbook, *Occupational Therapy: Overcoming Performance Deficits* (Christiansen & Baum, 1991), was published. Case studies in the text portrayed clients involved in crafts but other terms such as *hobbies* and *the arts* were used to describe them. The second edition (1997) mentions crafts incidental to their use as assessments such as the Draw-A-Person test, the Allen Cognitive Levels Screening, and Lerner's Magazine Picture Collage. Crafts are mentioned or discussed in newer publications related to mental health and pediatric practice (Bonder & Bello-Haas, 2009; Brown & Stoffel, 2011; Bruce & Borg, 1993, 2002; Case-Smith, 2010; Christiansen, 1994; Cottrell, 1996; Cynkin & Robinson, 1990; Drake, 2004; Early, 1993, 2009; Hellen, 2004; Henderson & Pehoski, 2006) but less so in those related to physical dysfunction (Pendleton & Schultz-Krohn, 2006; Radomski & Latham, 2008). This appears to be consistent with their current use in practice (Griffiths & Corr, 2007; Griffin, Greer, Everaert, & Struble, 2003; TeBeest, Kornstedt, Feldmann, Harmasch, & Kemnitz, 2001; Whittington, Weir, Powell, Mumbower, & Foster, 2010). The most common reasons given for the nonuse of crafts are insecurity about reimbursement, lack of time and resources, inability to do crafts personally, or lack of applicability to the therapeutic purpose (Griffin et al., 2003; TeBeest et al., 2001; Whittington et al., 2010). Some years ago, Barris, Kielhofner, and Watts (1988) attributed the diminishing discussion of crafts in occupational therapy "to the general devaluation of handmade objects in American culture."

So why is the use of crafts in occupational therapy still a topic to be explored? Are creative pursuits still viable treatment media in the age of shortened hospital stays, limited healthcare dollars, and technological revolution? As medical diagnostic and treatment technology has mushroomed, occupational therapy has been forced to appear more scientific, and crafts seem the very antithesis of this. Some therapists may view exercise and physical agent modalities as more consistent with our work-oriented culture, where crafts have come to symbolize a leisure time activity rather than real work. Many others, however, have long intuitively understood that crafts help restore skills in a multitude of areas. Some of the benefits cited by practitioners include improved problem solving, perceptual skills, motor skills, attention to task, increased self-esteem and sense of mastery, and more ease in communication and social skills (Amini, 2002; Griffiths & Corr, 2007; National Institute of Art and Disabilities, 2011). Clients are more motivated and become absorbed by creative activities, which facilitates faster achievement of goals (Griffin et al., 2003; McEvoy, 2007). Crafts can be easily graded, and clients like them because they have no requirement for disclosure of personal information and they are activities associated with "normal" rather than "unwell" people (Griffiths & Corr, 2007). Crafts are beneficial across contexts, promoting knowledge/skills, health/life balance, and culture/community inclusion (Pollanen, 2009).

More empirical evidence suggests that craft involvement has an impact on brain function. Crafts are able to naturally activate the spatial and intuitive functions of the nondominant side of the brain (Leask & Crow, 1997; Miller, 1988a, 1988b; Rosenfeld, 1988) and this fact is gradually being authenticated through research (Boucher & Bryden, 1997; Corballis & Beals, 1983; Herrmann, 1988; Thibodaux & Ludwig, 1988) as more is discovered about brain lateralization and localized specialization. The right hemisphere of the brain is linked to intuition, images and emotion, while the left hemisphere is responsible for analytical and detail-oriented tasks (Miller, 1988b). Since we know that leisure in general, and crafts in particular, involve expression of emotion and focused attention and skill, an outlet for the imagination and a more technical analysis of success (Olsen & Roarty-O'Herron, 2000), we infer that these occupations help integrate the function of both hemispheres (Flood & Phillips, 2007). In addition, a richly stimulating environment is thought to increase the number of neuronal connections in the brain (Cohen, et al. 2006). Miller (1988a) hypothesized that rehabilitation that addresses only physical problems may be less effective because the emotional component of recovery is neglected.

There is other documented evidence to show why crafts may actually be more efficient in rehabilitation than exercise or other activities (Lin, 1997; Stancliff, 1996). Lin (1997) found that occupational form affects performance; the brain is able to discern meaning from a familiar or purposeful activity because it makes perceptual and cognitive associations that may not exist with contrived or exercise-based activity. For example, placing small pegs in a pegboard has no memory base for most people, so the brain is unable to associate it with previous experiences or skills. Threading beads to make a necklace, however, may activate multiple pathways to stored perceptual and cognitive information because of its associations with certain sensory stimuli, past memories/experiences, and/or visualization of a final product. In another study, Thibodeaux and Ludwig (1988) found that subjects worked for longer durations on a sanding project without perceiving exertion when the wood piece was part of an end product, as opposed to sanding a free-standing (nonfunctional) board.

Research has shown that:

- Creative activities integrate left brain functions (verbal, analytical, detail-oriented) with right brain functions (intuitive, emotional, image-linked)
- Occupational form activates multiple areas of the brain through associations with previously stored information
- Purposeful activity reduces the perception of exertion

Crafts are part of the foundation of occupational therapy treatment; while some place more value on the use of technological methods—subconsciously or otherwise—this diminishes the complexity of what can be accomplished with the combination of hands and bodies, minds and spirits. The truth is that while the use of crafts in therapy has changed (Taylor & Manguna, 1991), many occupational therapists, treating clients with both physical and mental illnesses across the life span, do continue to use basic crafts or other creative activities in treatment (Griffin et al., 2003; Griffiths & Corr, 2007; Huebner, Custer, Freudenberger, & Nichols, 2006; TeBeest et al., 2001; Whittington et al., 2010). What may have started as a diversion from life's troubles or simply a means of humane treatment—then came to be seen as an agent of therapeutic change—can now be included as a means of enablement in occupational functioning (Polatajko, 2001). Crafts in particular help clients realize accomplishment through taking basic materials and processing, assembling, and forming them; they perceive that they can do the same with their lives. Crafts are a microcosm of life; one receives raw materials and through a series of efforts, waiting periods, and guidance, one creates a craft product—one lives a life. Successful completion of a craft—the generation of something completely new—may instill hope for other aspects of life (Amini, 2002; Olsen & Roarty-O'Herron, 2000; Perrin, 2001). The creative process mirrors the rhythm and structure seen in healthy, balanced occupation (Christiansen & Townsend, 2004). Crafts call on one's manual dexterity, attention to detail, and problem-solving ability; they provide tangible proof of self (Fidler & Velde, 1999). For adults, crafts offer an opportunity to make choices, exert control, and re-establish a productive role (Amini, 2002; Christiansen & Townsend, 2004; Schwartzberg, 2002). For children, they contain the important learning elements of play, such as repetition, experimentation, imitation, and active involvement (Chandler, 1997; Diffendal, 2002). They also enhance prevocational skills such as hand dexterity, concentration, the ability to follow directions, and creativity (Burkhardt, 2000; Cochran, 2010). For elders, crafts and other creative pursuits have been shown to have a positive effect on overall health (Cohen et al., 2006). Crafts require both physical and mental engagement on the part of the participant.

Crafts: A Microcosm of Life

The making of a craft project entails:

- Rhythm and awareness of time
- Structure and following rules
- Opportunities for control and making choices
- Occasional resistance to efforts
- Periods of activity alternated with periods of waiting
- Trial and error, and encountering novel situations
- Both mental and physical engagement
- Expression of likes, dislikes, and individual identity
- A productive role
- Opportunity for success, failure, and learning
- Creation of something transformed or new

While use of crafts should not be a blanket approach to occupational therapy treatment, it is important to retain them as a treatment alternative. They can provide more cultural and personal relevance than many other treatment choices and simultaneously address the more measurable components of function (Harris, 2008). Although other professions (e.g., recreational therapy) may utilize crafts in their repertoire of leisure activities, the treatment objectives are different. The purpose of any occupational therapy intervention should be to restore a person to some level of occupational wholeness, an integral part of one's sense of identity and community, health, and well-being. In addition, in order to maintain a client-centered focus, it should be neither static nor prescriptive (Hooper, 2010). Through careful activity analysis, creative activities allow occupational therapy to offer a unique intervention that both avoids duplication of services (Bissel & Mailloux, 1981) and meets clients' individual occupational needs (Hooper, 2010; Robinson, Kennedy, & Harmon, 2011). Neither occupational therapy nor its practitioners should live in the past; as a group we will continue to refine theory, and as individuals we will continue to develop our skills in choosing the best occupation or activity for each client. We should, however, hold on to that which is true and good from the inception of the profession. In an era where efficiency and outcome are the buzzwords, this book seeks to help crafts keep a voice in the ongoing "best practice" debate.

Discussion Questions

1. Describe the role of crafts or other creative activities in your own life, or in that of close friends or family.
2. Are crafts still relevant and useful in occupational therapy? Why or why not?
3. How can our profession continue to use crafts/creative media and maintain a respected place among healthcare professions?

References

Achternecht, E. H. (1971). *Medicine and ethnology: Elements and exercises.* Lawrence, KS: The University of Kansas Press.

Amini, D. (2002). Let's give a thumbs up for crafts. *Advance for Occupational Therapy Practitioners, 18*(23), 5.

Anthony, S. H. (2005). Dr. Herbert J. Hall: Originator of honest work for occupational therapy 1904-1923 (parts I and II). *Occupational Therapy in Health Care, 19*(3), 3-32.

Barris, R., Kielhofner, G., & Watts, J. (1988). *Occupational therapy in psychosocial practice.* Thorofare, NJ: SLACK Incorporated.

Bissel, J. C., & Mailloux, Z. (1981). The use of crafts in occupational therapy for the physically disabled. *American Journal of Occupational Therapy, 35*(6), 369-374.

Bonder, B. R., & Bello-Haas, V. D. (2009). *Functional performance in older adults* (3rd ed.). Philadelphia, PA: F. A. Davis.

Boserup, E. (1970). *Women's role in economic development.* London, UK: George Allen and Unwin.
Boucher, R., & Bryden, M. P. (1997). Laterality effects in the processing of melody and timbre. *Neuro-psychologia, 35*(11), 1467-1473.
Breines, E. B. (1995). *Occupational therapy activities from clay to computers: Theory and practice.* Philadelphia, PA: F. A. Davis.
Breines, E. B. (2008). Crafts in education: Once upon a time. *Advance for Occupational Therapy Practitioners, 24*(6), 15.
Brown, C., & Stoffel, V. C. (Eds.). (2011). *Occupational therapy in mental health: A vision for participation.* Philadelphia, PA: F. A. Davis.
Bruce, M. A., & Borg, B. (1993). *Psychosocial occupational therapy: Frames of reference for intervention* (2nd ed.). Thorofare, NJ: SLACK Incorporated.
Bruce, M. A., & Borg, B. (2002). *Psychosocial occupational therapy: Frames of reference for intervention* (3rd ed.). Thorofare, NJ: SLACK Incorporated.
Burkhardt, A. (2000). The application of activities to practice. In J. Hinojosa, & M. Blount (Eds.), *The texture of life: Purposeful activities in occupational therapy,* (pp. 129-158). Bethesda, MD: American Occupational Therapy Association.
Case-Smith, J., Allen, A. S., & Pratt, P. N. (2010). *Occupational therapy for children* (6th ed.). St. Louis, MO: Mosby.
Chandler, B. E. (Ed.). (1997). *The essence of play: A child's occupation.* Bethesda, MD: American Occupational Therapy Association.
Christiansen, C. (Ed.). (1994). *Ways of living: Self-care strategies for special needs.* Rockville, MD: American Occupational Therapy Association.
Christiansen, C., & Baum, C. (1991). *Occupational therapy: Overcoming human performance deficits.* Thorofare, NJ: SLACK Incorporated.
Christiansen, C., & Baum, C. (1997). *Occupational therapy: Enabling function and well-being* (2nd ed.). Thorofare, NJ: SLACK Incorporated.
Christiansen, C., & Townsend, E. (2004). *Introduction to occupation: The art and science of living.* Upper Saddle River, NJ: Prentice Hall.
Cochran, M. (2010). OT's creative principles help blind adolescents build skills. *Advance for Occupational Therapy Practitioners, 26*(22), 24.
Cohen, G., Perlstein, S., Chapline, J., Kelly, J., Firth, K., & Simmens, S. (2006). The impact of professionally conducted culturally programs on the physical health, mental health and social functioning of older adults. *The Gerontologist, 46*(6), 726-734.
Corballis, M., & Beals, I. (1983). *The ambivalent mind.* Chicago, IL: Nelson-Hall.
Cottrell, R. P. F. (1996). *Perspectives on purposeful activity: Foundation and future of occupational therapy.* Bethesda, MD: American Occupational Therapy Association.
Crepeau, E., Cohn, E., Schell, B.A. (Eds.). (2009). *Willard and Spackman's occupational therapy* (11th ed.). Philadelphia, PA: Lippincott Williams & Wilkins.
Cynkin, S., & Robinson, A. M. (1990). *Occupational health and activities health: Toward health through activities.* Boston, MA: Little, Brown and Company.
Danday, P. R. (1981). *Female power and male dominance: On the origin of sexual inequality.* Cambridge, UK: Cambridge University Press.
Diffendal, J. (2002). Kids, through the use of their hands.... *Advance for Occupational Therapy Practitioners, 18*(22), 12.
Drake, M. (2004). Working with elders who have psychiatric conditions. In S. Byers-Connon, H. Lohman, & R. Padilla (Eds.), *Occupational therapy with elders: strategies for the COTA* (2nd ed., pp. 269-279). St. Louis, MO: Elsevier Mosby.
Dunton, W. R. (1945). *Prescribing occupational therapy* (2nd ed.). Springfield, IL: Charles C. Thomas.
Early, M. B. (1993). *Mental health concepts and techniques for the occupational therapy assistant* (2nd ed.). New York, NY: Raven Press.
Early, M. B. (2009). *Mental health concepts and techniques for the occupational therapy assistant* (4th ed.). Philadelphia, PA: Lippincott Williams & Wilkins.
Eisler, R. (1987). *The chalice and the blade.* New York, NY: Harper and Row.
Fidler, G., & Velde, E. (1999). *Activities: Reality and symbol.* Thorofare, NJ: SLACK Incorporated.
Flood, M., & Phillips, K. D. (2007). Creativity in older adults: A plethora of possibilities. *Issues in Mental Health Nursing, 28,* 389-411.
Granziani, J. S. (1980). *Arabic medicine in the eleventh century as represented in the works of Ibn Jazlah.* Karachi, Pakistan: Hamard Academy Press.
Griffin, C., Greer, M., Everaert, C., & Struble, J. (2003). Arts and crafts, alive and well in OT? *Advance for Occupational Therapy Practitioners, 19*(12), 14.
Griffiths, S., & Corr, S. (2007). The use of creative activities with people with mental health problems: a survey of occupational therapists. *The British Journal of Occupational Therapy, 79*(3), 107-114.
Hambuger, P. (1943, September 25). The boys in maroon. *The New Yorker,* pp. 46-54.
Harris, E. (2008). The meanings of craft to an occupational therapist. *Australian Occupational Therapy Journal, 55,* 133-142.
Haworth, N. A., & MacDonald, E. M. (1946). *Theory of occupational therapy.* Baltimore, MD: Lippincott Williams & Wilkins.
Hellen, C. (2004). Working with elders who have dementia and Alzheimer's disease. In S. Byers-Connon, H. Lohman, & R. Padilla (Eds.), *Occupational therapy with elders: Strategies for the COTA* (2nd ed., pp. 254-268). St. Louis, MO: Elsevier Mosby.
Henderson, A. & Pehoski, C. (2006). *Hand function in the child: Foundations for remediation* (2nd ed.). St. Louis: Mosby/Elsevier.
Herrmann, N. (1988). *The creative brain.* Lake Lure, NC: Applied Creative Services.
Hocking, C. (2007). Early perspectives of patients, practice and profession. *The British Journal of Occupational Therapy, 70*(7), 284-291.
Holder, V. (2001). The use of creative activities with occupational therapy. *The British Journal of Occupational Therapy, 64*(2), 103-105.
Hooper, B. (2010). On arriving at the destination of the centennial vision: Navigational landmarks to guide occupational therapy education. *Occupational Therapy in Health Care, 24*(1), 97-106
Hopkins, H. L., & Smith, H. D. (1978). *Willard and Spackman's occupational therapy* (5th ed.). Philadelphia, PA: Lippincott Williams & Wilkins.
Hopkins, H. L., & Smith, H. D. (1988). *Willard and Spackman's occupational therapy* (7th ed.). Philiadelphia, PA: Lippincott Williams & Wilkins.
Hopkins, H. L., & Smith, H. D. (1993). *Willard and Spackman's occupational therapy* (8th ed.). Philadelphia, PA: Lippincott Williams & Wilkins.

Huebner, R. A., Custer, M. G., Freudenberger, L., & Nichols, L. (2006). The occupational therapy practice checklist for adult physical rehabilitation. *American Journal of Occupational Therapy, 60*(4), 388-396.
Kielhofner, G. (2004). *Conceptual foundations of occupational therapy* (3rd ed.). Philadelphia, PA: F. A. Davis.
Leask, S. J., & Crow, T. J. (1997). How far does the brain lateralize? An unbiased method for determining the optimum degree of hemispheric specialization. *Neuropsychologia, 35*(10), 1381-1387.
Lin, K. C. (1997). Enhancing occupational performance through occupationally embedded exercise: A meta-analytic review. *The Occupational Therapy Journal of Research, 17*(11), 25-47
MacKenzie, J. (1979). *The history of health and art of preserving it.* New York, NY: Arno Press.
McEvoy, D. (2007). If you want cooperation, go back to basics. *Advance for Occupational Therapy Practitioners, 23*(25), 45.
Merriam Webster (Ed.). (1994). *Merriam Webster's collegiate dictionary* (10th ed.). Springfield, MA: Merriam-Webster, Incorporated.
Miller, L. (1988a). The emotional brain. *Psychology Today, 22*(2), 34-42.
Miller, L. (1988b). Men without passion. *Psychology Today, 22*(12), 20-22.
Morgan, E. (1972). *The descent of women.* New York, NY: Stein and Day.
National Institute of Art and Disabilities. (2011). *Arts in aging resource list.* Retrieved from www.NEA.gov/Resources/Accessibility/rlists/ArtsAging.html.
Neistadt, M. E., & Crepeau E. B. (1997). *Willard and Spackman's occupational therapy* (9th ed.). Philadelphia, PA: Lippincott Williams & Wilkins.
Olsen, L. J., & Roarty-O'Herron, E. A. (2000). Range of human activity: Leisure. In J. Hinojosa, & M. Blount (Eds.), *The texture of life: Purposeful activities in occupational therapy*, (pp. 258-288). Bethesda, MD: American Occupational Therapy Association.
Pendleton, H. M., & Schultz-Krohn, W. (Eds.). (2006). *Pedretti's occupational therapy: Practice skills for physical dysfunction* (6th ed.). Philadelphia, PA: Elsevier
Perrin, T. (2001). Don't despise the fluffy bunny: A reflection from practice. *The British Journal of Occupational Therapy, 64*(3), 129-134.
Pinel, P. (1806). *Traite medico-philosophique de l'alienation mentale.* Paris, France: J. A. Brosson.
Polatajko, H. J. (2001). The evolution of our occupational perspective: The journey from diversion through therapeutic use to enablement. *Canadian Journal of Occupational Therapy, 68*(4), 203-207.
Pollanen, S. (2009). Craft as context in therapeutic change. *The Indian Journal of Occupational Therapy, 41*(2), 43-47.
Radomski, M. V., & Latham, C. A. T. (Eds.). (2008). *Occupational therapy for physical dysfunction* (6th ed.). Philadelphia, PA: Lippincott Williams & Wilkins.
Reilly, M. (1962). The Eleanor Clark Slagle lecture: Occupational therapy can be one of the great ideas of 20th century medicine. *American Journal of Occupational Therapy, 16*(1), 1-9.
Rich, A. (1976). *Of women born.* New York, NY: Bantam Books.
Robinson, K., Kennedy, N., & Harmon, D. (2011). Is occupational therapy adequately meeting the needs of people with chronic pain? *American Journal of Occupational Therapy, 65*(1), 106-113.
Rosenfeld, A. A. (1988). New images, new insights into your brain. *Psychology Today, 22*(11), 22-24.
Schwartzberg, S. (2002). *Interactive reasoning in the practice of occupational therapy.* Upper Saddle River, NJ: Prentice Hall
Sochen, J. (1974). *Herstory: A woman's view of American history.* New York, NY: Alfred Publishing Co.
Stancliff, B. L. (1996). Roundtable: Are arts and crafts a valuable modality? *OT Practice, 1*(10), 51-54.
Taylor, E., & Manguna, J. (1991). Use of treatment activities in occupational therapy. *American Journal Occupational Therapy, 45*(4), 317-322.
TeBeest, R., Kornstedt, K., Feldmann, C., Harmasch, L., & Kemnitz, S. (2001). *The use of expressive arts in various occupational therapy settings.* LaCrosse, Washington: University of Washington-LaCrosse.
Thibodaux, C. S., & Ludwig, F. M. (1988). Intrinsic movement in product oriented and non-product oriented activities. *American Journal of Occupational Therapy, 42*(3), 169-175.
Tracy, S. (1910). *A manual for nurses and attendants: Studies in invalid occupations.* Boston, MA: Whitcomb Barrows.
Whyte, M. K. (1978). *The status of women in preindustrial societies.* Princeton, NJ: Princeton University Press.
Whittington, D., Weir, M., Powell, A., Mumbower, S., & Foster, J. (2010). *Benefits and usage of therapeutic art modalities by occupational therapists in the aging population.* Unpublished Masters research project, University of Mississippi Medical Center School of Health Related Professions.
Willard, H. S., & Spackman, C. S. (1947). *Principles of occupational therapy.* Philadelphia, PA: Lippincott Williams & Wilkins.
Willard, H. S., & Spackman, C. S. (1954). *Principles of occupational therapy* (2nd ed.). Philadelphia, PA: Lippincott Williams & Wilkins.
Willard, H. S., & Spackman, C. S. (1963). *Occupational therapy* (3rd ed.). Philadelphia, PA: Lippincott Williams & Wilkins.
Willard, H. S., & Spackman, C. S. (1971). *Occupational therapy* (4th ed.). Philadelphia, PA: Lippincott Williams & Wilkins.

2

The Case for Crafts
Justification for Use in Occupational Therapy

Objectives

The student should be able to:

- Explain crafts and creative activities as occupation and their unique advantages in treatment
- Articulate both restorative and productive benefits of crafts
- Describe how crafts are both client centered and occupation based
- Describe how crafts can be used in assessment
- Cite numerous examples of current therapeutic use of crafts
- Cite examples of research supporting the therapeutic efficacy of creative media
- Understand how crafts can be incorporated into various occupational therapy treatment approaches or models

There seems no better time than now for a resurgence of crafts and creative media in occupational therapy. Craft fairs are common and well attended; hobby stores, knitting shops, and other suppliers are springing up everywhere; and home decorating and craft shows on television are hugely popular. High-end stores and magazines offer works of fine craftsmanship for sale and fair-trade craft programs are becoming increasingly common as a way of garnering income for individuals in developing countries (see Appendix II). The Internet has allowed crafters all over the world to share ideas and sell their wares (Breines, 2010; See Appendix II for a listing of craft idea websites). In spite of the proliferation of technology in every other aspect of life, crafting appears to be back in the mainstream.

In occupational therapy, the focal viewpoint is shifting back to occupation, and in healthcare in general, the trend is toward a client-centered practice. As a society, we are embracing diversity, and respect for cultural meaning and context is an expected component of treatment planning (Crowe & Hong, 2009). Although the value placed on scientific evidence and technology is still prominent, there is an emerging emphasis on holism, occupational engagement, cultural relevance, and quality of life. This chapter will discuss the applicability of crafts and other creative media within occupation-based, client-centered practice; provide examples and evidence of the benefits of craft use; and describe how creative endeavors blend with prevailing occupational therapy models of practice.

Tubbs, C., & Drake, M. *Crafts and Creative Media in Therapy, Fourth Edition (pp. 11-28).*

Fair Trade Crafts Websites

- www.globalcrafts.org
- www.tenthousandvillages.com
- www.crsfairtrade.org/crafts
- www.ananseviilage.com
- www.upavimcrafts.org
- www.globalexchangestore.org
- www.fairtradequilts.com
- www.fairtradefederation.org

Relevance to Contemporary Occupational Therapy Practice

Occupation, as it is now being defined in occupational therapy practice, is a highly individualized proposition. It is the core concern of the field of occupational science and encompasses all purposeful activities that make up one's life, going well beyond personal and economic survival, to include social, restorative, artistic- and culturally-meaningful pursuits. Those engaged in occupational science, either theoretically or in the practice of therapy, seek to understand the link between various occupations and the health and well being of both individuals and societies (Clark & Lawlor, 2009). The meanings of a given occupation are diverse and dynamic, dependent upon individual interests, culture, experience, and values (Crowe & Hong, 2009; Kielhofner, 2004; Pierce, 2001a; Rogers, 1996; Taylor, 2008). It has been demonstrated that tasks in their whole form elicit more efficient responses than tasks broken into parts (Ma & Trombly, 2001) and the aspects of occupation that differentiate it from discrete purposeful or enabling activities—meaning and contextual uniqueness—are in complete harmony with the use of crafts and other creative processes as intervention. While craft work in general is a universal occupation, its impact is individual in that no two projects are completed in exactly the same way or have the same meaning or expressive content for the participants.

Occupation is also uniquely human; animals, body organs and even machines can do an activity, but only human beings derive meaning and identity from the things they do (Kielhofner, 2004; Punwar & Peloquin, 2000). People seem to have an inner drive to engage in occupations far beyond the level of self-maintenance, which is too often the starting and stopping point in many traditional rehabilitation programs. We are intrinsically motivated to shape our identity through occupation as evidenced by artistic/cultural pursuits—including crafts—at all levels of society. Creative activities offer means of self-expression, role affirmation, and a "memento of efficacy" (Byrne, Raphael, & Coleman-Wilson, 2010; Glass, Mendes de Leon, Marottoli, & Berkman, 1999; Harris, 2008; Taylor, 2008). Components of crafts work are analogous to the challenges in daily life: having to wait; experiencing control or lack of control; encountering resistance to efforts and determining how much force is reasonable; and being aware of time. Crafts may provide needed escape, personal fulfillment, an alternative to spoken language (Fidler & Velde, 1999) or an alternative to destructive behaviors (Johnson, 2008). They help "impose order on the chaos" (p. 131) of pain or disability and change the focus from the past to the here-and-now and the potential for growth (Perrin, 2001; Pollanen, 2009). Creative activities foster our imagination, hold our attention, "lift our spirits," and provide a sort of reward for meeting the more mundane demands of our existence (Crabtree, 1998).

Humans instinctively value productivity as well, although meaningful productivity goes beyond prescribed job requirements to encompass personal satisfaction, pride of craftsmanship, and establishment of a unique identity. In the infancy of the profession, occupational therapists realized that clients gained dignity and meaning from both productive and aesthetic pursuits (Kielhofner, 2004; Reilly, 1962). Beyond productivity—and harder to measure—is the concept of pleasure. Occupational therapists intuitively know that an activity that is pleasurable is also one that is more arousing and engaging. In turn, a well-chosen activity that is engaging is more therapeutically effective (Caron, 2008). Productivity is goal focused and certainly well-suited to occupational therapy. Pleasurable productivity, however, is process focused and therefore can be even more transformative. Actions are more automatic, the client becomes totally absorbed, and the time passes quickly (Gaskill, 2010; Pierce, 2001a). One model suggests that leisure is most satisfying when it is completely absorbing; this is measured by the degree to which an activity is motivating, allows disengagement, and increases the participant's sense of internal control (Bundy, 2001). Leisure occupation can also be restorative, as opposed to productive, in nature (Pollanen, 2009). This includes quiet crafts such as needlework or ceramics. This quality is particularly beneficial to the client who is disorganized or depressed (Pierce, 2001a). A 1997 British study verifies this; elderly women stated that engaging in needlework gave them increased confidence and self-esteem; helped them cope with anxiety, depression, and pain; and gave them a way to meet and contribute to other people (Reynolds). Creative involvement can stabilize vital bodily functions such as heart rate and blood pressure, and some individuals may be more receptive to this form of "treatment" than to more medically-oriented ones (Flood & Phillips, 2007). An understanding of the importance of personal meaning, productivity, pleasure, and restoration as elements of occupation provides more than enough support for occupational therapists to not only continue, but to increase their use of crafts or other creative activities. This is not to say that every client will always choose a craft activity over another occupation, but it certainly justifies the craft as an equally valid option. Pride of craftsmanship, quality of experience, and a spirit of individuality are all by-products of creative pursuits, and are simultaneously all consistent with aims of occupational intervention (Pierce, 2001b). Client-centered practice demands that our intervention choices be the result of collaboration between client and therapist so that they are motivating and hold meaning for the participant (Perrin, 2001).

Substantiating Evidence

In today's highly competitive health care environment, rehabilitation professionals must justify their treatment approach through research; they must provide clear evidence of both functional outcomes and subjective benefit to the client. This is needed not only for reimbursement, but to convince the client that their time is wisely invested in a given therapy. The prevalence of creative activities as intervention should increase as we return to occupation-centered practice, but the marketplace will demand proof of their therapeutic worth. Crabtree (1998) specifically mentions the use of arts, crafts, and other creative endeavors as exemplary ways of infusing occupation into practice. He asserts that these occupations may hold more meaning for clients than our traditional (medical model) focus on independence and "function." Evidence from both occupational therapy and other fields is beginning to mount in favor of leisure and/or creative activities as a means of promoting health and reducing the effects of disability. The literature shows a high correlation between leisure and life satisfaction (Crepeau, Cohn, & Schell, 2009), perception of health (Wichrowski, Whiteson, Haas, Mola, Rey, 2005) and even survival (Glass et al., 1999). A 2002 study by Specht, King, Brown, and Foris looked at the importance of leisure (commonly including arts and crafts) for those with congenital disabilities. Study results showed that leisure involvement was often seen as a "turning point" in the lives of the respondents. They saw their ability to participate as an accomplishment and proof of their continued worth, and remarked on other benefits such as enjoyment, social connection, and physical health enhancement. For example, one participant cited his woodworking as a way to stay active, keep his hands "supple," achieve recognition, and increase his sense of self-worth. The authors suggest that leisure involvement is of particular importance for those who may not be able to meet the demands for traditional (i.e., productive) employment. The authors of a 1999 longitudinal study with elders also found similar results relative to overall health; subjects who participated in productive and social activities showed greater longevity than those who did not (Glass et al.). Viewed from this perspective, leisure is particularly important for older clients who are no longer involved in the productive world of work. It becomes a new, or more emphasized, expression of self-identity, and as such keeps them physically active and mentally engaged. An ongoing, population-based study, first presented in 2009, suggests that participation in cognitive activities—including crafts—decreases the risk for mild cognitive impairment with aging (Geda et al., 2009). *The Role of Occupational Therapy With the Elderly* (Rogers, 1996) emphasizes that avocational activities become especially meaningful as people age. Surveys show there is considerable continuity in leisure involvement, but older people may have to give up more physical activities, opting for those—such as crafts or other creative projects—that are less strenuous and/or can be done at home. While women tend to spend more time in creative leisure, occupational therapists have found crafts beneficial to both genders in improving task and interaction skills. A review of studies on the impact of creative activities with elders concluded that they are beneficial in anxiety reduction, coping with loss, increasing self-esteem and an internal locus of control, and general strengthening of neuronal connections in the brain. They may also have a role in the release of endorphins and regulation of hormone levels (Flood & Phillips, 2007). A 2001 study found that older adults who participated regularly in arts/creative activities had lower rates of medication use than those who did not (Hanna & Perlstein, 2008).

Other studies show the usefulness of various leisure activities as means to address overall health or specific skill deficits. A multidisciplinary group of researchers examined the effect of participation in a horticulture program on a group of cardiac patients. Those that took part in the intervention showed several positive outcomes, including a reduction in mood disturbance score, lowered heart rate, and an increase in interpersonal engagement (Wichrowski et al., 2005). A study with children demonstrated that use of a game—both meaningful and fun for the participants—facilitated the therapeutic goal of neck and back extension (Sakemiller & Nelson, 1998). A 2000 Canadian study looked at interventions used by occupational therapists to treat cognitive problems in individuals with traumatic brain injuries. Therapists listed crafts—including woodworking and card making—and the computer art program "Print Shop" as media used for all areas under consideration (Blundon & Smits, 2000). Occupational therapy students working in a homeless shelter found that participants in the creative arts program improved in their ability to follow directions and attention to detail, as well as socialization skills (Byrne et al., 2010). A recent case example touted the benefits of crochet, not exclusive to just motor demands of the activity. The participant, an eleven-year-old boy attending an inner city special education school, not only gained self-satisfaction from learning to crochet, but also gained skills related to its incorporation as a valuable occupation in his life. For example, his independence in community mobility and money management increased because he wanted to be able to ride the bus and independently shop for his supplies. He also learned to analyze patterns and choose those of which he felt capable. Over time, his motor skills improved as well (Cipriani, 2011).

While craft use in the clinic may seem at times to be waning, a thorough perusal of occupational therapy texts shows many examples of the employment of crafts or other creative media in case studies. Hasselkus' text (2002) cites a case of one of her own clients, describing his transformation from a dejected, troubled man to a happy man, well liked by others, through the use of wood carving and whittling in therapy. The client found that this occupation increased his self-esteem and gave his life a greater sense of meaning (Hasselkus & Dickie, 1994). Woodworking is also identified as a primary occupation in a case study in another text (Schkade & McClung, 2001). A case history in *Occupational Therapy Principles and Practice, Third Edition* (Punwar & Peloquin, 2000) describes the use of weaving with a female client with rheumatoid arthritis. She not only learned a skill that proved to be financially profitable, but also gained the strength and motion needed to feed herself. Early's text (2009) gives numerous examples of how to select crafts to meet various behavioral needs. Many current occupational therapy texts discuss the importance of creativity and leisure, including crafts. Hagedorn (2001) mentions the use of creative media in occupational therapy intervention. She asserts that the therapist should have a repertoire of both creative and practical skills, such as various types of needlework, ceramics, and expressive and dramatic arts. Hasselkus (2002) discusses creativity and its positive effects, which she finds well articulated in art therapy and gerontology literature. The use of creative media in occupational therapy is most healing when it is a bridge to, or a component of, the day-to-day living experience. Therapists often pride themselves on their ingenuity, but they should also build in opportunities for the clients to be creative, so they too can benefit from that same sense of satisfaction.

The eleventh edition of *Willard and Spackman's Occupational Therapy* lists leisure and play assessments and states that therapists "often" use games and crafts to increase manual dexterity, attention to task, social skills, and sense of self-efficacy and self-esteem; and that play and leisure activities can be used as rewards, means, or as an end in themselves (Creapeau, Cohn, & Schell, 2009). Punwar and Peloquin (2000) report that the past five years of occupational therapy writing contain a long list of creative interventions, including jokes/humor, cultural cooking, creative arts, ceramics, dancing, paper clip art, computer games, dramatic plays, leatherwork, Turkish knotting, macramé, magic, home improvement, beadwork, and horticulture. The sixth edition of Pedretti's *Occupational Therapy* text (Pendleton & Schultz-Krohn, 2006) has a chapter on leisure occupation and lists both its psychosocial and physical benefits. The authors describe the use of crafts in hand therapy (e.g., the employment of macramé, leather and woodworking) and state their usefulness not only in terms of motor improvement but in marking milestones of achievement. They also cite studies showing that purposeful activity increases a client's willingness to participate, and include arts and crafts as examples of purposeful activity. Another popular physical dysfunction text (Radomski & Trombly, 2008), states that the definition of leisure is varied but includes crafts. It lists desirable and therapeutic qualities of leisure: it is inherently satisfying, it is engaging and arousing, and it requires commitment on the part of the participant. The authors propose that use of leisure as intervention will gradually increase as treatment shifts from the hospital to the community setting and more emphasis is given to prevention (of illness) and promotion (of health). They even suggest that occupational therapists' use of exercise and physical agent modalities could be detracting from precious treatment time that could be used for a more holistic leisure experience. Other texts also reflect the value of leisure skill development as a meaningful occupation across the life span (Cottrell, 1996; Cynkin & Robinson, 1990; Early, 1993, 2009; Hinojosa & Blount, 2009). Arts and crafts are cited as important unifying elements of many cultures, and as such, relevant to rehabilitation (Royeen & Crabtree, 2006). As a key feature of one's ethnic identity, they may play an important role in promoting healing and restoring a sense of belonging.

There are abundant leisure and play assessment tools—many of which include crafts and other creative activities—indicating that this is still perceived as an important area for attention in occupational therapy. A few examples are the Idyll Arbor Leisure Battery 2001, the Canadian Occupational Therapy Measure, the Leisure Competence Measure, Assessment of Ludic Behaviors, Leisure Interest Profile for Adults, Leisure Interest Profile for Seniors, and the Experience of Leisure Scale. Additional examples of leisure assessment can be found in the text, *Measuring Occupational Performance* by Law, Baum, and Dunn (2005) and in *Occupational Therapy Assessment Tools: An Annotated Index*, edited by Ina Elfant Asher (2007). Other assessments use craft activities or components thereof to evaluate other nonleisure areas of function and specific motor, process, or interaction skills (Reynolds, 2008; Table 2-1). Practicing therapists who regularly incorporate crafts frequently refer to their value in assessment. Conversation comes more easily (Caron, 2008) and clients may be more comfortable sharing information about themselves than they might in a structured interview. In working with children, craftwork can help evaluate motor skills, but also impulse control, task perseverance, and the ability to follow directions (Diffendal, 2002). Therapists interviewed as part of a qualitative study stated they had the sense that they could learn much more about clients by observing them engage in a craft for a short period of time than they could learn "in weeks" using other methods (Schmid, 2004). Crafts sometimes have a unique ability to illuminate problems that go unnoticed during more routine activities. In the student observation example in Chapter 4, a postsurgical patient was given a model to complete because his therapist had identified dexterity deficits during his initial evaluation. As the patient worked on the model, however, it became obvious that he also had some previously undiscovered cognitive impairment. This surfaced during the craft because, unlike the self-care activities during which he had been observed, it was a novel activity. When the patient was called upon to perform in an unfamiliar problem-solving situation, he was not successful. Important safety implications could have gone overlooked had he not been challenged with this craft activity.

Personal testimonies and anecdotal evidence from practitioners also point out the multiple benefits of creative interventions. Cancer patients participating in a group mosaic project—part of an ongoing program of creative therapy designed to help patients cope with illness, connect with other patients, and explore their sense of self—spoke to the healing nature of the creative process (Taussig, 2005). One COTA in the United Kingdom commented on the therapeutic value of scrapbooking—a currently popular craft—as a way of expressing feelings and exploring the past, in addition to its more generalized benefits of improving fine motor and cognitive skills, for clients with both mental and physical disabilities (Johnson, 2005). An American student observed crafts use at its best while on fieldwork in New Zealand as she watched people learn "incredible things about themselves" through the use of creative activities. She found that clients were able to identify faulty behavior patterns in the craft workshop and see the application to their current situation of addiction (Wuller, 2005).

Numerous programs in occupational therapy are currently using crafts as their primary therapeutic approach. One facility in Pennsylvania provides work experiences for mental health clients through gardening, art, and the raising of angora rabbits. A group of occupational therapy students implemented a program that allowed participants to learn to make use of the angora fur through spinning and weaving, as well as making and marketing salable products. This occupation-based program was contextually appropriate and increased consumers' self-esteem and self-image (Scipio, Kisner, Vitiello, Silverman, & Salls, 2005). Another group of occupational therapy practitioners suggests the use of Harry Potter as a theme for inventing appealing children's activities. This approach allows children to participate in creating costumes, environments, and props that stimulate their imagination while addressing discrete problem areas (Sladyk, Berry, Brenner, Hengeveld, & Moisan, 2002). A program in New York implements "crafting" in a more functional sense. Therapists are using basic materials such as cardboard and PVC pipe to create adaptive equipment, giving them firsthand experience of the therapeutic value of building things with one's hands. They hope to

Table 2-1

ASSESSMENTS AND THEIR CRAFT COMPONENTS

	Beadwork	Ceramics	Cooking	Gardening	Leatherwork	Mosaic	Needlework	Paper Crafts	Woodworking
ADL Evaluation							✓		
Allen Cognitive Level Screening					✓	✓	✓		
Allen Diagnostic Module	✓				✓	✓	✓		✓
Assessment of Motor and Process Skills			✓						
Azima Battery		✓							
BH Battery						✓			
Build-a-City/Build-a-Farm								✓	✓
Carolyn Owens Activity Battery		✓							
Comprehensive Assessment Process						✓			
Comprehensive Evaluation of Basic Living Skills			✓						
Diagnostic Test Battery		✓			✓				✓
Fidler Activity Laboratory								✓	
Gillette Battery		✓				✓			
Goodman Battery		✓				✓			
Gross Activity Battery		✓							
IADL Checklists			✓				✓		
Interest Checklists			✓	✓	✓	✓	✓		✓
Jacobs Prevocational Skills Assessment			✓		✓				✓
Kitchen Task Assessment			✓						
Lafayette Clinic Battery								✓	
Magazine Picture Collage								✓	
Milwaukee Evaluation of Daily Living Skills							✓		
Nelson Clark's Clay Test		✓							
O'Kane Diagnostic Battery		✓							
Perkins Tile Task						✓			
Routine Task Inventory			✓				✓		
Scoreable Self-Care Evaluation			✓						
Shoemyen Battery		✓				✓			
Street Survival Skills Questionnaire			✓						
Tiled Trivet Assessment						✓			
Work Adjustment Program									✓

expand their program to include area students in the construction process as a means of addressing motor and prevocational skills (Hendrickson & Lesser, 2005). Therapists are finding the value of crafts in settings as diverse as homeless shelters, hospices, and adult day centers for those with developmental delays. The creative experience allows the individual to assume a productive or giving role that is otherwise lost due to their circumstances (Byrne et al., 2010; Hospice Education Institute, 2010; Winkle & Cobb, 2010).

Although it was during my occupational therapy education that I first learned of the use of "crafts" as a therapeutic medium, primarily utilized in mental health settings, it was not until I was a practicing therapist that I began to truly understand and appreciate the benefits of using craft activities for assessment as well as intervention.

First, crafts are an excellent and economical assessment tool. By having a client participate or engage in a craft activity, and depending on how the activity is set up, a therapist can assess several performance components with that one activity...fine motor (maybe even gross motor), strength, balance, activity endurance, initiation, sequencing, attention, direction following, problem solving, decision making, frustration tolerance, and coping skills. Thanks to the phenomenal work of Claudia Allen, we as clinicians know that performance in new or unfamiliar activities, such as crafts, can predict safety awareness and problem solving even outside of a clinical setting. In my many years of practice in a mental health facility, the Allen Cognitive Levels have often played a crucial role when working with an interdisciplinary treatment team to determine the most appropriate discharge setting for a client that is cognitively impaired.

Secondly, crafts can be used as meaningful productive activity in order to increase self-expression, self-esteem, adaptive coping skills, and healthy leisure routines. I felt the best way to expound on this was to share direct quotes from some of my clients when asked about participating in craft activities...

"They're FUN!" —N. B. (Female, age 31)

"They make me feel young again...and I can give them to my family as gifts." —K. G. (Female, age 27)

"It helps (me) to relieve stress, relax, and be creative." —R. L. (Female, age 48)

"I can create something on my own, it builds my morale, and it's terrific for me...it gets my mind off the jungle we're in." —C. M. (Female, age 48)

Overall, I feel that crafts can be a valuable means toward assessment as well as intervention in occupational therapy, regardless of the setting. I, personally, will continue to use craft activities when assessing clients in order to develop functional, realistic, and holistic treatment plans, and to empower my clients in the practice of healthy occupations.

Stacey L. Dupré, LOTR
Occupational Therapy Supervisor and Treatment Mall Coordinator
Eastern Louisiana Mental Health Services

Consumer interest in self-help and personal development also illustrates the benefit of crafts and creative involvement. The book, *Craft to Heal*, by Nancy Monson (2005), is a good resource for examples and discussion of the healing qualities of crafts. The author lists crafting experts, organizations, and retreat locations. Freelance writer Wendy Baker, by virtue of her personal experience in therapy, compiled a lengthy list of the benefits of arts and crafts. They are versatile, accessible, and can help form bonds between people. They can improve fine motor skills, provide diversion from pain, and inspire pursuit of a life-long hobby. Finally, they can provide affirmation, a sense of accomplishment and pride, and physical or psychic transformation for people struggling with disease or disability (Baker, 2005). A craft retailer in Massachusetts who provides work space for craft groups reports that she has observed that children seem to relax and communicate better with parents while doing crafts. She also relates the story of a friendship that formed between two cancer patients through their mutual enjoyment of crafts (LaGrossa, 2005). The New York Public Library has hosted a "Handmade Now and Then" class and one participant shared her story of teaching knitting to families of children in Mt. Sinai hospital as a means of relieving anxiety (Pigza, 2008). Even federal and local governments have acknowledged the health benefits of engagement in creative activities as evidenced by their funding of arts programs for the elderly (www.artandaging.org; www.NEA.gov/Resources/Accessibility/rlists/ArtsAging.html; www.NEA.gov/Resources). In New York City, retirement communities are being developed in collaboration with universities for intentional incorporation of arts programs, and the city of New York has allocated funds for senior arts programs at various existing cultural centers (Hanna & Perlstein, 2008).

Countless therapeutic recreation and social action programs utilize creative media with populations such as veterans (Lynch, 2009), women who are victims of domestic violence, incarcerated individuals (Johnson, 2008; Crochet Project, 2005), those with visual impairments/blindness (Cochran, 2010; Therapeutic Recreation Program, 2005; Michigan Department of Energy, Labor, and Economic Growth, 2005), and traumatized children in war-torn countries (Addis, 2010). These facilities and organizations cite all of the previously mentioned benefits of crafts: promotion of manual, cognitive and perceptual skills; establishment of valuable social roles and a sense of belonging; building prevocational skills; and fostering feelings of control and confidence. Another growing outlet for craftwork is that of altruism. People receive gratification through giving back to others or their community, and this role is often lost in the role of "patient." The reward of being able to do for others might be the motivation for a client who would otherwise have no interest in making a craft (Breines, 2009). There are numerous national and international organizations that solicit handcrafted items that could be completed as part of therapy. See Appendix II for a list of Web sites.

Crafting for Charity Web Sites

- www.craftbits.com/crafts/charity
- www.allfreecrafts.com/charity-crafts.shtml
- www.familycrafts.about.com/od/craftingforcharity/Crafting_for_Charity.htm
- www.craftsitedirectory.com/charities/index.html
- www.marthastewart.com/article/knitting-charity

Application to Theory

Another way of testing the relevance of crafts in occupational therapy is by reconciling their use with prevailing theoretical constructs of the profession. First considered is the occupational therapy paradigm, the encompassing perspective sometimes referred to as our professional "worldview." The contemporary paradigm of occupational therapy states that humans are occupational in nature, that occupational problems supersede skill deficits as a treatment focus, and that engagement in occupation is the core of therapy (Hooper, 2010; Kielhofner, 2004). Clients who are self-motivated or can be motivated by an occupational therapist to participate in activities and occupations will increase the probability of improving their functional ability and, more importantly, their state of well being. Under the paradigm umbrella of the profession fall the practice models, which are based on theory. A theory is a premise to explain or a speculation about a particular phenomenon. "Theory is not static, nor is it ever final" (Llorens, 1984). Humans are continuously changing and refining their conceptual thinking; likewise occupational therapy theory is evolving as therapists generate new ideas about the response to intervention and its relationship to human occupation. Theories relating to human behavior and function/dysfunction are derived from multiple disciplines and have been variously applied since the profession's inception. For example, Abraham Maslow, a humanist psychologist whose theories are frequently embraced by occupational therapists, developed a hierarchical scheme to depict levels at which humans satisfy their needs (Maslow, 1968). Figure 2-1 depicts this hierarchy as it might apply to the craft of leatherwork (Hinojosa & Blount, 2009).

Models of practice are based on concepts and principles about how to address particular problems (Reed, 1984). Many occupational therapy models have elements in common and therapists seldom base their treatment approach on only one. Some practitioners may have contributed ideas to more than one model and likewise, many models have multiple contributors. Of importance is that no occupational therapy model of practice, based on its beliefs about human activity, would exclude the use of crafts as a treatment medium, although some might use crafts as a means only and not as an end. The model used will affect

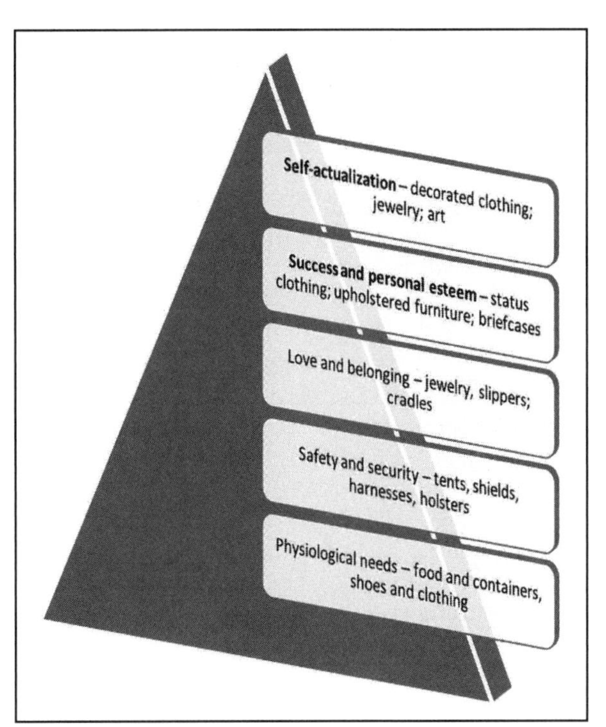

Figure 2-1. Leathercraft represented in Maslow's Hierarchy of Human Needs.

which crafts are offered, which tools are allowed, and/or the context in which they might be used. It could mean that the crafts chosen are not fully occupation based but are utilized merely to enhance specific performance skills. Even in this application, a craft may have the serendipitous effect of stimulating a client's overall interest in creative endeavors. The models and their underlying concepts and principles become very important to the individual therapist because they provide guidance in clinical decision making. For this reason, the student needs to have a basic understanding of commonly used models, be able to compare and contrast their underlying assumptions, and describe how each particular view of intervention plays a role in addressing occupational goals.

Authors reference different models in their books and articles, based on those which appear to have the most important and relevant ideas at the time of writing. Only a sampling of occupational therapy models is included in this text. They are based on information in recent occupational therapy texts (*Willard and Spackman's Occupational Therapy, 11th Edition*, Crepeau et al., 2009; Kielhofner's *Conceptual Foundations of Occupational Therapy, Third Edition*, 2004; Christiansen and Baum's *Occupational Therapy: Performance, Participation,and Well-Being, Third Edition*, 2005) and were chosen to represent the diversity of current approaches to practice. This section is intended to be illustrative only and not a stand-alone lesson on occupational therapy models. Whenever possible, previous "frames of reference" that relate to the model described here will be included so that the student can identify which theories have similar views and beliefs. See Table 2-2 for a summary of the models and their relationship to craft activities.

Neurologically-Based Models

Motor behavior and sensory processing and integration models are grouped together in this section, as all place great importance on neurological responses as determinants of human behavior. Human function is seen as a result of biological processes dependent on appropriate reception, perception, and integration of sensory input and/or integrity of connections within the central nervous system. Motor behavior, or output, is based on intact neurons and neurological wiring, chemical transport, and storage of information in the neurological system. Illness or defects in the brain's motor or sensory systems that interfere with processing or integration of input into the system or communication within the system may cause abnormal behavior. For example, if a person has unusual movement patterns, it is considered to be the consequence

Table 2-2

Occupational Therapy Models

Model	Therapy Emphasis	Activity Components	Craft Examples
Motor control (various)	Positioning, normal movement patterns, proprioceptive and tactile input	Weight bearing Bilateral Postural requirements	Rolling clay or dough Sawing or sanding Mixing/stirring
Sensory integration/ sensory processing	Multichannel sensory input	Variation in texture Visual interest Vestibular input	Papier mache Mixing (dough) with hands Leaf rubbing
Biomechanical	Strength, range of motion, endurance, positioning	Resistance Placement to facilitate reaching or specific grasp	Macramé Sawing, sanding Mosaics
Cognitive disabilities	Evaluation Task/environmental modification	Structured Procedural in nature Visual cues/samples	Wood kits Leather kits Tile mosaics
Cognitive retraining	Cognitive skill building, adaptive strategies	Structured Repetitious Cues or other memory aids	Tile mosaics Paper crafts Kits Cooking
Developmental	Meeting developmental milestones	Postural Grasp/dexterity Repetition	Beading Paper crafts Metal tooling
Occupational behavior	Client interest/ engagement Task competence Consistency with desired roles	Decision making/choice	

of neurological transmission problems which could in turn cause muscular imbalance or orthopedic (structural) distortion, and resulting ineffective behavior/performance in a given environment. Several well-known theories including neurodevelopmental treatment (Eggers, 1984); sensory integration (Ayers, 1987; Fisher, Murray, & Bundy, 1991; Van Deusen, 1993), Brunnstrom (Trombly, 1995); motor control and learning (Carr, Shepherd, Gordon, Gentile, & Held, 1987; Cohen, 1993; Crepeau et al., 2009; Montgomery & Connolly, 1991); and proprioceptive neuromuscular facilitation (Cohen, 1993; Trombly, 1995; Umphred, 1995) incorporate these general concepts. More recent formulations of motor behavior models take into account the influence of environment and goal orientation. Motor behavior is seen as self-organizing and relates to occupational form. Therefore, there is increased emphasis on tasks that are functional and meaningful, in addition to their role in modulating the sensory and motor experience (Kielhofner, 2004). Treatment using motor behavior models attempts to make an impact on the neurological system through positioning, normal movement patterns, and tactile and proprioceptive cues. Occupations may involve gross motor body movements, weight bearing, diagonal movement patterns, and controlled external sensory stimulation. Crafts that involve weight bearing, postural changes, and normal movement patterns are often considered most likely to achieve normal neural reactions. Sawing, sanding, rolling, rubbing, or mixing can be used to achieve goals in this model. Although a therapist might encourage or reject a craft activity based on its motor demands and/or sensory components, it is important that the client be given some choice. The client should be able to find meaning in the activity and be able to discern its purpose or goal in order to attain optimum performance.

Sensory processing theory suggests that behavior is determined in part by how a person perceives and then responds to various sensory stimuli. One model conceptualizes that, for a given individual, input of various types is perceived at particular thresholds, and that input is then managed according to the ability to self-regulate. This model, commonly associated with pediatric and mental health practice, proposes that some dysfunction or problem behaviors are related to a sensory processing imbalance. Because registration thresholds vary, some individuals may require intervention to attain the optimal amount and type of stimulation to maximize functional ability. As with the sensory integration model, the therapist must assess the client to determine sensory thresholds and the ability to regulate activities and environments accordingly (Dunn, 2009). Once this is determined, the therapist can then utilize activity strategies that best match those needs. Crafts and other creative activities offer a broad spectrum of sensory experiences and can be graded for duration, intensity, and degree of self-direction required or allowed. For example, a child having difficulty with schoolwork due to high proprioceptive threshold may benefit from a therapy session in which a craft involving polymer clay is used to provide input at a higher level. Because this craft is also somewhat abstract and variable in method, the child can more readily regulate the amount and duration of stimulation independently.

The sensory integration model is most often used with children, particularly those with mild to moderate learning or behavioral problems (Kielhofner, 2004). It proposes that graded sensory input leads to more normal integration of this input and thus facilitation of adaptive responses. In addition, the activities should be highly likely to create a successful experience, thereby forming new and more appropriate neural connections. The greater the inner drive to accomplish the activity, the greater the potential for effective neural organization and integration (Ayers, 1987; Baloueff, 2003). Because this model is most often applied in pediatric practice, it usually incorporates play, of which crafts, drama, or other creative experience can be a part. The therapist must first make a thorough assessment to determine which sensory experiences would be most therapeutic. The second step is to provide the child with choices to increase motivation, a sense of internal control, and use of imagination (Kielhofner, 2004). Crafts are excellent vehicles for providing a broad range of tactile, proprioceptive, and visual input, and successful experiences will simultaneously improve the child's self-esteem and sense of independence. It should be noted, however, that crafts rarely provide vestibular input, which is often an important part of sensory integration treatment.

Biomechanical Model

This model is concerned with the body's musculoskeletal ability to move and maintain postures. It focuses on joint range of motion; muscle strength and endurance; and the physiological, anatomical, and mechanical properties that underlie these capacities, including pain management. In its strictest application, there is no consideration of the influence of environmental, psychological, or cognitive factors on performance. The primary treatment aims in the biomechanical model are preventing deformity, maintaining/restoring musculoskeletal capacity, and compensating for limited motion (Kielhofner, 2004; Pedretti & Early 2001; Trombly & Randomski, 2002). Crafts or other creative processes might be used as means only in this model. The therapist might choose the activity based on its resistive or repetitive qualities or its range of motion demands. If a client is accustomed to participating in a particular craft or hobby, the therapist might provide assistive equipment, tool adaptations, or instruction in modified body mechanics to enable the client to continue this activity despite limitations in body structures or functions.

Cognitive Model

Cognitive models have generally been grouped into those that utilize compensatory approaches and those that use remedial approaches. Compensatory approaches rely on modification of the task or environment or use of external aids to improve function. Remedial approaches assume that discrete skills such as attention or sequencing can be improved through repetitious tasks, then combined and transferred to more functional activities (Toglia, Golisz, & Goverover, 2009). Occupational therapists have more recently conceptualized some models that utilize a combination of these two strategies. The commonly known cognitive disabilities model relies primarily on compensatory methods (Allen, 1985), while some of the newer models, such as the cognitive retraining model, employ both adaptive strategies and remedial training (Averbuch & Katz, 2005).

The cognitive disabilities model presumes that human behavior is a product of cognitive ability, and that this is demonstrated in the ability to learn, use language, and utilize and change material objects. Task analysis is a key component of this model. A given activity is carefully analyzed for process demands; the client's ability to perform that task then indicates the cognitive level at which they are functioning. According to this model, illness or dysfunction means inability to learn, with resulting limitations in task performance. This model assumes that cognitive impairment, including psychiatric disease, is caused, at least in part, by biological abnormalities. This model also assumes that therapy cannot change a cognitive disability that is caused by brain pathology (Allen, 1985; Bruce, 1994; Katz, 1992; Kielhofner, 1997).

One important function of the occupational therapist in the cognitive disabilities model is to assess a client's cognitive level by observing task performance, including the completion of craft activities. In treatment implementation, challenging clients with activities beyond their current functional level is avoided; craft materials and activities are chosen based on cognitive level. The client sometimes shows changes based on fluctuations in disease process, environmental changes, task repetition, or task modification. The therapist must be attentive to these changes and alter activities accordingly. (Earhart & Allen, 1988; Radomski, Dougherty, Fine, & Baum, 1994; Zemke, 1994). Some publications on cognitive disabilities name specific crafts that are appropriate for different cognitive levels (Earhart & Allen, 1988; Earhart, Allen, & Blue, 1993). The Allen Cognitive Levels Screening (ACLS) test involves leather lacing (see Figures 10-14 through 10-16 for illustrations of the stitches used). Verification of cognitive level is accomplished using craft projects in the Allen Diagnostic Module (Allen, Earhart, & Blue, 1992).

In the cognitive retraining model, the client may participate in simple, structured activities that require repetitive actions such as sequencing, visual scanning, or attention. At the same time, the therapist may also teach the client specific adaptations or strategies to improve performance. The activities utilized will gradually increase in complexity and the intervention will emphasize application of these new skills and strategies in necessary real-life tasks (Averbuch & Katz, 2005). Crafts could be used in this model to build and sharpen these discrete skills. Given the vast number of options, the therapist can easily select an appropriate project based on its requirement for attention, memory, sequencing, visual scanning, problem solving, and so on.

Developmental/Acquisitional Models

In the developmental/acquisitional models, humans are assumed to progress in an orderly way through various growth stages and learn specific skills along the way. The changes may be gradual and a person may show behaviors/skills from several different stages at the same time. Different theorists have described these stages with varying emphases and time parameters (Case-Smith, Allen, & Pratt, 1996; Gilfoyle, Grady, & Moore, 1990; Kramer & Hinojosa, 1993). Illness or dysfunction is shown by the absence of age-appropriate behaviors or skills. In other words, the ill or delayed client fails to pass through the expected stages of development or regresses from a higher to a lower stage. Dysfunction may be caused by neurological impairment, trauma, or environmental insufficiency; however the cause is not as important as the effect on developmental function. Dysfunction is defined as the failure to master or accomplish the life tasks expected for that particular stage of development.

Occupations such as crafts are thought of primarily as vehicles for attaining stage-specific behavior, for achieving mastery of a developmental stage and skill level (Crepeau et al., 2009). The treatment environment is arranged to maximize and promote development. For example, for a 5-year-old experiencing functional difficulties, appropriate life tasks might include such tasks as copying letters, coloring within lines, using scissors, constructing materials, and various group activities. An appropriate developmental environment would include materials such as wood; hammer and nails; clay; paper for copying words from large-print posters on the wall; and outline drawings of familiar objects to be colored, cut out, and pasted. Such activities would then be graded and carried out in dyads or small groups to accomplish the task of age-appropriate socialization and other behavior (Duncome, Howe, & Schwartzberg, 1988; Neistadt & Crepeau, 1997; Reed, 1984; Reed & Sanderson, 1983). The developmental models are used most frequently, although not exclusively, with children.

Occupational Behavior Models

Occupational behavior models are based on occupational behavior and the factors that impact it, and were developed in response to occupational therapy's renewed concern with occupational behavior and desire to return to occupation-based practice. Included in this group are the Model of Human Occupation (Keilhofner, 1995), Occupational Adaptation Model (Schultz & Schkade, 2003), The Canadian Model of Occupational Performance (Kielhofner, 2004), Ecology of Human Performance (Dunn, McClain, Brown, & Youngstrom, 2003), and the Person-Environment-Occupation Model (Stewart et al., 2003). These models grew out of and share several views on human activity and adaptation: humans are occupational in nature; environment has an effect on performance and vice versa; occupations are complex and meet intrinsic needs for organization, expression, and fulfillment; and dysfunction is the result of the inability of the person to adapt to changes in the environment and/or self. The recently added Kawa Model has a number of similarities to the previously listed approaches. Therapy should be based on the client's personal narrative and a dynamic give-and-take relationship between person and environment is assumed. Not only can the environment impact the individual, but the individual can influence and alter the environment as well. The client's life is visualized as a river and multiple factors can facilitate or hinder its flow. In this model, occupations have a collective as well as an individual nature (Byrne et al., 2010; Iwama, 2009). All of these models consider the unique and subjective experience of clients as they attempt to adapt; consequently, client-centered practice is a core concept in their application (Kielhofner, 2004).

The Model of Human Occupation was founded on the General Systems Theory (Kielhofner, 1995) and contends that occupation is essential to self-organization. Behavior is dynamic and dependent on context. Not only the treatment activity, but how the client feels about engagement in that activity, are important for change (Crepeau et al., 2009). This model states that human occupation is based on three subsystems: volitional, habituation, and performance. Each subsystem is equally important; however, they have fluctuating levels of influence. The volitional subsystem includes ideas about personal causation, values, and interests. The habituation subsystem encompasses habits and learned roles. The performance subsystem includes the skills needed for the person to perform an action or occupation. Concepts of cause and effect are important in this model, as they are related to a person's sense of self-efficacy and only the client can accomplish his or her own change (Kielhofner, 2004).

In all occupational behavior models, context is considered central to occupational performance since environmental interaction, in its broadest sense, is the essence of human occupation. Dysfunction is failure to successfully interact with the environment. In evaluating the client from an occupational behavior perspective, the therapist looks at the interaction between the client, the task, and the environment, at the same time realizing all of these components are dynamic. The client's goals, aspirations, and desires are central to treatment planning. The therapist then offers information and professional guidance in helping the client establish skills, make decisions, and adapt to cirumstances (Crepeau et al., 2009).

Therapy in these models is client centered; it is important for a client to choose his or her own activities/occupations (Early, 1993). Therapists should offer a range of options and encourage clients to choose an activity/occupation rather than assigning one. According to these models, all activities used in treatment should have relevance and meaning. Activities are best done in their whole form and not contrived (Kielhofner, 2004).

Occupations such as crafts provide a treatment milieu in which the client can explore and work with materials. The treatment setting provides a variety of craft samples and materials so that the client can make choices based on his or her interests, values, and past experience as well as the potential to achieve some mastery of the craft selected. Competence in a craft will result from development of skill in handling the materials, as well as continued motivation and formation of new habits. Concurrently, the client learns the role of worker or crafts person, thus experiencing a feeling of mastery of the clinical environment. It is this feeling of competence or mastery that can be transferred to exploration of the environment outside the treatment setting (Kielhofner, 2004). Any crafts or creative media are appropriate within these models. The primary requirement is that they are meaningful and provide the client with positive environmental—social, cultural, and physical—interaction experiences.

These theories would capitalize on a client's motivation toward any activity/occupation, which may or may not be a craft (Christiansen & Baum, 2005). If a craft or other creative project happens to be guiding the client toward mastery and generalizing to other tasks, as well as providing fulfillment, then it is an excellent therapeutic choice. In strict keeping with these models, however, the therapist would never compel a client to engage in a craft simply to work on a discrete performance skill.

Conclusion

Just as occupational therapists continually try to clarify and verify approaches to treatment, so too they seek to articulate an overarching vision for the profession. This vision must necessarily influence the choice of therapeutic tools. As we advance scientifically, we also reflect back on our founding philosophy. Suzanne Peloquin (2002) recently re-examined the autobiographical work of an early occupational therapy, *The Healing Heart* by Carlove and Ruggles, and its vision of "reaching for heart as well as hands." Most of the cases Ruggles relates in her book incorporated the use of crafts and compellingly illustrated their healing properties. Modern reviewers were able to easily discern both physical and emotional/psychological benefits of these activities so thoughtfully selected by Ruggles (Peloquin, 2002). While many of occupational therapy's current physical treatment approaches plainly reach for hands and bodies, it is questionable whether they also effectively reach for the heart. As Mary Reilly said so eloquently almost 50 years ago, "There is a long, perilous, and complex ladder to be scaled between neuromuscular efficiency and work satisfaction." The occupational therapy process should include "meaningful involvement in problem-solving tasks or creative performances, [teaching] the ability to experience pleasure in achievement and to tolerate the frustrations of struggle" (Reilly, 1962). The aim of this text is to demonstrate to the reader that crafts can indeed offer simultaneously pleasurable and instructional experiences and can play a role in the efficient restoration of occupational fulfillment.

Discussion Questions

1. Select one or more models of practice and describe how crafts/creative media would intersect with the corresponding assumptions regarding function/dysfunction and the purpose of therapy.
2. In what instances have you observed crafts used as part of a therapeutic or healing process (not necessarily in occupational therapy)?
3. From the information in this chapter, create a comprehensive list of the physical, psychological and social benefits of creative endeavors.

References

Addis, J. (2010). The art of participation. *World Vision magazine*, Winter 2010. Retrieved from http://www.worldvisionmagazine.org/stories/the-art-of-participation/.

Allen, C. K. (1985). *Occupational therapy for psychiatric diseases: Measurement and management of cognitive disabilities*. Boston, MA: Little, Brown and Company.

Allen, C. K., Earhart, C. A., & Blue, T. (1992). *Occupational therapy treatment goals for the physically and cognitively disabled*. Rockville, MD: American Occupational Therapy Association.

Asher, I. E. (Ed.). (2007). *Occupational therapy assessment tools: An annotated index*. Bethesda, MD: AOTA Press.

Averbuch, S. & Katz, N. (2005). Cognitive rehabilitation: A retraining model for clients with neurological disabilities. In N. Katz, (Ed.), *Cognition and occupation across the life span: Models for intervention in occupational therapy* (2nd ed., pp. 113-138). Bethesda, MD: AOTA Press.

Ayers, A. J. (1987). *Sensory integration and the child*. Los Angeles, CA: Western Psychological Services.

Baker, W. (2005). *Arts and crafts for recovery*. Retrieved from www.toydirectory.com/monthly/july2002/arts_for_recovery.asp.

Baloueff, O. (2003). Sensory integration. In E. Crepeau, E. Cohn, & B. Schell, (Eds.), *Willard and Spackman's occupational therapy* (10th ed., pp. 247-252). Philadelphia, PA: Lippincott Williams & Wilkins.

Blundon, G., & Smits, E. (2000). Cognitive rehabilitation: A pilot survey of therapeutic modalities used by Canadian occupational therapists with survivors of traumatic brain injury. *Canadian Journal of Occupational Therapy, 67*(3), 184-196.

Breines, E. B. (2009). Giving as motivation. *Advance for Occupational Therapy Practitioners, 25*(20), 6.

Breines, E. (2010). Crafts to computers (and back). *Advance for Occupational Therapy Practitioners, 26*(2), 10.

Bruce, M. A. G. (1994). *Cognitive rehabilitation: Intelligence, insight, and knowledge. AOTA self-study series: Cognitive rehabilitation*. Rockville, MD: American Occupational Therapy Association.

Bundy, A. C. (2001). Leisure. In B. R. Bonder, & M. B. Wagner (Eds.), *Functional performance in older adults* (2nd ed., pp. 196-217). Philadelphia, PA: F. A. Davis.

Byrne, P., Raphael, E. I., & Coleman-Wilson, A. (2010). Art as a transformative occupation. *OT Practice, 15*(5), 13-17.

Caron, N. (2008). The benefits of making a pen. *Advance for Occupational Therapy Practitioners, 24*(10), 28.

Carr, J. H., Shepherd, R. B., Gordon, J., Gentile, A. M., & Held, J. M. (1987). *Movement science: Foundations for physical therapy in rehabilitation*. Rockville, MD: Aspen Publishers, Inc.

Case-Smith, J., Allen, A. S., & Pratt, P. N. (1996). *Occupational therapy for children.* St. Louis, MO: Mosby.
Christiansen, C., & Baum, C. M., Eds. (2005). *Occupational therapy: Performance, participation, and well-being* (3rd ed.). Thorofare, NJ: SLACK Incorporated.
Cipriani, N. L. (2011). Kids get hooked: Crochet and contemporary occupational therapy. *OT Practice, 16*(5), 17-18.
Clark, F., & Lawlor, M. C. (2009). The making and mattering of occupational science. In E. Crepeau, E. Cohn, & B. Schell, (Eds.), *Willard and Spackman's occupational therapy* (11th ed., pp. 2-14). Philadelphia, PA: Lippincott Williams & Wilkins.
Cochran, M. (2010). OT's creative principles help blind adolescents build skills. *Advance for Occupational Therapy Practitioners, 26*(22), 24.
Cohen, H. (Ed.). (1993). *Neuroscience for rehabilitation.* Philadelphia, PA: Lippincott Williams & Wilkins.
Cottrell, R. P. F. (1996). *Perspectives on purposeful activity: Foundation and future of occupational therapy.* Bethesda, MD: American Occupational Therapy Association.
Crabtree, J. (1998). The end of occupational therapy. *American Journal of Occupational Therapy, 52*(3), 205-214.
Crepeau, E., Cohn, E., Schell, B.A. (Eds.). (2009). *Willard and Spackman's occupational therapy* (11th ed.). Philadelphia, PA: Lippincott Williams & Wilkins.
Crochet Project. (2005). *WRC horizons in treatment.* Retrieved from http://dhfs.wisconsin.gov/mh_wrcProfessional/Programs/Special Projects/crochet.HTM.
Crowe, T., & Hong, N. (2009). Culturally rich, meaningful occupations. *Advance for Occupational Therapy Practitioners, 25*(10), 8.
Cynkin, S., & Robinson, A. M. (1990). *Occupational health and activities health: Toward health through activities.* Boston, MA: Little, Brown and Company.
Diffendal, J. (2002). Kids, through the use of their hands.... *Advance for Occupational Therapy Practitioners, 18*(22), 12.
Duncome, L. W., Howe, M. C., & Schwartzberg, S. L. (1988). *Case simulations in psychosocial occupational therapy.* Philadelphia, PA: F. A. Davis.
Dunn, W. (2009). Sensation and sensory processing. In E. Crepeau, E. Cohn, & B. Schell, (Eds.), *Willard and Spackman's occupational therapy* (11th ed., pp. 777-790). Philadelphia, PA: Lippincott Williams & Wilkins.
Dunn, W., McClain, L. H., Brown, C., & Youngstrom, M. J. (2003). The ecology of human perfomance. In E. Crepeau, E. Cohn, & B. Schell, (Eds.), *Willard and Spackman's occupational therapy* (10th ed., pp. 223-227). Philadelphia, PA: Lippincott Williams & Wilkins.
Earhart, C. A., & Allen, C. K. (1988). *Cognitive disabilities: Expanded activity analysis.* Pasadena, CA: Catherine A. Earhart.
Earhart, C. A., Allen, C. K., & Blue, T. (1993). *Allen diagnostic module.* Colchester, CT: S & S Worldwide.
Early, M. B. (1993). *Mental health concepts and techniques for the occupational therapy assistant* (2nd ed.). New York, NY: Raven Press.
Early, M. B. (2009). *Mental health concepts and techniques for the occupational therapy assistant* (4th ed.). Philadelphia, PA: Lippincott Williams & Wilkins.
Eggers, O. (1984). *Occupational therapy in the treatment of adult hemiplegia.* Rockville, MD: Aspen Systems Corporation.
Fisher, A. G., Murray, E. A., & Bundy A. C. (1991). *Sensory integration: Theory and practice.* Philadelphia, PA: F. A. Davis Company.
Fidler, G., & Velde, B. (1999). *Activities: Reality and symbol.* Thorofare, NJ: SLACK Incorporated.
Flood, M., & Phillips, K. D. (2007). Creativity in older adults: A plethora of possibilities. *Issues in Mental Health Nursing, 28*, 389-411.
Gaskill, M. (2010). Cut-a-rug. *Today in OT, 3*(1), 20-21.
Geda Y. E., Roberts, R., Knopman, D., Pankratz, V. S., Christianson, T., Boeve, B., ... & Petersen, R. (2009). *Cognitive activities are associated with decreased risk of mild cognitive impairment: The Mayo Clinic population-based study of aging.* Abstract presented April, 2009.
Gilfoyle, E. M., Grady, A. P., & Moore, J. (1990). *Children adapt* (2nd ed.). Thorofare, NJ: SLACK Incorporated.
Glass, T. A., Mendes de Leon, C., Marottoli, R. A., & Berkman, L. F. (1999). Population based study of social and productive activities as predictors of survival among elderly Americans. *British Medical Journal, 319*, 478-483.
Hagedorn, R. (2001). *Foundations for practice in occupational therapy* (3rd ed.). Edinburgh, UK: Churchill Livingstone.
Hanna, G., & Perlstein, S. (2008). Creativity matters: Arts and aging in America. *Monograph, September*, 1-15.
Harris, E. (2008). The meanings of craft to an occupational therapist. *Australian Occupational Therapy Journal, 55*, 133-142.
Hasselkus, B. R., & Dickie, V. A. (1994). Doing occupational therapy: Dimensions of satisfaction and dissatisfaction. *American Journal of Occupational Therapy, 48*(2), 145-154.
Hasselkus, B. R. (2002). *The meaning of everyday occupation.* Thorofare, NJ: SLACK Incorporated.
Hendrickson, C., & Lesser, S. (2005). Building on possibilities. *Advance for Occupational Therapy Practioners 21*(9) 23-25.
Hinojosa, J., & Blount, M. (Eds.). (2009). *The texture of life: Purposeful activities in occupational therapy* (3rd ed.). Bethesda, MD: American Occupational Therapy Association.
Hooper, B. (2010). On arriving at the destination of the centennial vision: navigational landmarks to guide occupational therapy education. *Occupational Therapy in Health Care, 24*(1), 97-106
Hospice Education Institute. (2010), *Occupational therapy.* Retrieved from www.hospiceworld.org/book/occupational-therapy.htm.
Iwama, M. (2009). The Kawa model. *Therapy Times.* Retrieved from www.therapytimes.com/content.
Johnson, K. (2005). *The therapeutic value of scrapbooking.* Retrieved from www.seniority.co.uk/contributions/homeandhobbies/artsandcrafts.
Johnson, L. M. (2008). A place for art in prison: Art as a tool for rehabilitation and management. *Southwest Journal of Criminal Justice, 5*(2), 100-120.
Katz, N. (1992). *Cognitive rehabilitation: Models for intervention in occupational therapy.* Boston, MA: Andover Medical Publishers.
Kielhofner. G. (1995). *A model of human occupation: Theory and application* (2nd ed.). Baltimore, MD: Lippincott Williams & Wilkins.
Kielhofner, G. (1997). *Conceptual foundations of occupational therapy* (2nd ed.). Philadelphia, PA: F. A. Davis.
Kielhofner, G. (2004). *Conceptual foundations of occupational therapy* (3rd ed.). Philadelphia, PA: F. A. Davis.
Kramer, P., & Hinojosa, J. (1993). *Frames of reference for pediatric occupational therapy.* Baltimore, MD: Lippincott Williams & Wilkins.
LaGrossa, J. (2005). Crafts are back! *Advance for Occupational Therapy Practitioners, 21*(1), 15-17.
Law, M., Baum, C., & Dunn, W. (2005). *Measuring occupational performance: Supporting best practice in occupational therapy* (2nd ed.). Thorofare, NJ: SLACK Incorporated.

Llorens, L. A. (1984). Theoretical conceptualizations of occupational therapy: 1960-1982. *Occupational Therapy in Mental Health, 4*(2), 1-14.
Lynch, M. (2009). HHV supports creative expression as rehabilitative tool. *Journal of Rehabilitation Research & Development, 46*(7), xiii-xxi.
Ma, H. I., & Trombly, C. A. (2001). The comparison of motor performance between part and whole tasks in elderly persons. *American Journal of Occupational Therapy, 55*(1), 62-67.
Maslow, A. (1968). *Toward a psychology of being* (Rev. ed.). New York, NY: Van Nostrand.
Michigan Department of Energy, Labor, and Economic Growth (2005). *Occupational therapy/crafts.* Retrieved from www.michigan.gov/lara/0,1607,7-154-28077_28313_33124-110976--,00.html.
Monson, N. (2005). *Craft to heal.* Tucson, AZ: Hats Off Books.
Montgomery, P. C., & Connolly, B. H. (Eds.). (1991). *Motor control and physical therapy: Theoretical framework and practical applications.* Hixson, TN: Chattanooga Group, Incorporated.
Neistadt, M. E., & Crepeau, M. B. (1997). *Willard and Spackman: Occupational therapy* (9th ed.). Philadelphia, PA: Lippincott Williams & Wilkins.
Pedretti, L., & Early, M. B. (Eds.). (2001). *Occupational therapy: Practice skills for physical dysfunction* (5th ed.). St. Louis, MO: Mosby.
Peloquin, S. M. (2002). Reclaiming the vision of "reaching for hearts as well as hands." *American Journal of Occupational Therapy, 56*(5), 517-526.
Pendleton, H. M., & Schultz-Krohn, W. (Eds.). (2006). *Pedretti's occupational therapy: Practice skills for physical dysfunction* (6th ed.). Philadelphia, PA: Elsevier
Perrin, T. (2001). Don't despise the fluffy bunny: A reflection from practice. *British Journal of Occupational Therapy 64*(3), 129-134.
Pierce, D. (2001a). Occupation by design: Dimensions, therapeutic power, and creative process. *American Journal of Occupational Therapy, 55*(3), 249-259.
Pierce, D. (2001b). Untangling occupation and activity. *American Journal of Occupational Therapy, 55*(2), 138-146.
Pigza, J. (2008). *Craft therapy, then and now.* Retrieved from http://drupal02.nypl.org/blogs/2008/06/07/craft-therapy-then-and-now.
Pollanen, S. (2009). Craft as context in therapeutic change. *The Indian Journal of Occupational Therapy, 41*(2), 43-47.
Punwar, A. J., & Peloquin, S. M. (2000). *Occupational therapy principles and practice* (3rd ed.). Philadelphia, PA: Lippincott Williams & Wilkins.
Radomski, M. V., Dougherty, P. M., Fine, S. B., & Baum, C. (1994). *Case studies in cognitive rehabilitation. AOTA self-study series: Cognitive rehabilitation.* Rockville, MD: American Occupational Therapy Association.
Radomski, M. V., & Trombly, C. A. (Eds.). (2008). *Occupational therapy for physical dysfunction* (6th ed.). Philadelphia, PA: Lippincott Williams & Wilkins.
Reed, K. L. (1984). *Models of practice in occupational therapy.* Baltimore, MD: Lippincott Williams & Wilkins.
Reed, K. L., & Sanderson, S. R. (1983). *Concepts of occupational therapy* (2nd ed.). Baltimore, MD: Lippincott Williams & Wilkins.
Reilly, M. (1962). Occupational therapy can be one of the great ideas of the 20th century. *American Journal of Occupational Therapy, 16*(1), 87-105.
Reynolds, F. (1997). Coping with chronic illness and disability through creative needlecraft. *British Journal of Occupational Therapy, 60*(8), 352-356.
Reynolds, F. (2008). Expressive media used as assessment in mental health. In B. J. Hemphill-Pearson, (Ed.), *Assessments in occupational therapy mental health: An integrative approach* (2nd ed., pp. 81-96), Thorofare, NJ: SLACK Incorporated.
Rogers, J. C. (1996). Ability and disability: The performance areas. In K. O. Larson, R. G. Stevens-Ratchford, L. Pedretti, & J. Crabtree, (Eds.), *ROTE: The role of occupational therapy for the elderly* (pp. 230-262). Bethesda, MD: American Occupational Therapy Association.
Royeen, M., & Crabtree, J. L. (2006). *Native Americans. From culture in rehabilitation: From competency to proficiency* (pp. 131-150). Upper Saddle River, NJ: Pearson/Prentice Hall.
Sakemiller, L. M., & Nelson, D. L. (1998). Eliciting functional extension in prone through the use of a game. *American Journal of Occupational Therapy, 52*(2), 150-157.
Schkade, J., & McClung, M. (2001). *Occupational adaptation in practice: Concepts and cases.* Thorofare, NJ: SLACK Incorporated.
Schmid, T. (2004). Meanings of creativity within occupational therapy practice. *Australian Occupational Therapy Journal, 51*(2), 80-88.
Schultz, S., & Schkade, J. K. (2003). Occupational adaptation. In E. Crepeau, E. Cohn, & B. Schell, (Eds.), *Willard and Spackman's occupational therapy* (10th ed., pp. 220-223). Philadelphia, PA: Lippincott Williams & Wilkins.
Scipio, A. J., Kisner, J. L., Vitiello, A. V., Silverman, L., & Salls, J. (2005). The craft is back at Angora Gardens. *OT Practice, 10*(13), 20-22.
Sladyk, K., Berry, C., Brenner, C., Hengeveld, T., & Moisan, M. A. (2002). Harry Potter: Occupational therapy's new magic wand. *OT Practice, 7*(18), 13-18.
Specht, J., King, G., Brown, E., & Foris, C. (2002). The importance of leisure in the lives of persons with congenital disabilities. *American Journal of Occupational Therapy, 56*(4), 436-445.
Stewart, D., Letts, L., Law, M., Cooper, B. A., Strong, S., & Rigby, P. J. (2003). The person-environment-occupation model. In E. Crepeau, E. Cohn, & B. Schell, (Eds.), *Willard and Spackman's occupational therapy* (10th ed., pp. 227-233). Philadelphia, PA: Lippincott Williams & Wilkins.
Taussig, V. (2005). Healing through creative mosaics. *Advance for Occupational Therapy Practitioners, 21*(22), 17.
Taylor, J. B. (2008). *My stroke of insight* (p. 114). New York, NY: Viking Penguin.
Therapeutic Recreation Program. (2005). *Lighthouse for the blind.* Retrieved from www.lhb.org/services/arts-recreation-center.shtml.
Toglia, J. P., Golisz, K. M., & Goverover, Y. (2009). Evaluation and intervention for cognitive perceptual impairments. In E. Crepeau, E. Cohn, & B. Schell, (Eds.), *Willard and Spackman's occupational therapy* (11th ed., pp. 739-768). Philadelphia, PA: Lippincott Williams & Wilkins.
Trombly, C. A. (Ed.). (1995). *Occupational therapy for physical dysfunction* (4th ed.). Baltimore, MD: Lippincott Williams & Wilkins.
Trombly, C. A., & Radomski, M. V. (Eds.). (2002). *Occupational therapy for physical dysfunction* (5th ed.). Baltimore, MD: Lippincott Williams & Wilkins.

Umphred, D. A. (Ed.). (1995). *Neurological rehabilitation* (3rd ed.). St. Louis, MO: Mosby.

Van Deusen, J. A. (1993). *Body image and perceptual dysfunction in adults*. Philadelphia, PA: W. B. Saunders.

Wichrowski, M., Whiteson, J., Haas, F., Mola, A., & Rey, M. (2005). Effects of horticulture therapy on mood and heart rate in patients participating in an inpatient cardiopulmonary rehabilitation program. *Journal of Cardiopulmonary Rehabilitation, 25*(5), 270-274.

Winkle, M. Y., & Cobb, A. L. (2010). Plotting next steps: Transitions for adults with developmental disabilities. *OT Practice, 15*(21), 13-16.

Wuller, C. (2005). *Occupational Therapy New Zealand.* Retrieved from www.international.colostate.edu/intled/internships/internships_ceceliawuller.htm.

Zemke, R. (1994). *Task skills, problem solving, and social interaction. AOTA self-study series: Cognitive rehabilitation.* Rockville, MD: American Occupational Therapy Association.

□ □ □ □ □ □ □ Section II

How to Use Crafts

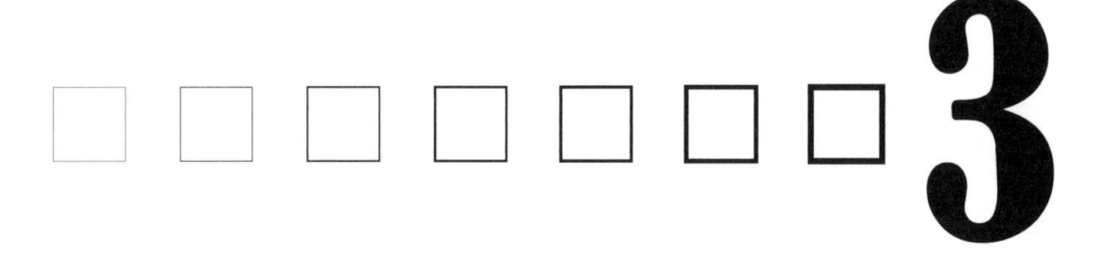

Analyzing and Grading Crafts and Creative Media

Objectives

The student should be able to:

- Understand the historical context of activity analysis in occupational therapy
- Know common components of, and be able to complete, an activity analysis for a given craft activity
- Explain the difference between grading and adaptation relative to therapeutic application
- Know basic *International Classification of Functioning* definitions and relate them to the *Occupational Therapy Practice Framework*

Analysis Activity

Occupational therapy is a "doing" profession; clients should be involved in doing activities that comprise or lead to desired occupational engagement. The profession of occupational therapy continues to struggle to define and differentiate the words *occupation* and *activity*, and the authors of the most recent edition of the *Occupational Therapy Practice Framework (OTPF)* have chosen to use them interchangeably (American Occupational Therapy Association [AOTA], 2008). The term *activity analysis*, however, is one that all therapists recognize, and understand as the breakdown of a task or occupation into disparate parts in order to determine the skills needed for, and the barriers to, its performance. This process is rooted in the theories of Frederick Taylor and Frank and Lillian Gilbreth that suggested a detailed breakdown of an industrial task into the motions and implements necessary to accomplish it most efficiently (Kuhaneck, Spitzer, & Miller, 2010). Prior to World War II, although therapists considered postures and other activity demands, "occupational therapy" meant making something, and numerous other factors were considered such as compatibility of craft with diagnosis (both performance and medical factors), cost/availability of materials, and the usefulness of the end product (Hocking, 2007). Following World War II, however, there was a greater emphasis on physical dysfunction rehabilitation as a role of occupational therapy, and *activity analysis* was coined as a descriptive term for part of the occupational therapy process; here, as in other fields, the focus was on motions and strength needed for a task. Occupational therapists dissected the physical aspects of work activities so that veterans could be specifically trained to enable their participation in these activities, and subsequently used tools such as goniometers and dynamometers (Pierce, 2001). During this time, the phrase activity analysis began to be used in texts written by American occupational therapists (Willard & Spackman, 1947) but the term was not used globally until the 1960s (Council on Physical Medicine of the American Medical Association, 1947; Department of the Army, 1951; Fidler & Fidler, 1963; MacDonald, 1960; Scullen, 1956; Willard & Spackman, 1963). Although L. J. Haas published an approach to task analysis that included consideration of an activity's social and emotional aspects as early as 1925 (Kuhaneck et al., 2010), the concept of considering other, possibly less measurable, aspects of an activity/occupation—such as the psychological, social, and economic—gained acceptance only gradually.

Many different methods of activity analysis have been developed since 1960. As practice issues have evolved over the decades, including physical versus psychosocial focus and emergence of specialty practices, different analyses developed for each area of expertise. The trend toward holistic thinking, however, was reflected in 1988 with the development of one integrated activity analysis form (Hopkins & Smith, 1988). Still, within an area of specialization in occupational therapy, the corresponding activity analysis may have a somewhat different organizational focus and call for slightly different information. Some authors even suggest the use of an adapted activity analysis in implementing administrative decisions as well as clinical ones (Punwar & Peloquin, 2000). A systems theorist might assert that the overall value of an activity cannot be discerned from the analysis of its parts (Kielhofner, 2004) and the sums of the parts may not be equal to the whole in terms of its essential nature or meaning to the performer. An activity can be examined as an endeavor that a client wants to learn or resume, or as a means of accomplishing a therapeutic purpose (Fidler & Velde, 1999). It can also be analyzed relative to a particular frame of reference and in this case the therapist will be most interested in the factors relevant to that approach.

Newer texts describe environmental and social/cultural aspects as equally important to the motor and cognitive demands (Crepeau, Cohn & Schell, 2009; Pedretti & Early, 2006). This occurred as a result of, or in conjunction with, the development of the *OTPF*, (AOTA, 2002, 2008) and the reaffirmation of client-centered evaluation and treatment. The *OTPF* (see Appendix IV) replaced the earlier codified occupational therapy language known as Uniform Terminology (AOTA, 1994), and was designed to be more consistent with the *International Classification of Functioning (ICF)* developed by the World Health Organization in 2001. The activity analysis described in this chapter is based upon the revised 2008 *OTPF* (AOTA, 2008) and can be used with any of the theoretical models outlined in Chapter 2. More experienced therapists rarely complete full activity analyses in written form but are continually engaged in this process mentally as the therapy session proceeds (Kuhaneck et al., 2010) Students benefit from completing multiple detailed activity analyses as they seek to become proficient at assessment of clients and adaptation of tasks.

Similarly to the *OTPF*, the *ICF* differentiates body structures and functions, and distinguishes between activity completion and participation. Impairment, defined as a problem with structure and/or function, does not necessarily imply inability to do an activity (execute a task). Likewise, inability to do a specific activity does not have to preclude participation in the larger sense (involvement in a life situation). The *ICF* seeks to integrate both medical and social models of health; therefore it considers not only the individual, but the environment as well. The environment can be a barrier or a facilitator, and this can occur either through the presence of certain factors, or through their absence. For example, the presence of a ramp is a facilitator for someone in a wheelchair; absence of a negative stereotype is also a facilitator. The *ICF* also differentiates between performance and capacity. Capacity is the predicted ability of a person to execute a task based on a standard procedure and environment; performance is what the person actually does, which may be accomplished through an adapted procedure and/or environment.

These concepts are entirely consistent with the philosophy of occupational therapy. It is not difficult to see how "participation" in *ICF* terms equates with "occupational functioning" in the *OTPF*. Satisfactory occupational functioning can be achieved regardless of an impairment or activity limitation. Like the *ICF*, the *OTPF* considers environment, or context, to be a highly important variable. Occupational therapists use the process of activity analysis to determine not only how, but where and when adaptations can be made to maximize occupational competence, an important factor in occupational identity. Hence, the primary aim of adaptation is to change the activity so that a client can continue to participate in a valued occupation (Kielhofner, Forsyth, Kramer, Melton, & Dobson, 2009) or in *ICF* terminology, to enable participation despite a limitation.

Table 3-1

GRADING

Ideas for grading/remediation-craft as a means:

- Have client participate in planning or materials preparation
- Increase or decrease the number of steps
- Place/remove a time requirement
- Increase/decrease resistance
- Place objects to facilitate reach or postural changes
- Increase/reduced number of tools/supplies available
- Change the number of choices available
- Change the design
- Have client participate in clean up

Adaptations to enable participation/compensation-craft as an end:

- Alter the method
- Use enlarged or reshaped handles
- Reduce the number of steps/complexity
- Provide a stabilizing surface
- Provide extra lighting or magnification
- Use adapted tools (e.g., electric scissors)

Grading is similar to adaptation, but has a subtle difference in meaning. Grading, as used by occupational therapists, may be clarified by Merriam Webster's (1994) definition of *gradual*, which comes from the same root word:

Gradual (adj.): 1. Proceeding by steps or degrees; 2. Moving, changing, or developing by fine, slight, or often imperceptible degrees.

A recent text on activity analysis defines grading as "to arrange or position in a scale of size, quality, or intensity" (Hersch, Lamport & Coffey, 2005). Grading generally refers to structuring an activity such that the challenge or demand will gradually increase and thereby facilitate improvement in a client's function. Given these definitions, adaptation versus grading might be likened to compensation versus remediation, respectively. For example, the client may use sanding blocks of gradually decreasing size to work on increasing grip strength (grading); another client, for whom woodworking is a preferred occupation, may use an adapted sanding block to compensate for the (permanent) inability to grasp.

There is no one correct way to grade an activity; see Table 3-1. Any modifications made should take into account a client's values, developmental or functional level, and occupational history. Both processes—adapting or grading—may involve changes such as the number of steps, arrangement of the work area, tools or techniques used, time allotted, and complexity of the completed project. See Table 3-1 for some general suggestions; the Practice Framework section on Activity Demands may also stimulate some helpful ideas. Some clients may resist doing an activity in any other than the "normal" way, and this wish should be respected as long as safety is not compromised (Hersch et al., 2005). Activity modifications suggested in this text include ideas that could be considered adaptation OR grading, depending on the therapist's or client's ultimate objective. In some instances this involves choosing a simpler (or more complex) project from a given craft category. For example, for a client interested in sewing but limited by a motor or visual impairment, the therapist may choose a plastic canvas coaster project instead of a counted cross stitch wall hanging. The therapist must ensure, however, that this substitute activity will retain its intrinsic value to the client. Some authors discourage the use of contrived activities or using only parts of whole activities; the grading or adaptation process should maintain realism and relevance for the participant as much as possible (Hersch et al., 2005; Kielhofner, 2004). While the most meaningful activities are those in which the client has previously participated, the individual may also find purpose in a novel activity when its potential for enabling a future goal is made clear (Velde & Fidler, 2002). When discussing problems in occupational functioning, the therapist should take care to instill in the client the belief that a solution for their constraints exists (Bontje, Kinébanian, Josephsson, & Tamura, 2004); this fosters a sense of hope and increases motivation to participate. Incidentally, therapists themselves should adapt or grade their therapeutic interactions styles as needed to maximize client performance.

In practice, many clients improve, but some deteriorate. A craft that the client may have accomplished or been proficient in at an earlier period may need to be simplified. This concept is central to the practice of occupational therapy—to match or adapt the activity to the client. By approaching each craft with the certain knowledge that it can be made simpler or more complex as needed, the therapist can be confident in allowing a client to choose a craft with personal meaning and then adapting it to actual ability. Applying knowledge of activity demands, including modification, will also assist the therapist in writing clear, measurable goals that can be achieved using any craft in this text. These goals should be discussed and established with clients as a way for them to evaluate their own level of capability. This offers an excellent opportunity to discuss how the short-term objectives of a craft project can be related to long-term occupational goals and the grading process can be used to demonstrate the small steps clients must take to achieve true independence.

Activity analysis has been central to occupational therapy treatment for over 60 years, and though areas of emphasis have changed over time, it is still important to go through the process of calculating the requirements of a task and its potential benefits for a client. Although Barris, Cordero, and Christiansen (1986) implied that a therapist could analyze and modify an activity without knowing how to do it, this seems improbable. Realistically, the therapist must have a thorough knowledge of how an activity is done regardless of the ability to actually do it. He or she should be familiar with the properties of the materials and the methods and sequence of the process in order to implement organized and consistent experiences (Taussig, 2004). Based on the holistic philosophy of occupational therapy, an activity analysis cannot exist without a client in mind. In analyzing a craft activity for use in treatment, the therapist should first consider client goals and interests. Second, the therapist should think about factors that will influence a client's success with the activity. Unlike with an exercise or enabling activity, the client will have an expectation of outcome and may be displeased if the end product is unattractive or unfinished. Included in factors to consider are the quality of the materials, the number of steps, wait time, and the amount of creativity required. For example, some materials, such as clay or wax, are more forgiving than others, such as metal or leather. Some have sensory components such as texture or odors that may be objectionable to clients. Some projects require precision, such as trying to replicate a design, while others will be acceptable with a rough, rustic or abstract look, such as handmade paper or a scrap fabric wreath. If a project requires gluing or painting, this usually means waiting until it dries before going on to the next step and will require that the client can tolerate this delay. Some clients will lack the ability to conceptualize and will need a specific pattern to follow, color suggestions, or may prefer a project that needs no decoration at all, such as a basic wood project. Although crafts may well be used as a means to an end rather than as end in themselves, clients will find them unsatisfying if they dislike the look of what they create.

Because cultural and personal context cannot be ignored in the activity analysis, the format in this text uses a hypothetical client. This is critical to the occupational therapist's quest to emphasize the unique meaning and relevance of an activity to an individual, above and beyond its generic purpose or goal. The activity analysis form (see Appendix III) was developed for crafts and activities presented in this book. It uses the same vocabulary as the *OTPF* (AOTA, 2008), though not necessarily in the same sequence. For example, the performance contexts and patterns are early in this activity analysis form because they guide the user to look first at the global world of the client and the "fit" of the activity within a typical routine. This is followed by a description of the activity and its demands, then continues to include performance in areas of occupation, performance skills, and client factors. Throughout the form, if the *OTPF* terms do not apply to crafts or other creative media, they are not included.

While this activity analysis form is intended to be holistic in its approach, that is, it encompasses "all aspects of a client's health" (Christiansen & Baum, 1997), it allows the user to distill the activity from several perspectives (e.g., objects or space needed to perform it) or fit with existing roles and cultural values. To break something apart is the antithesis of holistic; however, time is of the essence in the modern health care system, so this form allows therapists to use only those parts necessary for each individual client. The experienced occupational therapist has neither time nor need to complete a comprehensive activity analysis on every treatment activity. A periodic review of the form, however, would serve as a beneficial refresher on clinical reasoning. Practicing therapists will want to consider whether they are using the craft as a means to achieving another goal or as an end in itself. If the activity is to be a therapeutic means, the therapist may be more interested in sections IV, V, VI, and X. Sections VIII and XI cover some overlapping information; VIII deals with applied performance skills, while XI deals with their more discrete components. The occupational therapy student should complete this form for different activities and clients as often as is feasible until the process comes naturally. The student/therapist is encouraged to fill in all the information called for after each word or phrase. If the information asked for is not applicable to the craft activity, the therapist should write "N/A" (not applicable) in that space. Although this text is not intended to replace a comprehensive volume on activity analysis, a blank version of this sample activity/occupation analysis form is located in Appendix III. The form contents have been adapted from Drake, 1999; Hersch et al., 2005; and the AOTA *OTPF*, 2008. The therapist can consult these references if there is confusion about the meaning of any terminology. By approaching each craft with a view of possible modifications, a therapist can match an activity/occupation with the treatment needs of a broad spectrum of clients. When knowledge of process and creativity are used in this endeavor, crafts can offer satisfaction at almost any functional level.

The following is a completed sample of a typical activity analysis using the form in Appendix III and is based on the case study below. It is not inclusive of every item of the *OTPF*, but is rather tailored with application of crafts in mind. In the chapters that follow, examples of simple and more complex approaches for each craft category are included. To determine the most therapeutic level of challenge, the therapist must first become proficient at activity/occupation analysis.

Case Study

Stephanie was admitted to an adolescent inpatient psychiatric facility at her parents request after repeated problems at school, lost friendships, and an increasing inability to control her behavior at home. Stephanie, 15, was the second oldest of five children in her close Catholic family. Approximately 1 year ago, she was diagnosed with type I diabetes and put on a strict diet along with the insulin pump. Stephanie's parents, strong believers in personal responsibility and self-control, monitored their daughter closely. After a "honeymoon" period of faithfully following her diet, Stephanie began to rebel. She was sneaking food both at school and at home, having temper tantrums, and falling behind in her schoolwork. The more her parents tried to control her, the worse her behavior became. Stephanie seemed unable to gain any solace from her siblings or friends and became isolative and angry. Her parents finally reached the realization that they needed professional help.

Prior to her diagnosis, Stephanie had enjoyed reading, cooking and shopping with her friends. At school, she was a member of the girls' volleyball team, the yearbook staff, and several academic honoraries. With her family, she particularly found pleasure in cooking and decorating for holidays, as well as going on family trips and outings. The occupational therapist gleaned this information by interviewing both Stephanie and her parents. She also evaluated Stephanie using the Internal/External Locus of Control Scale and the Adolescent Role Assessment. Results revealed that she perceived a high degree of external control and that she felt incompetent in many of her previously valued roles. She felt that her disease compromised her contribution to her family and that her enjoyment of cooking, eating, and celebrating was lost. She felt she had no control over her own actions, her health, or circumstances around her. Loss of perceived role competence was heading Stephanie toward clinical depression. Due to a lack of enough characteristic symptoms, however, the psychiatrist ultimately gave her a diagnosis of Adjustment Disorder.

Together, the therapist and Stephanie agreed that she needed to work on more positive coping strategies, renew social participation, and independently manage her diet.

The occupational therapist tried having Stephanie join the coping skills group, but she failed to complete the assignments and was uncommunicative during the discussions. Since Stephanie liked cooking and holiday decorating, the therapist decided to offer her the opportunity to do crafts. From the choices offered, Stephanie chose to make a candle. She stated she liked burning candles at home in her room, especially those with different fragrances. Stephanie began by making a container candle in a small canning jar. Once the therapist gave her the instructions, she was able to complete the activity independently. She even cleaned and put away the tools and equipment she had used. The next day, she asked if she could make another candle before she was discharged. The therapist thought that since Stephanie had shown a high degree of competence in the first project, she might try something more difficult. She gave her a book with instructions for other projects and allowed her to choose her next one. Stephanie chose a layered, molded pillar candle. She was able to gather all the needed supplies, and using just the written instructions, completed the candle independently. The therapist provided only supervision and occasional experienced advice. Stephanie was thrilled with the finished product and stated she was going to give it to her best friend. Later that day, the therapist overheard her talking with her mother about wanting to get some candle making supplies for home. She said it took her mind off wanting to cook and eat "forbidden" foods. The therapist also knew that it had helped restore her sense of competence and control.

I. **Name of activity/occupation:** Making a layered candle

A. Brief description—A candle will be made from a block of paraffin by melting and pouring into a milk carton mold

B. Major steps (include time required for each):

1. Begin to heat paraffin—Place paraffin chunks (about 1 pound) in a coffee can; place coffee can in a pan of hot water on the stove; keep burner on a low setting (*10 minutes*)
2. Prepare the mold—Cut and clean the milk carton (1 pint size); make a small hole in the bottom (*5 minutes*)
3. Prepare the wick—Cut the wick a few inches longer than the mold; soak it in melted paraffin, straighten, let dry (*10 minutes*)
4. Insert the wick through the hole in the bottom of the mold, leaving a tail of about one inch; seal the hole with mold seal; tape the wick tail to the bottom (refer to Figure 14-2 in Chapter 14; *1 minute*)
5. From the top, pull the wick taut and wrap it around a dowel or pencil which has been placed across the top of the mold; tape to hold (refer to Figure 14-1 in Chapter 14; *1 minute*)
6. Continue to melt paraffin until it reaches 160 degrees; add one teaspoon of stearin (unless already contained in paraffin compound) and stir (*10 minutes*)
7. Using hot pads or other protection, pour paraffin into mold about 1/3 full (*1 minute*)
8. Return paraffin to water bath, add yellow dye, stir
9. When it returns to 160 degrees, pour into mold about 2/3 full (*5 minutes*)
10. Return paraffin to water bath, add yellow, blue, and stir
11. When it returns to 160 degrees, pour into mold almost full (*5 minutes*)
12. Let cool for 10 to 15 minutes; insert pointed tool down around wick and fill any depression created with a little more hot wax; use a funnel if necessary
13. Let cool completely, then tear away mold (*1 hour*; can speed cooling time by placing in an ice water bath)

C. Precautions: Hot stove burner, hot paraffin and container, sharp tool (awl, ice pick)

II. **Performance contexts and environments (for a hypothetical client)**

A. Personal

1. Age/gender—15 year old female
2. Residential status—Lives at home with parents
3. Socioeconomic status—Middle class family
4. Educational status—10th grade student

B. Social
   1. Support system—Close knit family
   2. Social group membership—School friends, church friends

C. Cultural—Cultural norms, ethnicity, customs, beliefs (American Caucasian; family relationships, hard work, self-reliance highly valued)

D. Physical—Treatment setting
   1. Space available, furniture arrangement—Clinic kitchen; table and 4 chairs in middle with walking space around
   2. Lighting, ventilation, temperature—Florescent lighting; centrally heated and cooled; non-opening windows
   3. Appliances, equipment—Sink; stove/oven; fully stocked kitchen (pots, pans, utensils, etc.)

E. Temporal
   1. Time of day—10 a.m.
   2. Amount of time needed, multiple sessions?—1 hour session; will return before lunch to tear off mold

F. Virtual (Computer use, etc.)—N/A

III. Performance patterns

A. Habits (Does the activity utilize or reinforce useful habits?)—Yes; similar to cooking; must observe similar rules and safety precautions

B. Routine (Does the activity have an established sequence?)—Yes; some steps could be eliminated (adding color) but order must stay the same

C. Roles (Is the activity consistent with customary roles of the client?)—Yes, because she enjoys both cooking and decorating

D. Rituals—Candle use is common in the client's Catholic faith

IV. Therapeutic application

A. Treatment goal, relation to occupational performance—To renew leisure involvement as a means of coping; to have a positive experience by following rules/recipes

B. Appropriate population/general skills needed
   1. Age range, diagnostic group—10 years and up; may not be appropriate for some geriatric clients; useful for multiple diagnostic groups, including mental health and physical dysfunction
   2. Motor skills—Must be able to maintain and change postures; must have short distance mobility and ability to reach from one surface to another; must have gross coordination and manipulation skills for pouring; must have strength to lift and carry container of paraffin (< 1 pound) short distances; must be able to work at a consistent pace since material needs to be at certain temperature for certain operations
   3. Process (cognitive, sensory, emotional) skills—Must be able to attend for at least 5 minutes at a time (longer steps involve some waiting times); must be able to use tools appropriately and ask for assistance if needed; must sequence activity in the correct order and be spatially oriented; must be able to respond to environmental cues due to safety risks; must be able to adjust behavior for a positive outcome
   4. Communications skills—Solitary activity, but may have to interact with therapist

C. Activity demands
   1. Nonexpendable tools and equipment; source and cost:
      - Stove, hot plate, electric skillet, or other heat source, $20 minimum
      - Cooking pot, $5
      - Awl, ice pick, or barbeque skewer, $2
      - Funnel, $2
      - Scissors, $2
      - Small dowel or pencil, less than $1
      - Measuring spoon for stearin, $1 or less

2. Expendable materials and supplies; source and cost:
    - Paraffin, $1 ($1 per pound)
    - Wicking, $10 (for 100 yards)
    - Dye, $1
    - Stearin, $2 (may already be in wax compound)
    - Tape, $1
    - Mold sealer, $3 (can use low-cost modeling clay)
    - Water, no direct cost
3. Space requirements—2- x 4-feet counter area
4. Sequencing and timing—Accurate timing necessary; melted paraffin will harden quickly
5. Acceptable criteria for completion—Candle that will burn

D. Preparation
1. By whom—Client or therapist (or therapist assistant or aide)
2. Steps and time required—Gather materials, break paraffin into chunks if necessary, 15 minutes
3. Placement of tools and materials—Placed within reach on counter area

E. Sensory or psychological stimulation anticipated—There will be odors of melting wax; heat; olfactory stimulation if scents are used; could possibly trigger memories

V. Therapeutic modification/method of instruction

A. Opportunities for grading
1. Sequence, duration, procedures—Could make one-color candle, container candle; sequence would remain the same; would eliminate one or more steps, shorten time
2. Working position—Could be completed in sitting, especially with movable heat source such as an electric skillet; would need way to reach up to sink for water in double boiler
3. Tools (position, size, shape, texture, weight)—Use differently sized/shaped containers for melting wax; use blunt-ended tool for stirring, poking around wick after filling
4. Materials (position, size, shape, texture, weight)—Could begin with smaller (or larger) chunks of paraffin; could eliminate additives; may attach wick to larger tool for dipping if unable to hold onto wicking. Could melt existing candle and reuse its wick.

B. Opportunities for adapting
1. Orthotics, prosthetics—Splinting for functional wrist/hand position
2. Assistive devices, technology—Adapted handle scissor (or knife) for cutting wick; two-handled pan, or adapted cup ring around can, for melting wax; pot stabilizer; adapted faucets at sink or knobs on stove, or knob turner.
3. Preventative
    a. Energy conservation/joint protection—Teach to lift and carry containers with palms instead of fingers; enlarged or adapted handles to minimize grasp requirements; gather materials before starting to minimize mobility demands
    b. Positioning/body mechanics—May work in sitting; instruct in posture, body mechanics during reaching
    c. Activity balance/wellness—Could be used as a hobby, means of relaxation; use of candle can also be related to relaxation sessions

C. Method of instruction
1. Tactile, verbal, visual cues (type and frequency), verbal, visual, written; visual sample at beginning of task; verbal and written, intermittent throughout
2. Teaching-learning environment—Will allow teaching opportunities about the importance of following directions/prescribed sequences, adhering to time parameters; adhering to measure parameters (amounts, temperatures)
3. Group versus individual, group member-assisted—An individual activity; could instruct or assist others

VI. Therapeutic qualities

A. Energy patterns (pacing, attention to task)—Pacing is important; wax must be poured at certain temperatures, allowed to harden a specified time

B. Activity patterns

1. Structured versus unstructured—Structured
2. Repetitive—No
3. Expressive/creative—Yes; allows for some creative additions such as colors, scents, mold shapes, etc. but these are not required
4. Tactile (equipment, materials, persons)—Touching, handling wax; hot container

VII. Areas of occupation (which and why?)

A. IADL—Yes, in similarities to cooking

B. Education—Following rules, directions, schedules; maintaining attention

C. Work—Following rules, directions, schedules; maintaining attention; working at a consistent pace

D. Play—No

E. Leisure—Yes, this could be a hobby

F. Social participation—Indirectly; candles might be used at social occasions

VIII. Performance skills required

A. Motor and praxis skills

1. Client position/posture—Upright, sitting, or standing
2. Postural control—Required due to hot materials
3. Position changes, ambulation—Minimal position change, primarily trunk rotation; ambulation not required, could substitute wheelchair mobility; must carry (hot) item short distances
4. Trunk and limb ROM—Trunk rotation, minimal flexion; upper extremity ROM needed, largest range requirement is in elbows; 75 degrees shoulder flexion, 30 degrees abduction; 30 degrees to 120 degrees elbow flexion; 30 degrees wrist extension; full pronation, neutral supination
5. Strength—Must lift paraffin container from hot water; requires upper extremity strength
6. Muscle tone—Hypertonia or reflexes could compromise safety in handling hot wax
7. Endurance—Endurance for about one hour for a minimally exertive task; could sit to rest during waiting periods
8. Coordination—Gross coordination required for pouring; fine coordination for preparing mold and if decoration is added
9. Manipulation—Must pick up wax pieces, handle wick, hold tools; needs tip-to-tip pinch, lateral pinch, cylindrical grasp
10. Praxis—Steps must be done in sequence and with appropriate timing using familiar actions such as lifting, pouring, cutting

B. Sensory-perceptual skills

1. Pacing/timing—Must follow prescribed sequence
2. Proprioception—Must be able to determine correct body position and postural changes needed and grade upper extremity actions such as grasp strength
3. Visual—awareness of spatial relationships required for mold preparation and pouring of wax
4. Auditory—N/A
5. Tactile—Hot/cold sensation necessary for safety

C. Emotional regulation skills

1. Controlling emotions/frustration tolerance—Necessary for safety; needed in the event of a less than optimal outcome
2. Task persistence—Necessary for safety and acceptable end product
3. Responding to feelings of others—N/A
4. Using coping/relaxation strategies—Probably not necessary

D. Cognitive skills

1. Judging—Must recognize need for assistance and safety considerations such as handling hot/sharp objects

2. Selecting—Must be able to choose appropriate tools and supplies
3. Sequencing—Must be able to continue and terminate activity, with or without cueing and adhere to correct sequence
4. Problem solving—Must be able to adapt as needed and manage unexpected situations such as spills; may need cueing to anticipate mistakes
5. Attention to task—Must be able to attend for at least 5 minutes at a time without redirection and must be goal directed
6. Organizing (Must find, gather, and replace tools and materials; with or without assistance)—Organize work space, and know when to initiate and terminate each step of the activity

E. Communication and social skills
1. Body language and position—N/A, unless interacting with therapist
2. Personal space, appropriate contact—N/A, unless interacting with therapist
3. Exchanging information—Must ask for assistance (if needed) in an acceptable manner; verbal ability not mandatory
4. Maintaining appropriate relationships—N/A, unless interacting with therapist

IX. Client factors—Specific skill requirements

A. Global mental functions
1. Must client be fully oriented? No
2. Must client have a stable personality, behavior? Yes
3. Must client have motivation? Impulse control? Yes

B. Specific mental functions
1. How much attention, memory are needed? Attention of 5 minutes at a time; 1 hour memory
2. Must client be able to interpret all sensory stimuli? Yes
3. Will thought disorders interfere? Yes
4. What language ability is required? None
5. Are executive functions needed? Yes, to plan, anticipate problems
6. Is calculation ability required? No
7. What motor planning skills are needed (is task familiar or novel)? Novel
8. Must client have intact body image, concept? No

C. Sensory functions and pain
1. How much visual acuity and what types of visual perception are needed? Fair acuity, good depth perception, fair figure-ground discrimination
2. How much hearing is needed? None
3. How much balance is needed? Good
4. Must client perceive and respond to pain? Yes
5. Does client need to be able to discriminate other sensory stimuli (e.g. taste, smell, touch, body movement, temperature)? Body movement and temperature

D. Systems function
1. What is client diagnosis/diagnoses? Adjustment disorder
2. Will the activity have an effect on respiration, blood pressure, or other cardiac function? No
3. Will the activity have an effect on digestive, metabolic, endocrine, or excretory functions? No
4. Will the activity have an effect of skin, hair, or nails? Could burn skin

E. Neuromuscular/motor function—See Part VIII Motor Skills, A, B, and C

X. Miscellaneous psychosocial considerations

A. Does the craft provide the opportunity to discover what is? Is it valuable to the client? Yes; could stimulate a discussion of uses of candles, memories, etc. (e.g., could bring up church, holidays, birthdays, gift-giving occasions, favorite colors, scents)

B. Could the craft contribute to self-esteem? Yes. How? By resulting in a product that many people would find attractive and might purchase from a store

C. Does the craft offer opportunities for affective expression?
   1. Hostility/aggression (i.e., motions such as hammering, tearing, piercing) No
   2. Sadness (i.e., slow movements) No
   3. Happiness (i.e., pride, hope, laughter) Yes; pride in end product; stimulation of positive memories
   4. Loving (i.e., stroking, holding) No

D. Does the craft provide opportunities for testing reality of the client's own perceptions/beliefs (i.e., is my behavior/perception/belief normal?) Yes, since there is a concrete end product that will or will not "work"

E. Is there an opportunity to develop leadership skills while doing the craft?—Yes, if instructing others

Discussion Questions

1. How much (or how little) choice should you allow a client in choosing a craft? How would you deal with an insistent client who has chosen an activity you believe to be much too difficult?
2. Is continuous, physical engagement in a task necessary for therapeutic benefit? How would you handle a situation in which the client is spending a great deal of time on design or discussion of a project that you had chosen to address a motor function?
3. How much can you adapt or grade an activity without losing its meaning entirely? How can you relate this to the concepts of purposeful activity versus occupation?
4. Imagine you have chosen a craft to facilitate a client's attention to task and other cognitive processes. You are pleased with the client's initiation and perseverance during the activity, but the client complains that their creation is "ugly." How do you respond? How do you reconcile your focus on process with the client's focus on end product?

(Adapted from Hagedorn, 2001)

References

American Occupational Therapy Association. (1994). Uniform terminology for occupational therapy (3rd ed.). *American Journal of Occupational Therapy, 48*(11), 1047-1054.

American Occupational Therapy Association. (2002). Occupational therapy practice framework: Domain and process. *American Journal of Occupational Therapy 56*, 609-639.

American Occupational Therapy Association. (2008). Occupational therapy practice framework: Domain and process (2nd ed.). *American Journal of Occupational Therapy, 62*(6), 625-683.

Barris, R., Cordero, J., & Christiaansen, R. (1986). Occupational therapist's use of media. *American Journal of Occupational Therapy, 40*(10), 679-684.

Bontje, P., Kinébanian, A., Josephsson, S., & Tamura, Y. (2004). Occupational adaptation: The experiences of older persons with physical disabilities. *American Journal of Occupational Therapy, 58*(2), 140-149.

Christiansen, C., & Baum, C. (1997). *Occupational therapy: Enabling function and well-being* (2nd ed.). Thorofare, NJ: SLACK Incorporated.

Council on Physical Medicine of the American Medical Association. (1947). *Manual of occupational therapy.* Chicago, IL: American Medical Association.

Crepeau, E., Cohn, E., Schell, B.A. (Eds.). (2009). *Willard and Spackman's occupational therapy* (11th ed.). Philadelphia, PA: Lippincott Williams & Wilkins.

Department of the Army. (1951). *Occupational therapy.* Washington, DC: U.S. Government Printing Office.

Fidler, G. S., & Fidler, J. W. A. (1963). *Communication process in psychiatry: Occupational therapy.* New York, NY: The MacMillan Co.

Fidler, G. S., & Velde, B. P. (1999) *Activities: Reality and symbol.* Thorofare, NJ: SLACK Incorporated.

Hagedorn, R. (2001). *Foundations for practice in occupational therapy* (3rd ed.). Edinburgh, UK: Churchill Livingstone

Hersch, G., Lamport, N., & Coffey, M. (2005). *Activity analysis: Application to occupation* (5th ed.). Thorofare, New Jersey: SLACK Incorporated.

Hocking, C. (2007). Early perspectives of patients, practice and profession. *The British Journal of Occupational Therapy, 70*(7), 284-291.

Hopkins, H. L., & Smith, H. D. (1988). *Willard and Spackman's occupational therapy* (7th ed.). Philadelphia, PA: Lippincott Williams & Wilkins.

Kielhofner, G. (2004). *Conceptual foundations of occupational therapy* (3rd ed.). Philadelphia, PA: F. A. Davis Co.
Kielhofner, G., Forsyth, K., Kramer, J. M., Melton, J., & Dobson, E. (2009). The model of human occupation. In E. Crepeau, E. Cohn, & B. Schell (Eds.), *Willard and Spackman's occupational therapy* (11th ed.). Philadelphia, PA: Lippincott Williams & Wilkins.
Kuhaneck, H. M., Spitzer, S. L., & Miller, E. (2010). *Activity analysis, creativity, and playfulness in pediatric occupational therapy.* Sudbury, MA: Jones and Bartlett Publishers.
MacDonald, E. M. (1960). *Occupational therapy in rehabilitation.* London, UK: Bailliere, Tindall, and Cox.
Merriam Webster (Ed.). (1994). *Merriam Webster's collegiate dictionary* (10th ed.). Springfield, MA: Merriam-Webster, Incorporated.
Pedretti, L., & Early, M. B. (Eds.). (2001). *Occupational therapy: Practice skills for physical dysfunction* (5th ed.). St. Louis, MO: Mosby.
Pierce, D. (2001). Untangling occupation and activity. *American Journal of Occupational Therapy, 55*(2), 138-145.
Punwar, A. J., & Peloquin, S. M. (2000). Occupational therapy: Principles and practice (3rd ed.). Philadelphia, PA: Lippincott Williams & Wilkins.
Scullen, V. (1956). *Occupational therapy manual for personnel in the New York state department of mental hygiene.* Albany, NY: State of New York Department of Mental Hygiene.
Taussig, V. (2004). Keeping crafts alive in mental health. *Advance for Occupational Therapy Practitioners, 20*(16), 14.
Velde, B., & Fidler, G. (2002). *Lifestyle performance: A model for engaging the power of occupation.* Thorofare, NJ: SLACK Incorporated.
Willard, H. S., & Spackman, C. S. (1947). *Principles of occupational therapy.* Philadelphia, PA: Lippincott Williams & Wilkins.
Willard, H. S., & Spackman, C. S. (1963). *Occupational therapy* (3rd ed.). Philadelphia, PA: Lippincott Williams & Wilkins.
World Health Organization. (2001). *International classification of functioning.* Retrieved from www.who.int/classifications/icf/en/.

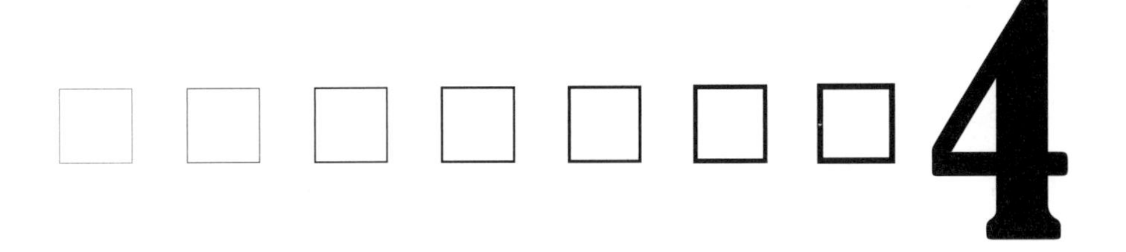

Documenting the Use of Crafts and Other Creative Media

Objectives

The student should be able to:

- List the purposes of documentation
- Explain how documentation of creative media use is consistent with the general purposes of documentation
- Describe how crafts can be used in assessment and give examples of assessments that include crafts
- Describe how to make skilled intervention evident in documentation of crafts/creative media use
- Describe how to incorporate the *Occupational Therapy Practice Framework* (*OTPF*; American Occupational Therapy Association [AOTA], 2002) terminology in documentation of creative media
- Verbalize a basic understanding of how craft as an occupation is consistent with the occupational therapy domain and process
- Effectively report on the therapeutic use of a craft using the SOAP format

Documenting the use of crafts or other creative media is really no different than documenting any other treatment approach. The therapist must consider both the purposes of documentation and the structure and language to best achieve them. Some therapists downplay the use of crafts in their reports, fearing they will be seen as juvenile or unscientific and therefore unworthy of reimbursement. This attitude has no doubt contributed to the decline in the use of crafts in occupational therapy, making the roles of this and other rehabilitation professions less distinct from one another (Holder, 2001; Hooper, 2010). While occupational therapists in the United States have been forced to balance between providing optimum treatment and producing revenue, overemphasis on objectivity and function—to the exclusion of the subjective experience—may compromise the holistic client-centered approach (Jongbloed & Wendland, 2002). Activities with greater personal meaning may cause a patient to be more fully invested in the therapy process. In addition, having a patient engage in a craft can allow the therapist to assess performance skills applicable to many aspects of daily function (Schmid, 2004). While a patient can often perform habitual activities with little difficulty, the novelty of completing a craft may illuminate deficits in areas such as problem solving, recognition of errors, capacity for learning, and the ability to anticipate consequences of actions (Allen, Earhart, & Blue, 1992; Taussig, 2004).

Tubbs, C., & Drake, M. *Crafts and Creative Media in Therapy, Fourth Edition (pp. 43-50).*

This chapter will explain how to document the use of crafts and other creative activities as skilled therapeutic interventions utilizing accepted terminology, how to relate this to broader goals related to daily occupation, and how a therapist might use crafts as a means of assessment. In addition, this chapter will provide examples of how the *OTPF* is useful for guiding clinical reasoning and documentation and how this universal occupational therapy terminology can be applied to crafts just as easily as to other media and methods (AOTA, 2008). If the clinician can demonstrate the utility of crafts and other creativity-based approaches in providing skilled assessment and intervention, their unique contribution for the restoration of occupational goals may be revitalized.

In completing all types of documentation, occupational therapists must consider who will have access to and utilize their reports. Clients' information is available to multiple audiences, including the clients themselves. Therapy reports may be read by insurance reviewers, teachers, parents, or others who may not be familiar with specific occupational therapy terminology or the occupational therapy approach in general. It is important to identify the special professional skill and yet make it easy for the reader to understand (Glomstad, 2005). Therapists document for a number of reasons, and each plays a role in the accurate reporting of the therapeutic use of crafts. The first purpose is communication and management of client care (Borcherding, 2005). Historically, even before the era of third-party payers, occupational therapists needed to make clear to the physician their intentions in having a client make something. The emphasis was on preparing the client to rejoin the workforce, and therapists felt compelled to prove their value (Hocking, 2007). A client's performance in a craft activity can relay valuable information about safety, ability to follow directions, or motor skill, for example. Abilities and deficiencies in completing a craft are likely to help predict performance in other areas of function. In the school setting, a child's participation in a craft activity may have educational relevance, for instance the ability to copy a shape, or use scissors, or stay on task for a given length of time.

A second, and much emphasized, reason for documentation is third-party reimbursement (Borcherding, 2005). Because Medicare and Medicaid require that therapy services be "medically necessary" and that the client has a need for "skilled intervention" (Lemke, 2004), occupational therapists have come to believe that they will not be reimbursed for using crafts as therapeutic agents. Some authors suggest that therapists should "de-emphasize" the media in documenting treatment (Borcherding, 2005), but this could prove to be a double-edged sword. A more generic approach to recording information about a therapy session may actually result in increased scrutiny and uncertainty about the uniqueness or value of a service. In an increasingly technological environment, some therapists have simply become uncomfortable with the term *crafts* (Drake, 1999). If, however, the treatment choice is based on sound clinical reasoning and is well articulated, the skills gained through participation in crafts or other creative activities can certainly fulfill Medicare's requirements of being "meaningful, utilitarian, and sustainable over time" (Allen et al., 1992). One therapist reported that she had never had a payment denial for using crafts because she consistently documented the component skills (of the craft) in relation to clients' functional goals (Sorenson, 2010). Occupational therapists must be persistent and clear in documenting the use of crafts if they are ever to be fully legitimized (Taussig, 2004). For example, ability to sand on a wood project for 15 minutes may translate into the strength and endurance necessary to complete a stated occupational goal such as independence in a home care activity; or working on a hand sewing activity can strengthen the skills needed for buttoning, without the client having to button and unbutton over and over (Bergman, 2010). Documenting in this way will show a consistency between goals, treatment selection based on skilled activity analysis, and outcome. This consistency is important to payers but should be a primary concern of the therapist as well. Occupation-specific changes should be the focus of long-term goals (Amini, 2005) and some component of those long-term goals should be evident in all treatment activities. In documenting use of creative media, it is important to show that clients are learning or gaining a skill, and not that the therapist is simply "giving" them or "helping" them complete a project (Glomstad, 2005). Using crafts should not mean less work on the part of the therapist—he or she must be both physically and mentally present (Diffendal, 2002). Keep in mind that payers will not reimburse for time spent in preparation of materials and if treatment is carried out in a group setting, the therapist may want to note communication/interaction goals in the progress report (Drake, 1999). In summary, documentation that demonstrates a client-centered focus, occupational goals, and clear justification for treatment choice is the best practice and should be sufficient for any reimbursement source.

All therapy notes, once submitted, become part of a legal document, another reason to be clear and accurate in reporting what takes place in therapy (Borcherding, 2005; Sames, 2010). If the occupational therapist couches craft use in nonspecific terms, it becomes harder—not easier—to defend. Lawsuits are often adjudicated years after the event took place, so any vagueness in the record will come back to haunt the writer. Again, the therapist will be well served by emphasizing component skills and relating them to other areas of occupation (Amini, 2005). Another function of documentation is its use in accreditation, quality improvement, and ongoing administrative decision making (Borcherding, 2005). If the therapist is able to show clinical reasoning in the effective use of crafts in the clinic, this may actually guide the entire facility toward a more occupation-centered focus. When clients find meaning in their therapeutic regimen, they tend to have more positive perceptions of the facility, the therapist, the treatment, and the outcome. Administrators and payers alike look for outcomes that show improved occupational performance, role competence, client satisfaction, improved health/wellness, and increased quality of life (Clark & Youngstrom, 2003), and participation in leisure/creative activities can certainly have an impact on all these areas. A new therapist may find that he or she can actually change the culture of a clinic by introducing creative media where they had not been used before.

A final reason for clinical documentation and record keeping is research (Borcherding, 2005). Occupational therapists have long held that leisure participation, creative pursuits, and other productive activities facilitate improvement in physical, cognitive, and psychological functioning (Fidler & Velde, 1999), and that creative involvement is an important component of health maintenance—a stated objective of health maintenance organizations. Payers tend to discount anecdotal evidence, however, and in light of the current dearth of research in this area, they may see crafts as merely diversion and thus the domain of less costly facilities such as adult day care and recreational centers. In other words, to continue to be seen as a legitimate profession, occupational therapy must provide solid research to verify the value of our contribution. This research will be impossible without clear and honest documentation of therapeutic techniques. In order to remain a viable profession, occupational therapists must demonstrate that purposeful, meaningful, occupation-based activity—the stated domain of practice—is an indispensable component of successful rehabilitation.

Participation in crafts provides an ideal means of assessment in that the therapist can ascertain abilities in areas vital to everyday occupation, such as strength and dexterity, judgment and safety awareness, task persistence, and interaction with others. Consider the following example provided by a fieldwork student:

Observation Paper—"Mr. J: Building a Wooden Model of a Boat"

Mr. J's long-term goals are independence and safety in all self-care tasks. Two weeks ago Mr. J fell in the bathroom of his hospital room and was discovered by the OT, who found him very confused and seemingly oblivious to the situation. Prior to that incident, Mr. J's therapy had focused on basic ADL and improving fine motor skills.

Today, as Mr. J participated in a fine motor activity, he did not seem to have any recollection or insight regarding his prior mental state. When the OT praised him for his progress with fine motor skills, he denied that he ever had difficulty in this area.

Today's fine motor activity was to build a wooden boat model. The kit included a paintbrush, glue, paint, and 14 small wooden pieces but was missing the step-by-step instructions. Mr. J was left to build the boat his own way by copying the picture of the finished model on the outside of the box.

Several things struck me as I observed Mr. J performing this activity: 1) Mr. J was determined to put the complete structure together before gluing it. At first, I thought this was a wise choice since it's important to make sure one knows where all the pieces belong before applying permanent adhesive. The issue came when the smaller pieces would not stay in place, and Mr. J kept repositioning these dry, unglued pieces to no avail. Even though it was clear that he had figured out the model, it appeared that he would have continued for hours to try to get it to stay perfectly in place without glue. He needed a verbal cue to begin the gluing process. 2) There were two pieces on the model that were similarly shaped but slightly different in size. Twice, we had a conversation about these pieces. The larger piece went toward the front of the boat and the smaller piece went in back. Because these two pieces did not affect the architectural integrity of the model, it really did not matter that he ended up gluing each in the wrong spot. Yet, because it had been discussed and he had switched to the appropriate position twice before, it is unsettling that he still missed it by the end. 3) Mr. J was very conservative with the glue and had an extremely steady hand using the brush to paint the glue on the tiniest pieces. He was very precise and methodical with his movements.

4) At the end of the activity, when the OT asked if he wanted to paint the boat, he said no. He explained that had he wanted to paint it, he would have done so before gluing it together. 5) During clean up, he immediately wanted to put the structure back into the small box that initially contained the kit. He gave no attention to the fact that the glue had not dried, and that placing the model into a confined space might cause the pieces to come apart.

I admired the way the therapist communicated with the patient. She was never condescending and gave verbal cues in the form of a question, such as "What do you think you can do to make it so those smaller pieces will stay in place?" During clean up, she explained that it is customary for the rehab department to recycle the paintbrushes and paints to use again and asked if he would do this for her. He replied, "This paintbrush is a single-use brush. If I was the manufacturer and had intended for the paintbrush to be reused, I would have included some acetone with the kit." Throughout therapy, he used flowery rhetoric to justify his mistakes. Everything he did seemed to be "on purpose" and suggestions from the therapist were met with the response of "it could also be done this way" (the way he was doing it).

Megan Slay Wood, OT student, 2011

The client in the above scenario had identified impairment in fine motor skills but participation in a craft activity revealed cognitive deficits that had gone unnoticed during more routine, familiar tasks. In this instance, the craft served as an informal, observation-based assessment. Over the years, crafts have also been a component of a number of structured occupational therapy assessments. These are noted as appropriate in the corresponding craft chapters, and listed comprehensively in Chapter 2 (see Table 2-1). For some clients, completing a craft may feel less intimidating than a performance-based assessment and may reduce the sense of being scrutinized (Taussig, 2004). The way a client approaches a craft may provide insight into problem behaviors and serve as a predictor of future performance in tasks outside a clinic setting (Allen et al., 1992; Glomstad, 2004; Taussig, 2004). Impairment-focused assessments may miss the "big picture" but craftwork can demonstrate how the brain, body, and emotions are working together (Glomstad, 2004).

Documentation of the use of creative media can and should consistently demonstrate skilled intervention and client progress toward measurable outcomes relevant to long-term occupational goals. Crafts, by their nature, are well suited to these requirements: they follow a specific structure, have a definable end product, and require hands-on participation of the client. Using craft activities to enable the client to see how their habits interfere with goal attainment is most certainly skilled treatment. Another way to demonstrate skilled intervention is through the use of task analysis. Information gained through task analysis can be used in modifying an activity to maximize safety and capacity, as well as to show its relationship to more long-term, occupational goals. For example, a long-term goal of independent dressing has fine motor components that might be improved by completing a mosaic; or independence in simple meal preparation could be addressed through a creative group cooking project.

Documentation should always highlight the client's response to treatment; this includes the level of assistance needed, when the assistance is needed, and the client's subjective experience. The amount and type of assistance needed in crafts is likely to parallel that needed for other occupational activities. The ability of a client to deal with an unfamiliar or unexpected situation may become evident through the process of a creative construction. Craft involvement can give the therapist a good idea of the client's environmental awareness and recognition of mistakes and safety hazards (Allen et al., 1992). Awareness of a client's preferences and dislikes is necessary in order to make treatment as meaningful and motivating as possible, and enjoyment—or rejection—of a particular craft might also indicate a client's chance of success in other pursuits. A thorough occupational history will help in choosing and justifying treatment, as well as in setting achievable goals.

The 2008 *OTPF* (see Appendix IV), an updated replacement for Uniform Terminology (AOTA, 1994), renews emphasis on the profession's use of occupation. The overarching role of the occupational therapist is in "supporting health and participation in life through engagement in occupation" (AOTA, 2008). According to the *OTPF*, the general roles of the occupational therapist are to create or promote (wellness), establish or restore (function), modify (activities or environments), and prevent (injury or illness) (AOTA, 2008; Sames, 2010). The use of crafts is consistent with fulfillment of these roles and should be documented as such. The *OTPF* provides a helpful guideline in terms of how to view performance and the language used to report it.

Seen in this way, and not as a boundary-limiting practice, the *OTPF* can actually ease the process of documenting treatment plans, interventions, and outcomes. It can also aid in clinical reasoning, the process used in selecting and structuring treatment activities.

Completing an activity analysis as illustrated in Chapter 3 will also aid in effective documentation. Using terminology consistent with the *OTPF*, the therapist can communicate the steps and skills involved in the activity, then relate these components to occupational goals. For example, working on a hand-built ceramic piece may increase intrinsic hand muscle strength and motor control, facilitating the occupational goal of keyboarding. The ability to reduce barriers to performance by isolating and honing specific skills in disparate tasks is the occupational therapist's area of expertise and should be routinely documented.

The following cases illustrate the use of the above concepts and terminology in both clinical reasoning/treatment planning and documenting a client's participation.

A male client, who has had a stroke and is being treated on an inpatient rehab unit, would like to pursue the craft of fly tying consistent with his hobby of fishing. The client has a mild nondominant hemiparesis. The occupation of this client, in this example, is fishing. The activity to support participation is fly tying. Initially, the areas of occupation would be considered. Fly tying for this man would be a leisure activity because it is associated with his long-time hobby of fly fishing. The performance skills that a therapist might consider in making a treatment plan would include primarily motor and praxis, sensory-perceptual, emotional regulation, and cognitive. Motor skills that would be particularly relevant include coordination and strength and praxis. Sensory and cognitive skills of greatest importance might be visual, tactile and position perception; selection of tools; sequencing of steps; and problem solving. In consideration of performance patterns, the occupational therapist would want to ensure that the activity reinforced useful habits—for example, regular engagement in activity, correct motor patterns—and that the activity was consistent with pre-morbid routines and roles.

The performance contexts for this man would include the rehab gym, where he is participating in occupational therapy treatment (physical context); his age (63), gender, and socioeconomic status (personal context); his developmental stage (temporal context); his roles as retiree, husband, and grandparent (social context); and his customs and values (cultural context). Taken together, these contexts would indicate that this is an appropriate activity choice. Fly tying is likely to be a valued occupation for a retired male who has previously enjoyed fishing with his wife and grandchildren. The current physical context is a suitable, though not familiar one for this activity. In choosing assessments to determine this client's capacity for fly tying, the therapist would choose assessments that address these areas of occupation and underlying performance skills. In so doing, the therapist considers the activity demands of fly tying and specific client factors that may have an impact on performance. The therapist would determine what tools and space were needed; the steps/sequencing of the task; and what motor, cognitive, sensory, and interaction skills were required. The therapist would note whether or not the client had adequate body functions and structures to complete the activity, and if not, whether or not adaptations or accommodations could be made. Examples of body functions the client might need are distal joint mobility, tactile and proprioceptive senses, pain perception, sustained attention and memory, visuospatial perception, and praxis. In this example, the therapeutic activity and the occupational goal happen to be the same.

Another example might be a female child, diagnosed with mental retardation and autism, who lives in a developmental center and is learning to hold scissors in preparation for participation in the facility's classroom education program. The inability to successfully hold the scissors interferes with the occupational areas of education and play.

Performance skills that might be considered for intervention to enable this student are motor and praxis skills of posture, range of motion, and fine and gross coordination; sensory skills of visual perception and proprioception; emotional regulation skills of managing frustration and task persistence; and cognitive skills of attention, organization, and following directions. The therapist will be concerned with the student developing age appropriate roles and habits.

Performance contexts for this student might include her age; gender; and level of mental, emotional and social development. It might also include where the intervention takes place, including the toys and furniture present, as well as the people that will be present at the time of treatment and in follow-up care. The background of this student and caregivers, along with the "culture" of the developmental center; are also important contextual factors. Health care facilities develop their own traditions and mores over time, which are usually a blending of several elements, including the ethnicity, socioeconomic status, and attitudes and beliefs of the staff; administrative policies; and the ethos of the surrounding community.

If this is a typical residential center, many of the direct-care workers may be young and single, or single parents; their income and/or work schedule may limit time or resources needed to engage in arts and crafts at home with their own children, if they have them. Consequently, in considering the cultural performance context, the therapist would recognize that it might be unrealistic to expect these staff members to provide experiences for this student that they do not provide for their own children or with which they are unfamiliar. Since carry-over from treatment sessions is a priority, the therapist should choose an activity with a practical connotation and cultural significance or value such as cutting out paper dolls and clothes. This choice would be age and gender consistent and might be viewed as a form of play (familiar) rather than a craft (less familiar). Regardless of the activity chosen, the occupational therapist must consider the ability of both the facility and the child to meet the activity demands, such as time requirements, social demands, and required actions. The therapist might write short-term objectives to address client factors such as sustained attention, visual/spatial awareness, behavioral regulation, body image, muscle strength, and eye-hand coordination. These objectives might utilize the completion of the craft as a way of measuring improvement, for example: "Client will cut paper doll clothes, staying on the lines 50% of the time, with moderate verbal cueing to visually attend to task." Or "Client will correctly identify paper doll body parts 75% of the time, after rehearsal with therapist during cutting." The short-term objectives of increased attention to task, ability to follow directions, or improved fine motor skills can then be related to long term occupational goals such as independent scissor use and completion of assignments, both of which are necessary to participate in education (adapted from Drake, 1999).

As evidenced by the preceding examples, areas of occupation, performance skills, and client factors sections of the *OTPF* can help the therapist to select appropriate problems upon which to focus. The performance patterns, context(s), and activity demands sections can guide the therapist in choosing specific activities. In thinking about goals, the therapist might use the areas of occupation to suggest terminology for formulating the occupational goals, and performance skills or client factors to focus on areas that can demonstrate measurable improvement in the short term. Taken all together, the *OTPF* and thorough knowledge of activities will provide a treatment rationale consistent with the client's life situation, personal goals, and capabilities. This approach to treatment planning and documentation will work with crafts as well as with any other treatment modality.

Realities of time constraints and productivity demands will not permit documentation of the entire process of clinical reasoning. The therapist must decide which factors are implied or assumed and which must be articulated. At a minimum, the therapist must clarify what skills/deficits were being addressed, what skilled intervention was provided—including task or environmental modification—and how the client responded. The assessment portion of the note may be the place to relate discrete tasks to the long-term functional goals. Using the first of the preceding examples, a progress note might look like the following:

S: "This is really making me anxious to go fishing again."

O: Client attended OT for 45 minutes this a.m. Client participated in a fly tying activity to work on attention to task, fine motor dexterity, and to facilitate return to a preferred hobby. Therapist placed some materials to client's left to encourage visual scanning; occasional verbal cueing needed. Therapist cued client to visually attend to affected hand in holding hook; client responded by adjusting calibration of left hand. Client was able to correctly sequence task and required no cueing for attention, organization, or tool use. Client exhibited moderate difficulty with bilateral coordination, no problem manipulating with right hand. Client completed two flies during session and expressed pleasure with his end products.

A: Client is showing improvement in left upper extremity fine motor skills, attention to task, and task organization. He continues to have some left visual scanning and bilateral coordination deficits. Skill improvement will facilitate client's performance in self-care and meal preparation tasks, as well as resumption of a preferred hobby. STG: Client will complete all grooming independently, within a reasonable time, without cues to locate needed items.

P: Continue the initial treatment plan.

The following is a second example, based on the student observation of Mr. J described earlier in the chapter. Obviously, there is more than one way to write a technically correct note, but here the purpose is to convey important information about a client's functional ability and potential safety concerns to the entire treatment team. In this instance, the session became more evaluative than remedial. Note that use of a craft is mentioned but the emphasis is on the performance skill level and its impact on daily occupations.

Name: Mr. J
Diagnosis: Brain injury secondary to fall; S/P MVA w/ persisting RUE pain and internal injuries
Date: xx/xx/xx

S: Patient denies any memory of having fine motor difficulties.

O: Pt participated in 40-minute OT session today to work on fine motor skills and increasing activity level and endurance. Pt was given a multistep craft activity to complete that required following directions, consistent attention to task, and task persistence, as well as bilateral FM skills. Pt required verbal cues to go from the first to the second step of the project. Pt incorrectly placed at least one piece despite multiple cues by the therapist for correct placement. Pt exhibited precise and steady hand function during the task and was able to physically place pieces without assistance. As Pt exhibited planning deficits, therapist used questions to facilitate performance, (e.g. Pt intended to place glued model back into the box before it had dried, which would have caused it to come apart). Pt verbally responded to suggestions, but denied their usefulness, e.g. stating "yes, but it could also be done this way." Pt consistently justified his actions, even when they were contrary to project directions or had an undesired outcome. Pt was able to finish activity w/o requesting a rest break.

A: Pt demonstrates significant improvement in fine motor skills. Pt exhibits difficulty with executive functioning skills such as problem-solving and anticipating consequences of actions, but demonstrates no insight regarding these deficits. This could pose safety risks during daily activities. Pt has physical ability to be independent with routine self care but cueing may be needed. Supervision at home is recommended.

Plan: Implement activities to facilitate executive function and to improve insight into deficits in order to increase safety, especially when novel situations are encountered.

Signed ________________________________

Although most therapists intuitively acknowledge the therapeutic quality of creative activity, they must recognize that this quality can also exist in the absence of skilled intervention. In this instance, the craft is more diversional in nature and would not fall within the domain of occupational therapy (Burson, 2002). On the other hand, if selected, implemented, and documented properly, the inclusion of crafts in the occupational therapy treatment repertoire should only enhance the value and viability of the profession. Occupational therapy faces aggressive competition in the health care workforce; its practitioners must demonstrate that they are uniquely qualified to use occupation therapeutically. In fact, no other profession claims to use "occupation" or to work toward occupational performance (Pierce, 2001). This approach cannot be realized in other than a client-centered way, which is the new direction of health care. To shift the occupational therapy domain into that of other professionals, or to adopt treatment techniques just because they are currently popular, is to deny its most singular professional strength (Youngstrom, 2002). In addition, this would ultimately be a disservice to clients, who would at best receive duplicated services, or at worst, would be robbed of opportunities for enhanced healing and personal growth.

If occupational therapists will consistently and accurately measure and document baseline and progressive levels of function—regardless of the therapeutic activity—they can justify their services (Glomstad, 2005). Through documentation, occupational therapists are called upon to articulate a rationale for the therapy they provide, show the relation of this service to outcomes, and to reflect professional reasoning and judgment (Clark & Youngstrom, 2003). Practitioners must strive to effectively communicate and treat from a uniquely occupational therapy perspective to ensure their rightful place in the health care services continuum.

Discussion Questions

Utilize the following case study to complete the questions that follow. Details of the client's performance have been omitted to encourage the student to think through the task demands, including areas that might be especially challenging, and to imagine ways that the activity could be graded or adapted.

Naomi is a 16-year-old student who suffered a traumatic brain injury in a four-wheeler accident. She has impairment in multiple cognitive areas including memory, attention to task, initiating and terminating tasks, organization, and problem solving. She also exhibits incoordination in her right upper extremity; fine motor activities are particularly difficult. The occupational therapist has decided to have Naomi make a scrapbook that will also serve as a daily journal. The therapist will offer her a selection of tools and materials to use, as well as visual samples. She plans to have her work on the scrapbook for 15 to 30 minutes each day, gradually reducing the amount of structure and verbal cueing provided.

1. Add details about Naomi's life; then relate her personal areas of occupation, roles and habits, and performance contexts to this craft activity.
2. Add details about Naomi's possible performance relative to task demands and write a SOAP note. Be sure to include how this activity might relate to long term occupational goals.
3. How might you grade or adapt this activity? Add this information to the SOAP note to document skilled intervention.

References

Allen, C. K., Earhart, C. A., & Blue, T. (1992). *Occupational therapy treatment goals for the physically and cognitively disabled.* Bethesda, MD: American Occupational Therapy Association.

American Occupational Therapy Association. (1994). Uniform terminology for occupational therapy (3rd ed.). *American Journal of Occupational Therapy, 48*(11), 1047-1059.

Amercian Occupational Therapy Association. (2008). The occupational therapy practice framework: Domain and process (2nd ed.). *American Journal of Occupational Therapy, 62*(6), 625-683.

Amini, D. (2005). The test of occupation-based goal writing. *Advance for Occupational Therapy Practitioners, 21*(14), 13.

Bergman, S. The use of needle crafts in occupational therapy. *TQS Articles.* Retrieved from www.thequiltshow.com/os/articles.php/articles_id/26.

Borcherding, S. (2005). *Documentation manual for writing SOAP notes in occupational therapy* (2nd ed.). Thorofare, NJ: SLACK Incorporated.

Burson, K. (2002). Personal communication on AOTA mental health listserv on 4/10/02.

Clark, F. C., & Youngstrom, M. J. (2003). Guidelines for documentation of occupational therapy. *American Journal of Occupational Therapy, 57*(6), 646-649.

Diffendal, J. (2002). Kids, through the use of their hands.... *Advance for Occupational Therapy Practitioners, 18*(22), 12.

Drake, M. (1999). *Crafts in therapy and rehabilitation* (2nd ed.). Thorofare, NJ: SLACK Incorporated.

Fidler, G., & Velde, B. (1999). *Activities: Reality and symbol.* Thorofare, NJ: SLACK Incorporated.

Glomstad, J. (2004). A birdhouse in the hand. *Advance for Occupational Therapy Practitioners, 20*(6), 17

Glomstad, J. (2005). The keys to getting paid. *Advance for Occupational Therapy Practitioners, 21*(3), 19-20.

Hocking, C. (2007). Early perspectives of patients, practice and profession. *The British Journal of Occupational Therapy, 70*(7), 284-291.

Holder, V. (2001). The use of creative activities with occupational therapy. *British Journal of Occupational Therapy, 64*(2), 103-105.

Hooper, B. (2010). On arriving at the destination of the centennial vision: Navigational landmarks to guide occupational therapy education. *Occupational Therapy in Health Care, 24*(1), 97-106.

Jongbloed, L., & Wendland, T. (2002). The impact of reimbursement systems on occupational therapy practice in Canada and the USA. *Canadian Journal of Occupational Therapy, 69*(3), 143-152.

Lemke, L. (2004). Defensive documentation: Managing medicare denials. *OT Practice, 9*(16), 8-12.

Pierce, D. (2001) Occupation by design: Dimension, therapeutic power, and creative process. *American Journal of Occupational Therapy, 55*(3), 249-259.

Sames, K. (2009). Documentation in practice. In E. Crepeau, E. Cohn, & B. Schell (Eds.), *Willard and Spackman's occupational therapy* (10th ed.). Philadelphia, PA: Lippincott Williams & Wilkins.

Schmid, T. (2004). Meanings of creativity within occupational therapy practice. *Australian Occupational Therapy Journal, 51*(2), 80-88.

Sorenson, J. (2010). Documenting occupation-based treatment. *Advance for Occupational Therapy Practitioners, 26*(18), 7.

Taussig, V. (2004). Keeping crafts alive in mental health. *Advance for Occupational Therapy Practitioners, 20*(16), 14.

Youngstrom, M. J. (2002). Introduction to the OT practice framework: Domain and process. *OT Practice,* CE1-CE8.

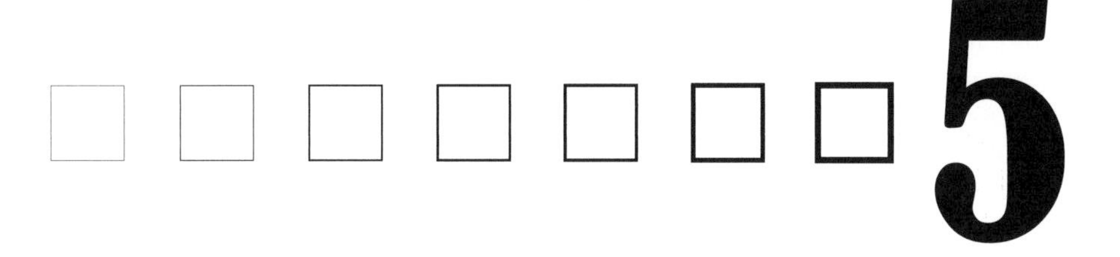

Using Crafts and Creative Media in Practice

Objectives

The student should be able to:

- List the basic steps of treatment planning
- Describe elements of clinical reasoning used in choosing crafts or other creative activities in treatment
- Explain both advantages and disadvantages of using kits
- Describe various strategies to ensure the greatest effectiveness in the therapeutic application of crafts

The Occupational Therapy Process and Pragmatic Reasoning

The occupational therapy process has several steps: screening and evaluation, treatment planning, implementation of treatment, and re-evaluation (Christiansen & Baum, 1997). Elements of discharge planning are also present in each step. Since a therapist cannot make decisions about appropriate treatment until a client's functional level has been determined, choosing activities for a client occurs during the treatment planning stage following evaluation. A common approach to treatment planning is to list the client's problems, prioritize them, and collaboratively compose long-term goals for those considered to be most important and/or achievable through intervention. Long-term goals are often thought of as the outcome expected in 3 months to 1 year (Kettenbach, 1995). To be considered a client-centered process, this obviously must include as much client input as possible. Short-term objectives—those that could reasonably be achieved in a shorter time frame—are then established for each long-term goal. The last step in treatment planning is usually to list activities that could help the client accomplish the short-term objectives and thus take steps in the direction of achieving long-term occupational goals.

The reasoning behind the activity choices that make up treatment plans is the rationale, more commonly called clinical reasoning (Christiansen & Baum, 1997; Crepeau, Cohn, & Schell, 2003; Sabonis-Chafee & Hussey, 1998). In an article in the *American Journal of Occupational Therapy*, Schell and Cervero (1993) propose that clinical reasoning is a part scientific, part narrative process. The scientific component is systematic and highly cognitive, based on data collection and hypothesis testing. The narrative component,

Tubbs, C., & Drake, M. *Crafts and Creative Media in Therapy, Fourth Edition (pp. 51-60).*

however, is improvisational and intuitive, and based on a client's values, beliefs, and subjective experience. Other influences on clinical reasoning are the treatment environment and the therapist's own paradigm. These interactive elements of reasoning should apply to all activity selections, including the various creative media (Schell & Cervero, 1993). For example, a therapist might initially consider a macramé project for a client with osteoarthritis in the shoulders. This choice is based primarily on data collection (scientific component), that is, the client has limitations in upper extremity range of motion and endurance, and the activity demands of macramé include repetitive reaching. Upon discussion, however, the therapist discovers that the client perceives this as a dated craft with an undesirable end product (narrative component); the therapist must now reconsider to generate other options that still address the identified problems. Other influences on the activity choice may be clinic demands and resources that restrict the time or materials for this project (environmental); or the therapist's potential embarrassment at having the client work on such a project in a busy clinic (personal paradigm).

In another instance, the client's religious and cultural mores may affect activity choice. For example, Islamic law discourages artistic pursuits that replicate human form, as in photography or painting. Other crafts, such as woodworking and weaving, though, have a strong historical relevance to Arab culture and also result in functional objects. Thus, the therapist can still choose a craft activity and grade for motor, cognitive, and sensory aspects while retaining motivation and meaning for the client (Ahmad, Alsharif, & Royeen, 2006). From a psychosocial perspective, the therapist might consider Maslow's hierarchy of needs (see Figure 2-1). For example, in using a cooking activity, a client might learn basic skills to fulfill the need for nourishment (physiological need), might decorate valentine cupcakes to share with others at the facility (love and belonging), or might learn an artistic style of food presentation (self-actualization). The actual tasks may all be similar, but they are done for vastly different reasons. The special skill of the occupational therapist is to identify and balance these myriad components to make the most therapeutic choices.

Above all, the therapist should consider the interests and motivating factors of the client. In a study some years ago, therapists offered elderly clients a choice between a functional art activity and a rote exercise. Each activity called for shoulder range of motion, and the researchers hypothesized that more of their subjects would choose painting. In the resulting data, the overall percentage of difference was in fact insignificant, but the women subjects chose the painting activity two to one. Obviously, more played into the decision than the researchers had anticipated (Mullins, Nelson, & Smith, 1987). In a more recent study involving the use of music as pain management technique, subjects who were able to self-select the music played realized the greatest benefit (Mitchell, MacDonald, & Knussen, 2008). In a 2007 survey of mental health occupational therapists, recurrent themes emerged among those who used crafts, including the necessity of client choice and client interest in activity selection (Griffiths & Corr, 2007). In summary, the activity must be desirable from the client perspective. Crafts are no more a blanket therapy solution than are exercises or other modalities; the therapist is not a prescriber but rather a guide (Perrin, 2001). An expedition guide does not choose the destination for the tourist, but rather finds a way for the tourist to arrive at the destination selected. In the same way, effective therapists must first ascertain the "destination" the client hopes to reach, and then employ their expertise in getting them there.

In summary, the therapist must have a rationale for using crafts or other creative media as their treatment choice. There is both research and anecdotal evidence (see Chapter 2) to suggest the value of this type of activity over less individualized approaches—such as exercise or physical agent modalities—but therapists must be able to clearly articulate their reasoning to maintain credibility. The following questions may help the therapist through this reasoning process:

- What goal or objective do I expect the client to accomplish through this activity?
- Can I/the client relate this activity to broader, occupation-based treatment goals?
- What new skills might this activity help the client learn?
- Could this activity help the client develop new and productive habits?
- Does this activity capitalize on the client's strengths?
- Is this activity consistent with the client's culture, gender, and age?
- Is the client satisfied with this activity?
- Is this activity an appropriate use of the client's time?

- Can this activity be graded/adapted to best suit the client's abilities and limitations?
- Will the client's projected length of stay allow enough time to complete this activity?
- Will I have enough time to assist the client when necessary?
- Does the clinic contain the space and materials needed to complete this activity?
- Have clients been successful with similar activities in my past experience?
- Can I explain how this activity fits within the model(s) of practice I am using?

Although not an exhaustive list, these clinical reasoning questions will provide some guidance on whether or not an activity—in this case, a craft or other creative project—is indeed a viable option. The therapist and client can select from several options that are diverse in outcome but similar in process or therapeutic quality. Again, this calls for experienced activity analysis and clarity of treatment objectives.

Once the therapist has decided to incorporate crafts and creative media into treatment, he or she needs to consider elements such as client abilities and interests, contextual factors, and characteristics of the activity itself. Factors relative to the client include gender, age, "natural" inclinations (especially for children), whether or not solitary or group activity is preferred, barriers and facilitators in daily life, and aspects that satisfy emotional needs or provide a sense of self-efficacy. Considerations relative to the activity include level of challenge, cost, time required, sensory components, and whether it is best done individually or in a group (Kuhaneck, Spitzer, & Miller, 2010).

Therapists who wish to use crafts will also have to deal with pragmatic issues such as cost, time, and space. No matter how much one may be enthused about using creative media, practical clinical constraints will likely limit the scope of possible activities. For example, in a community-based setting, where participants may attend over an extended period of time, long-term projects or those that require larger equipment investments may be feasible. On the other hand, in more medically oriented settings with a shorter average length of stay, craft choices may be constrained by time. If time and/or cost are the primary limitations, the therapist could consider having the client/client's family supply the materials, or bring an unfinished project from home (Amini, 1999). Use of prepared kits is another common way that occupational therapists have traditionally managed some of these issues. Both advantages and disadvantages of using kits will be discussed in more detail below.

Using Kits

The development of reimbursement systems for occupational therapy services has radically changed our ideas about what we can and should do for our clients. Most third-party payers set limits on the number and kind of treatment sessions they will reimburse. Prior to the 1970s, payment systems were such that most occupational therapists were able to provide treatment without concern for chargeable units, billing codes, and therapy caps. As insurance companies and Medicare began to pay an additional fee for therapy above and beyond the per diem charge, billing systems and documentation requirements began to change. Therapists had to document more carefully to justify to the insurance company why a client needed a given type, frequency, and duration of treatments (Sames, 2009). Professional and ethical questions naturally arose: "If this client doesn't have insurance to pay for my services or supplies, shall I provide services anyway, or charge other clients with insurance more in order to be able to do so?" Or, "Shall I not do activities that require supplies, since I know insurance will not pay for them?" Or, "Will the insurance company perceive my treatment to be worthy of payment? Or, "Is my job performance to be measured by the improvement in my clients or by how much money I can make in the department?"

These questions are more relevant than ever, but may come as a shock to new therapists with an idealistic view of the health care system. They may assume that federal and private resources are limitless and that all services, supplies, and equipment should and will be covered. Insurance will generally cover face-to-face contact with clients doing specific types of treatment. More often than not, though, when a therapist is preparing materials for a session, that therapist is not earning money for the department; that is, there is no chargeable client treatment. This pressure to produce revenue may cause a therapist to choose a kit rather than grading an activity up to a more complex task by using basic craft materials. Ironically, kits are usually more expensive and when used in volume, may offset any savings realized by the decreased time spent in preparation. At one time, a registered occupational therapist may have delegated materials preparation to a certified occupational therapy assistant (COTA). However, COTAs' time is also chargeable and they often have their own caseloads and work largely independently of the therapist. Nonetheless, a recent student research survey showed that therapists who work with COTAs are more likely to use crafts than those who do not (Whittington, Weir, Powell, Mumbower, & Foster, 2010). Some therapists may also have therapy technicians or volunteers prepare materials since their services are not chargeable. Supervision or instruction may still be needed, however, to avoid waste. Consequently, prepared kits continue to be a frequently chosen alternative.

Assuming the occupational therapist has decided to use crafts in the treatment repertoire—reimbursement issues aside—numerous factors, including arguments both for and against the use of kits, should be considered in their implementation. Based on our earliest professional writings, it is apparent that occupational therapists used materials that had at least some amount of preparation before they were incorporated into an occupational therapy activity. Of course, there was the stray therapist who may have learned a unique skill, such as finding and preparing her own ceramic clay, but the profession as a whole benefited from the specialization of materials and tools typical of the industrial age. Use of crafts, like other media, should be consistent with the prevailing cultural norms and practices; consequently, the use of kits does not necessarily detract from the benefit of using crafts and is not a betrayal of the profession's foundational beliefs. Kits are widely available (see Appendix I) and selection in both type and complexity is vast, especially when purchased online or from a catalog. Alternatives expand even more if the therapist is willing to start from scratch, but the array of things necessary to have on hand may be space- or cost-prohibitive. One option would be to offer a limited selection of craft activities for which a common set of supplies could be kept; a clinic with a small number of craft choices is better than one with none at all.

Space is another issue that may determine whether or not a therapist uses kits. In the early days of occupational therapy, when hospital stays were longer and revenue production was of little or no significance, it was important to have many different craft choices available so clients confined long term would not get bored with one category of craft. Hospital stays in almost all types of treatment settings have been substantially reduced. The inventory of craft projects is necessarily smaller and less storage space may be allocated; kits generally take up less space than a reasonable amount of basic raw materials. Space is a particularly important factor for therapists working in home care. A home health therapist can only utilize what can be carried from place to place, unless the items are already in the client's home. This may be another instance where the therapist must limit craft choices, unless the client is willing to furnish some of the materials and tools.

Cost is another factor with similar trade-offs in the decision to use kits or not. In general, kits are more costly but the initial expense of stocking a variety of basic supplies may not fit as well in some clinics' budgeting schemes. In choosing to employ crafts in therapy, the therapy manager/administrator must accept the fact that reimbursement sources will pay for neither supplies nor kits. This uncompensated cost must be accommodated for in other ways. In instances where occupational therapists do not have administrative support for this treatment approach, they sometimes elect to spend their own money to buy desired items. The fact that time spent in preparation of raw materials is also nonreimbursable may weigh in favor of kits as well; however, the determined therapist can do this preparation before or after normal working hours or use alternative time-management strategies.

If using crafts as a means of assessment, kits are most appropriate to ensure consistency. The Allen Diagnostic Module, part of a standardized cognitive assessment that utilizes a very specific set of craft projects, is probably the best-known example of this application (Earhart, Allen, & Blue, 1993). Use of a kit also allows the therapist to observe whether or not a client can read and follow written directions, or whether he or she can copy a provided sample. Completion of a craft from raw materials may provide too many variables to prove valuable or efficient in assessment.

A final—and most vital—factor to consider is that of the "fit" with the client's desire and customary approach to tasks. A therapist inexperienced in crafting may feel more comfortable using kits, but the more the craft corresponds with the client's perception of normal occupation, the more effective it will be in accomplishing the rehabilitation goals. For example, if a client does intricate woodworking as a hobby or career, that individual is unlikely to be happy with a kit for a birdhouse or a stool. Alternatively, if a client is unfamiliar with a craft or does not perceive him or herself to be creative, then a kit may be more suitable. The therapist must also have firmly in mind the therapeutic purpose of the craft. If fostering creativity and decision making is the focus, a kit may be less useful. Kits necessarily limit variation and independent thinking. If, on the other hand, the therapeutic focus is on following directions, staying on task, or a specific motor skill, a kit may be perfectly appropriate. In either case, use of a craft is certainly preferable to many other, less occupation-based activities.

In summary, there are multiple factors to consider when deciding whether to use a kit or start from scratch when using crafts in the clinic. Space, cost, choice and availability, therapist time, and therapeutic aim will all play a part in this decision. A clinic may also opt to stock some basic supplies and a few frequently used kits. And, since craft materials are rarely reimbursable, it is also important that the occupational therapist be able to articulate to his or her supervisor the benefits of this media. See Chapters 2 and 4 for evidence of benefits and documentation suggestions.

General Tips for Using Crafts

The following suggestions should help the client get the most out of craftwork; they will also help the therapist avoid some common pitfalls.

Preparation

- Be able to relate the craft to longer term goals, both for documentation and for the client/family. Some therapists have confided that one of the biggest obstacles to their use of crafts is the inability to articulate their relevance to occupational goals and resulting concerns about reimbursement (TeBeest, Kornstedt, Feldmann, Harmasch, & Kemnitz, 2001; Whittington et al., 2010). For example, having a client plan and implement a simple tile mosaic design may teach or reinforce skills to plan a simple budget or weekly menu. Or the ability to thoroughly sand all the pieces of a wood project may translate into the increased endurance needed to complete a home cleaning task.
- Consider recycled or scrap material alternatives to minimize cost. As is mentioned in numerous sections in the following chapters, many attractive and useful craft items can be made with materials that are often simply discarded. For example, old greeting cards can be used in collages or to cover (decoupage) boxes or other containers. Whole books are devoted to projects made with scrap fabric (or other materials) and are readily available via the Internet (see Resources, Chapter 14). Crafts do not have to be costly.
- Practice grading down projects; occupational therapy practitioners, especially students, sometimes overestimate a client's skills. Every occupational therapy student has had the experience—in spite of the most careful planning—of an implemented activity resulting in utter failure. The more alternative approaches you have in mind at the outset, the less likely this is to happen.
- If the craft project requires preparation prior to the treatment session, be sure to allow for this in your schedule. Materials may need to be gathered, paints mixed, the area protected from spills, and so on. Also take into account the time needed for instruction. Therapists usually utilize crafts that they already know how to do, so it is common to underestimate how long it will take to explain it to the client. Time for clean up will of course depend on the activity. In any case, whether you want the client to assist or you plan to do it all yourself, the time needed to clean the area and the tools used will need to be considered in planning. In fact, when choosing crafts in general, ensure that you have the required solvents or other agents as well as the equipment, such as sinks or containers, needed for clean up.
- If the project requires individual design/creativity, be prepared with some suggestions or ideas. Clients who are unaccustomed to doing creative activities and/or those with cognitive dysfunction may need guidance, or even a design to copy, when initiating an art or craft project. For example, if the task is to make simple greeting cards to give to friends or family, you may want to provide stencils or stamps in case the client cannot conceptualize his or her design. Some individuals are naturally creative, but others are not.
- Be aware of literacy requirements; not all clients can read but may not necessarily let you know this. If you notice that a client is stalling in initiating or continuing an activity, it may be due to inability rather than disinterest. It is easy to forget that a significant percent of adults have less-than-functional reading skills.

- If something can be spilled, it probably will be. Be sure to cover the client and the working surface if needed.
- Make sure there is adequate time to complete the project. A half-finished project is discouraging to both client and therapist and trivializes the value of the activity.

Implementation

- Have a sample. Clients tend to do much better and experience less frustration when they know what their end product should look like. Inability to perform the activity without a visual sample, however, may provide some clues about cognitive function.
- Have an attractive sample. A client will be less inclined to want to do the activity if they anticipate an undesirable product.
- Offer a choice if possible. This gives the client a greater sense of control in the therapy session and allows them to express personal interest and individuality. Again, inability to make a choice—when options are offered—gives the therapist insight into cognitive skills.
- Be sure you can do the activity yourself; if you expect your client to complete the project from written directions, make sure you have read and can follow them. Failure to do this can result in a largely wasted therapy session. Do not assume that the client will be able to figure it out independently.
- Offer suggestions rather than criticism during the process. Be kind but not condescending in your evaluation of the finished product. Having clients do crafts may require extra patience on the part of the therapist, especially if he or she is an experienced crafter. Allow the client to learn through trial and error and make their own design choices when appropriate to the therapeutic goals. While indeed "beauty is in the eye of the beholder," the client is often realistic in their self-assessment and may find it disconcerting if the therapist is overly complimentary.
- Use professional judgment about when to intervene, and how much or how little assistance to give. This will be heavily dependent on the goal to be accomplished. For example, if the activity objective is to improve fine motor skills, the therapist may allow the client to struggle a bit. On the other hand, if the objective is to relearn a desired crafting occupation, the therapist may need to provide more help so the client is not disappointed with the outcome.
- Encourage conversation during craftwork. You will often get more information from a client when they are engaged in an activity rather than being interviewed. Working on a project relieves one from having to make continual eye contact. You can further increase the comfort level by working on a project at the same time so the client doesn't feel that he or she is being continually scrutinized.
- For projects that need to dry or be continued in another session, be sure to have adequate and secure space. Counter space in a clinic is often limited, so be aware of this ahead of time and respect the space needs of coworkers.
- Mark projects, finished or not, with the client's name or initials for later identification. Assume that clients will want to keep the articles they have made. If projects have been done in a group setting, it is easy to forget what belongs to whom. You might also consider displaying finished items if space permits and clients are agreeable to it.
- Always clean tools thoroughly as soon as possible after the session ends; count tools before and after if necessary. Tools will have a much longer life if they are well cared for, doing so will reduce the overall cost of using crafts as a modality. Losing tools also unnecessarily adds to the cost of craft use. In certain settings, (e.g., mental health facilities) ensuring that patients do not leave with tools is an important safety practice as well.
- Involve the client in set up and clean up; this can be a valuable teaching technique, so don't do it all yourself just to save time. Again, this will be dependent on the objectives of the activity.

For Groups

- Look for opportunities for clients to lead. This becomes especially valuable when leading a group of clients with varying levels of ability. An individual might be bored or feel insulted when asked to do an activity that is too simple, but if encouraged to help a fellow participant, may instead feel a sense of worth and importance.
- Make sure the number of participants is feasible. Consider the space available, the amount of assistance they might need, and feasibility of meeting activity objectives. Nothing creates chaos quite like not have enough eyes and hands to adequately assist all the members of a craft group.
- Be aware of how much interaction is required by the activity and group members' tolerance for this. In pediatric or mental health settings, part of the activity goal may be learning to share, but the therapist must be sure all participants are capable of a minimum level of the behavior required.

Discussion Questions

Utilizing the case studies from the craft chapters, consider and discuss application of the suggestions in the previous "General Tips for Using Crafts" section. For example:

1. Should the activity be done in a group or individually?
2. How much preparation time/completion time is required?
3. How could/should the activity be graded?
4. How much creativity is needed?
5. Could the activity be done more cheaply?
6. What other crafts or creative activities might fulfill the same therapeutic purpose?

(Adapted from Banks, 2000; Melville, 1998; Posthuma, 2002)

Resources for Diverse Populations

Ethnic or Cultural

The American Boy's Handy Book: What to Do and How to Do It, Centennial Edition
By Daniel Carter Beard and Noel Perrin
David R. Godine, Centennial edition, 2010
A classic do-it-yourself for kids; crafting, science projects, mechanics and more.

Great Craft Projects From Around the World
By William Reid
J. Weston Walch, Publisher, 2000
Folk art; includes masks and kites.

Classic Origami
By P. D. Tuyen
Sterling Publishing Co., Inc., 2005
Vietnamese author relates this art to his Vietnamese childhood. He discusses the origins of this craft and current trends. Thorough, clear sequential drawings of the process for the 26 animals that are listed in the index.

The Kids' Multicultural Craft Book
By Roberta Gould and Sarah Rakitin
Williamson Publishing, 2003
Brief historical/geographical information and crafts from Central and South America, Africa, Europe, the Pacific, and North America.

Brown Bag Ideas From Many Cultures
By Irene Tejada
Sterling Publishing, 1993
Creative activities using common household materials.

Southwestern Arts and Crafts
By Nancy Krenz and Patricia Byrnes
The Sunstone Press, 1979
Contains Mexican and Indian crafts, recipes, music, and dance for kindergarten through sixth grade.

The Craftsman in America
By The National Geographic Society
Special Publications Division, 1975
Historic as well as modern crafts developed in America. Not a how-to book.

West African Weaving
By Venice Lamb
Gerald Duckworth and Co., Ltd., 1975
Tribal maps show origins of various weaves. Many photos of weavers at work.

African Crafts and Craftsmen
By René Gardi
Van Nostrand Reinhold Company, 1969
Large print and wonderful photographs of a variety of crafts, from raw materials to finished products from across the African continent.

Disabled and Special Populations

Gardening Projects for Horticultural Therapy Programs, 2004
By Hank Bruce
Several other accessible/therapeutic gardening books are available from the American Horticultural Therapy Association, www.ahta.org.

National Agrability Project
http://www.agrabilityproject.org/

Making Things: The Handbook of Creative Discovery
By Ann Sayre Wiseman
Little Brown and Co., 1997
A collection of 125 innovative projects for children, such as weaving, macramé, bread-dough sculpture, sandcasting, puppets, costumes, games, toys, and art. Illustrated with line drawings with color accents. Includes an index.

Therapeutic Crafts: A Practical Approach
By Cynthia Johnson, Kathy Lobdell, Jacqueline Nesbitt, Marjorie Clare
Thorofare, NJ: SLACK Incorporated, 1996

Expressive Arts for the Very Disabled and Handicapped for All Ages
By Jane C. Cohen
Charles C. Thomas, Publisher, Ltd., 1995

Accessible Gardening for People With Disabilities: A Guide to Methods, Tools, and Plants
By Janeen R. Adil
Woodbine House, 1994

Arts and Crafts for the Physically and Mentally Disabled
By Elaine and Loren Gould
Charles C. Thomas Publishers, 1978
An extensive presentation of the implementation of craft programs for the disabled institutionalized client. It describes planning, coordinating, motivating, and utilizing patients, available space, time allocation, equipment, staff, personnel, and volunteers with detailed craft project descriptions.

Crafts for the Very Disabled and Handicapped
By Jane G. Kay
Charles C. Thomas, Publishers, 1977
Many inexpensive and simple crafts. Decorations for both Jewish and Christian holidays.

Disabled Village Children
By David Werner
Hesperian Publications, available from www.hesperian.org
Creative ideas for crafts, activities and equipment with a minimum of resources

Pastimes for the Patient, Revised Edition
By Marguerite Ickis
A. S. Barnes and Co., Inc., 1966
This text contains chapters on nature crafts such as plants, terrariums, bird crafts, chip carving, leather, drawing and painting, weaving and fibers, and music, as well as others.

References

Ahmad, S. O., Alsharif, N. Z., & Royeen, M. (2006). Arab Americans. In M. Royeen, & J. L. Crabtree (Eds.), *Culture in rehabilitation: From competency to proficiency* (pp. 181-202). Upper Saddle River, NJ: Pearson Prentice Hall.

Amini, D. (1999). Hands and crafts: Traditional OT. *Advance for Occupational Therapy Practitioners* print archives, posted on 8/9/1999.

Banks, B. (2000). *Activities for older people.* Woburn, MA: Butterworth Heinemann.

Christiansen, C., & Baum, C. (1997). *Occupational therapy: Enabling function and well-being* (2nd ed.). Thorofare, NJ: SLACK Incorporated.

Crepeau, E., Cohn, E., & Schell, B. A. (2003). *Willard and Spackman's occupational therapy* (10th ed.). Philadelphia, PA: Lippincott Williams & Wilkins.

Earhart, C. A., Allen, C. K., & Blue, T. (1993). *Allen diagnostic module.* Colchester, CT: S & S Worldwide.

Griffiths, S., & Corr, S. (2007). The use of creative activities with people with mental health problems: A survey of occupational therapists. *British Journal Of Occupational Therapy, 70*(3), 107-114.

Kettenbach, G. (1995). *Writing soap notes* (2nd ed.). Philadelphia, PA: F. A. Davis.

Kuhaneck, H. M., Spitzer, S. L., & Miller, E. (2010). Activity analysis, creativity, and playfulness in pediatric occupational therapy. Sudbury, MA: Jones and Bartlett Publishers.

Melville, S. (1998). *Crafts for all abilities.* Tumbridge Wells, Kent, UK: Search Press, Ltd.

Mitchell, L. A., MacDonald, R. A. R., & Knussen, C. (2008). An investigation of the effects of music and art on pain perception. *Psychology of Aesthetics, Creativity, and the Arts, 2*(3), 162-170.

Mullins, C. S., Nelson, D. L., & Smith, D. A. (1987). Exercise through dual-purpose activity in the institutionalized elderly. *Physical and Occupational Therapy in Geriatrics, 5*(3), 29-39.

Perrin, T. (2001). Don't despise the fluffy bunny: A reflection from practice. *The British Journal of Occupational Therapy, 64*(3), 129-134.

Posthuma, B. W. (2002). *Small groups in counseling and therapy: Process and leadership* (4th ed.). Boston, MA: Allyn & Bacon.

Sabonis-Chafee, B., & Hussey, S. M. (1998). *Introduction to occupational therapy* (2nd ed.). St. Louis, MO: Mosby.

Sames, K. (2009). Documentation in practice. In E. Crepeau, E. Cohn, & B. Schell (Eds.), *Willard and Spackman's occupational therapy* (10th ed.). Philadelphia, PA: Lippincott Williams & Wilkins.

Schell, B., & Cervero, R. (1993). Clinical reasoning in occupational therapy: An integrative review. *Amercian Journal of Occupational Therapy, 47*(7), 605-609.

TeBeest, R., Kornstedt, K., Feldmann, C., Harmasch, L., & Kemnitz, S. (2001). *The use of expressive arts in various occupational therapy settings.* LaCrosse, Washington: University of Washington-LaCrosse.

Whittington, D., Weir, M., Powell, A., Mumbower, S., & Foster, J. (2010). *Benefits and usage of therapeutic art modalities by occupational therapists in the aging population.* Unpublished Masters research project, University of Mississippi Medical Center School of Health Related Professions.

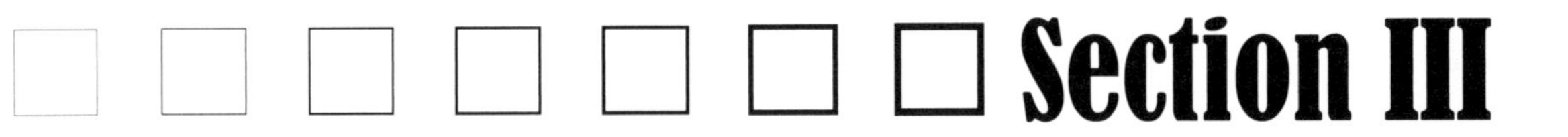

Section III

Crafts in Application

Traditional Occupational Therapy Crafts

Modern and Domestic Crafts

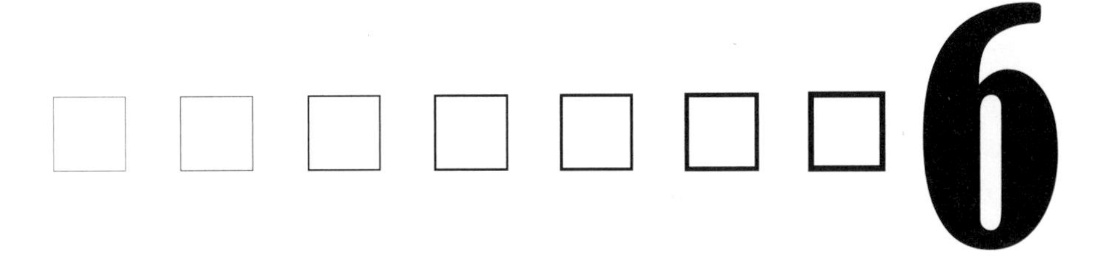

Mosaic and Glass Crafts

Objectives

The student should be able to:

- Discuss historical/cultural examples of mosaic work
- List basic supplies and materials needed to do mosaics and simple glass crafts; and know how to complete and grade a basic project
- Explain advantages and limitations of mosaic activities in therapy
- List precautions of mosaic and glass craft activities
- Articulate ways of using mosaic and simple glass craft activities with various client populations

Introduction

Mosaic, a surface decoration made of assembled small pieces called tesserae, is an ancient craft, probably originating in the Middle East about 5,000 years ago. It became an important art form in many cultures and countries, including Greece, Egypt, Italy, Mexico, France, Thailand, Jordan, and America. Mosaic was probably first used as floor and wall decoration, but was eventually incorporated into thrones, temple columns, and jewelry (Lapidus, 1977). Mosaics became very popular during the early Christian era, perhaps because they were durable and could be used to make murals depicting sermons in pictures at a time when most people were unable to read. To create the mural, the artist pressed small pieces of colored glass, ceramic fragments, and stone into fresh plaster or concrete following a preconceived design. It was necessary to work quickly, doing only a small area at a time. Modern materials make this process easier, but design complexity and tesserae size are still the chief determinants of difficulty. In therapy applications, the process generally consists of gluing down the tiles or other pieces, then filling spaces in between with grout. Mosaics can also be done with no space between tiles, which eliminates the need for grout (Department of the Army, 1971; Moseley, Johnson, & Koenig, 1962; *Reader's Digest*, 1979).

One attraction of this craft for today's therapist is that small mosaic projects can be completed within an abbreviated hospital stay. For grouted projects, however, at least two sessions will be necessary, as the glue must dry completely before the grout can be applied. The basic supplies needed for mosaic work are the tiles—usually glazed ceramic or glass—or other tesserae material, a mounting surface, glue, and grout,

Tubbs, C., & Drake, M. *Crafts and Creative Media in Therapy, Fourth Edition (pp. 63-74).*

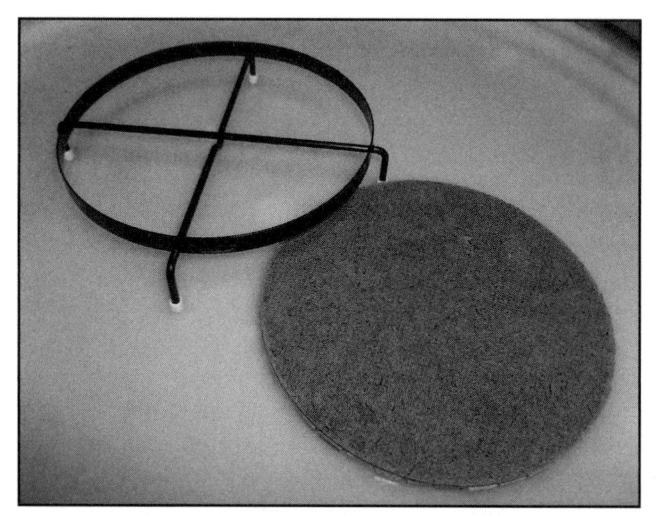
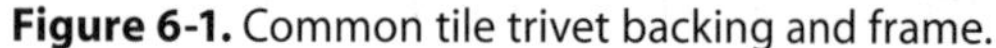

Figure 6-1. Common tile trivet backing and frame.

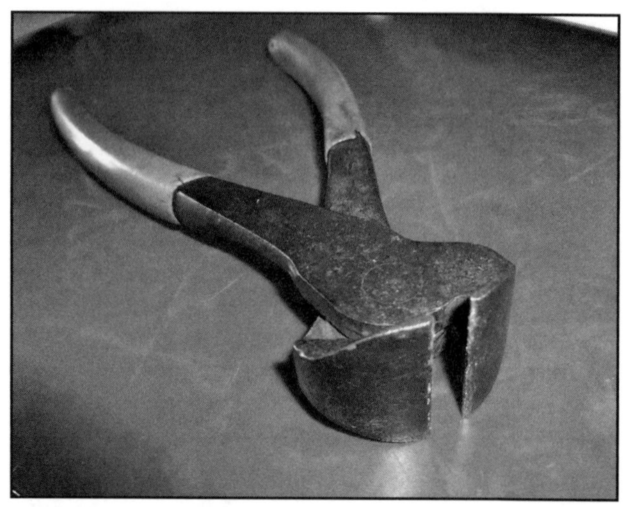

Figure 6-2. Tile cutter.

along with tools for spreading and cleaning, usually a sponge and blunt wooden implement such as a tongue depressor. A float is necessary for spreading grout in larger projects such as tabletops. Tile trivets, which come in a variety of shapes, are a common mosaic project. Trivet are often made using metal frames into which a backing is placed. The metal trivets purchased through craft suppliers have a masonite board on which to mount the tile (Figure 6-1). Some clinics simply cut their own backboards out of thin plywood-like material. In the event the client does not complete the tiling, the therapist may choose to save the metal frame for another project. Tile top boxes are another choice available in most craft catalogs. Many other less structured tiling projects are currently popular including mosaic flowerpots, vases, candleholders, and outdoor decorations, and such substrate objects are readily available in retail stores. Mosaic material need not be limited to ceramic tile, but can incorporate glass, stones, broken pottery or dishes, or natural materials such as seeds or beans. In longer-term facilities, residents can attempt more challenging mosaic projects such as table tops, jewelry boxes, trays, picture frames or pictures (*Better Homes and Gardens*, 1966; Janitch; 1973, Lapidus, 1977). Grout is available from craft suppliers, but it can also be purchased in larger quantities and in a selection of colors from hardware or home improvement stores.

Mosaic work has several qualities that make it useful therapeutically. It requires few tools, is not especially messy, and the various steps make it useful in assessing or treating diverse skill areas such as size and color discrimination, ability to make decisions, fine motor manipulation, spatial awareness, ability to follow directions, and ability to organize and carry out a plan.

Stained glass work, also used decoratively for over 6,000 years (*Reader's Digest*, 1979), has a similar patchwork appearance. In addition to employing a different process, stained glass works are usually made up of larger pieces and are designed to allow light to pass through. One author wrote a moving account of her recovery from a stroke. She found that her favorite hobby—making stained glass—was all breakthrough activity and one on which she wanted to expend her limited energy. Being a neuroanatomist, she chose to make a stained glass brain and found that its fabrication improved her stamina, balance and equilibrium, manual dexterity, and cognitive processing (Taylor, 2008). Constructing stained glass is an involved procedure that is seldom used as a treatment modality, but the occupational therapist may utilize a simple substitute such as glass painting or etching that will approximate a stained or frosted glass appearance using a much simpler process.

Special Considerations and Precautions

Mosaic work is generally a safe activity. Few tools are required and use of kits and precut tiles eliminates the need for a tile cutter (Figure 6-2). If a tile cutter is used, the client should be protected from flying shards by cutting inside a bag, or under a table or other shielding surface. If using glass tiles, be aware of sharp edges. Some commercially available glass pieces are smooth, but some types have rougher edges, so these, as well as any glass that is cut or broken by the crafter, should be handled with gloves. Gloves should also be worn when working with grout since the sanded forms are abrasive and some grout compounds contain allergenic chemicals (Biggs, 1999). Glass etching cream used in alternative glass decorating projects is caustic to skin and gloves are advisable for this process as well. Dust from the grout may present a hazard for clients with respiratory problems. Etching creams and some glass paints may also cause odors or respiratory irritation that some clients cannot tolerate.

When preparing to grout a mosaic piece, be sure that the glue is dry so that pieces will stay in place. When working with grout, it is important to mix to the correct consistency and allow adequate drying time. Grout that is too thin will crack as it dries and grout that is too thick will be difficult to smooth into spaces. It is also important to gently wipe off as much excess grout as possible while it is still wet. Dried grout on top of the tiles or glass not only creates extra work, but may mar the appearance of the finished product. In cleaning grout residue from the tile, always use a blunt instrument (e.g., such as a tongue depressor) that will not scratch the surface and be careful not to gouge into the grout spaces. Leftover mixed grout as well as residue from dry grout should be discarded into a trash receptacle, never washed down a drain. The grout will eventually harden and could cause plumbing problems. While it is safe to wash off small amounts from containers or implements in the sink, if mosaic work is done frequently, a sink with a plaster trap is advisable.

If the mosaic construction is to be used in an outdoor or wet application, epoxy glue is necessary and grout sealer is recommended. Spacing of greater than 1/4 inch between tiles requires sanded grout for durability; unsanded grout should be used to fill smaller spaces. Thicker grout or prepared mastic will be needed for mounting tiles on a vertical surface. Masonite is a satisfactory backing for small projects, but larger ones will require a thicker backing such as plywood (Lapidus, 1977).

Cost may be an issue for some mosaic projects, but this craft can be done inexpensively as well. Use of broken dishes or other scrap or natural materials significantly reduces the cost.

Project—Tiled Candle Holder

Plan It

This project can be made with a recycled glass candle container/jar but the therapist should be sure that any container used is heat tolerant. Mastic works well for adhering tiles to a vertical surface; it can be purchased in hardware or home improvement stores and will keep for months if the lid is kept sealed. This project will take at least two sessions since the glue must dry completely before the grouting can be done.

Get Ready

Supplies

- Paper and pencil for drawing the design (optional)
- An assortment of ceramic tiles in various shapes, sizes, and colors
- A large-mouth glass container
- Mastic or tacky glue (common white glue will not hold well enough on a vertical surface)
- Grout
- Grout additive (optional)
- Water
- Grout sealer or liquid floor wax (optional)

Tools

- Small bowl for mixing grout, preferably disposable
- Larger bowl to hold water for cleaning sponge
- Tongue depressor or other mixing stick
- Spatula or small grout float
- Tile cutters (optional)
- Sponge

Time required: Two 30- to 45-minute sessions

Approximate cost: $1 to $2

Do It

Process

1. Have the client plan the design and choose the tile colors based on size and shape of container. Random or geometric pattern designs are much easier than creating a picture and are recommended for the beginner.
2. If tiles need to be cut to fit, the client should put on goggles before using the tile cutters (see Figure 6-2). Cut the tiles inside a paper or plastic bag, or with hands under the table, protecting self and others from flying fragments. Some clients may need to have their tiles cut for them.
3. Glue the pieces down individually; the tiles should not extend above the edge of the container. Avoid using too much glue; if it squeezes up into the spaces, it will interfere with the grout. If necessary, use tweezers to remove or replace tiles in interior areas of the design. Allow space of 1/16 to 1/8-inches between the tiles. Consistency in spacing will produce the most attractive end product (Cheek, 1998), although this will be more challenging with irregularly shaped pieces. Use a ruler as a guide if necessary, but make sure the space is wide enough for the grout to be applied between the tiles. Some suggest standing a nickel or dime between tiles to ensure uniform spacing.
4. Continue gluing until the design is completed. Allow the glue to dry thoroughly.
5. Mix the grout according to package directions; the mixture should be the consistency of creamy peanut butter. Be sure to mix enough to do the entire project at once and be prepared to use it immediately, as the mixture dries out relatively quickly.
6. Pour or scrape the grout mixture with the spatula onto the tiles. Use the spatula, fingers, or tongue depressor to push the grout down into all the crevices. Be sure to grout all the way to the edge; any residue on the rim can be cleaned off later. Make sure to smooth all spaces and eliminate any air pockets or cracks. Gloves are recommended when handling grout since it contains both chemicals and abrasives (Biggs, 1999).
7. With the flat side of a barely damp sponge, lightly rub the excess grout off the tiles, being careful not to rub it out of the cracks.
8. Allow grout to dry slowly overnight. Place a damp cloth or paper towel over it so that it will not dry too quickly and create cracks. Cracking is hard to repair satisfactorily without digging out the whole seam and regrouting.
9. When the grout is completely dry, rub any remaining grout film off the tiles with a dry or slightly damp sponge. Well-cleaned tile edges define and improve the appearance of the finished product (Figure 6-3).
10. Apply the grout sealer if desired. Liquid floor wax can be used as a grout sealer (Biggs, 1999; Department of the Army, 1971; Moseley, Johnson, & Koenig, 1962; *Reader's Digest*, 1979; VanZandt, 1973).

Change It

Vary the activity by using a different container or different tile. Or place tiles right next to each other, that is, eliminate the space for grout. To grade this activity down, tiling can be done on flat, horizontal surface, such as a basic trivet or on the glass inside a small picture frame. Or use the faux stained glass technique described next. To grade this activity up, a number of elements can made more challenging, such as using a larger container, using smaller tiles, or creating a more complex or pictorial design. If the mosaic is done on a horizontal surface, the creator can also lay out the full design before gluing, then remove and glue one tile at a time. Two or three tiles will need to be removed initially to allow working space without disturbing or losing the entire design. This method requires good fine motor control and patience.

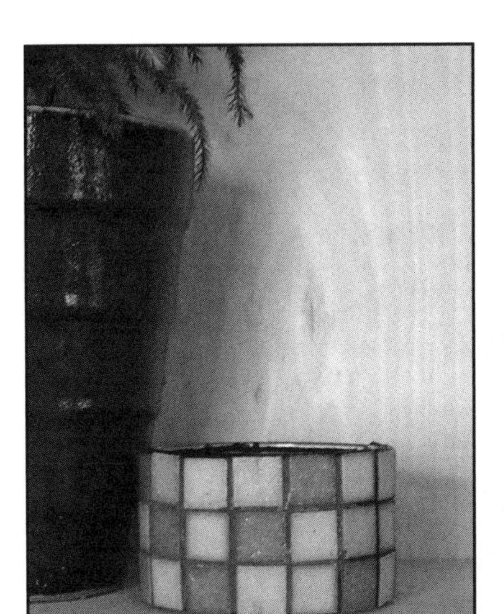

Figure 6-3. Tiled candle holder.

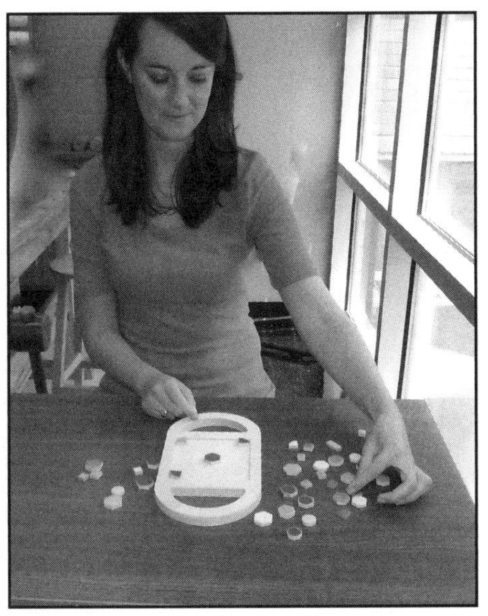

Figure 6-4. Mosaic work can facilitate visual scanning and visual discrimination skills

Document It

The following are examples of documentation of performance skills or relevance of mosaic work to areas of occupation:

- "With occasional cueing to turn head to compensate for visual field deficit, the client was able to locate correct colors of tiles from a container placed on the left side." (Figure 6-4)
- "After completing tile mosaic project, client showed improvement in other fine motor activities such as buttoning and handling make-up tools."
- "During the tile mosaic activity, the client repeatedly replaced and removed tiles, demonstrating difficulty with decision-making and task termination."

Faux Stained Glass Container

Supplies

- A large-mouth glass container OR small picture frame with glass
- Glass paint
- Tube "leading"

Tools

- Marking pen
- Paint brush

Process

1. If desired, first draw the design on paper corresponding to container or frame glass size.
2. Place picture under glass and trace design onto glass with marking pen.
3. Squeeze glass "leading" from tube over design marking.
4. Paint within spaces with glass paint. Let dry (Figure 6-5).

Use of the tube leading product requires grip strength and a fairly steady hand, so the client may want to experiment on scrap material first. Also consider that the leading will require several hours of drying time before the glass painting can be done.

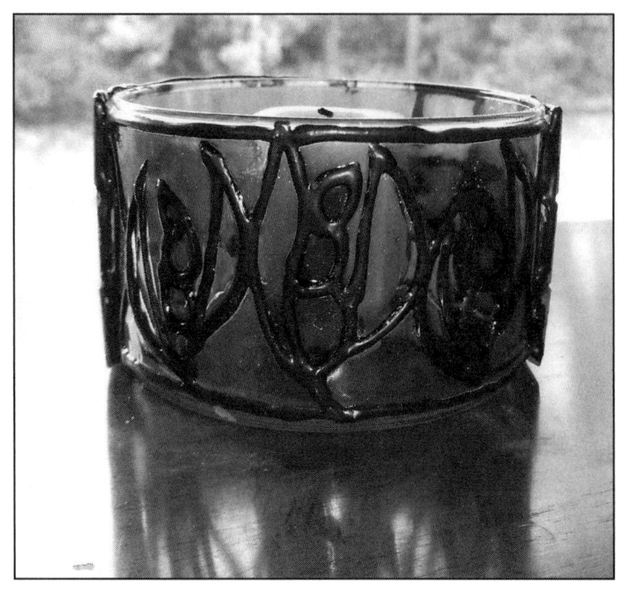

Figure 6-5. Faux stained glass.

Other Ideas and Grading

Possibilities for mosaic projects are plentiful. Broken pieces of colorful plates can cover a tabletop, flowerpot, or lamp base. Create a picture on a wooden background using dried beans, whole cloves, pumpkin seeds, and so on. The natural colors of these materials will create pictures with subtle shading and an earthy look. Tear or cut small squares of colored paper to use as "tiles" for a group mural. You can also create small, attractive, and inexpensive mosaics using eggshells. First, hard boil and dye the eggs. Peel the egg, keeping pieces as large as possible. After thoroughly cleaning the back and drying the pieces, place them onto glued areas. Gently press to crack, then use a finger or small pointed tool to slightly separate the pieces. Continue to fill in according to the planned design. For this method, use clear-drying glue; no grouting is necessary. Ceramic pieces or glass beads can also be used to embellish objects without completely covering the surface. Use painting or other techniques, then add tiles as special visual features. Mosaics can also be made with colored sand, shells, wood, cork, or using mixed media to create a more three-dimensional effect. For a simple children's activity, have them place small plastic beads inside a form, then iron, to make mosaic-like pictures.

As mentioned in the introduction section, etching and painting are two ways of decorating glass that are feasible for use in therapy. Painting can be done with products specially formulated for glass or with basic acrylic paints. Some glass paints come in multiple colors and mimic the look of stained glass; others produce a frosted or etched appearance. Another idea is to cover parts of a glass container (e.g., a wine bottle) with tape or stickers then coat the exposed glass with a contrasting color of acrylic or interior latex paint. After the paint dries, remove the adhered material to reveal the design (Wasinger, 2009). Glass etching is also a simple process and some creams come with pre-cut design stencils; the maker can also create his or her own design using masking tape to cover nonetched areas. Before using any paint or etching products, the therapist should read labels to verify directions for application, cleaning, and food use precautions. Inexpensive drinking glasses, clear glass candleholders or vases (new or leftover), and glass plates are good bases for these projects, and an assortment is available in most dollar stores. Virtually any clear glass objects, including windows and mirrors, can be embellished with these methods. For those on shoestring budgets, a similar translucent glass look can be achieved by gluing white or colored tissue paper on the outside of a glass jar.

Mosaics can be varied in so many ways that the therapist need not feel confined to the traditional trivet project. Some alternatives and grading suggestions have already been introduced in previous sections. One of the most obvious ways to grade a mosaic project is by size. You can use an article as small as a coaster or one as large as a tabletop as a substrate for a tiling project. Mosaic work can be made physically simpler by using larger tesserae, by doing mass placement, or by eliminating spaces between tiles. Gluing on a flat, horizontal surface is easier than on a contoured or vertical surface. The indirect method of gluing (arrange

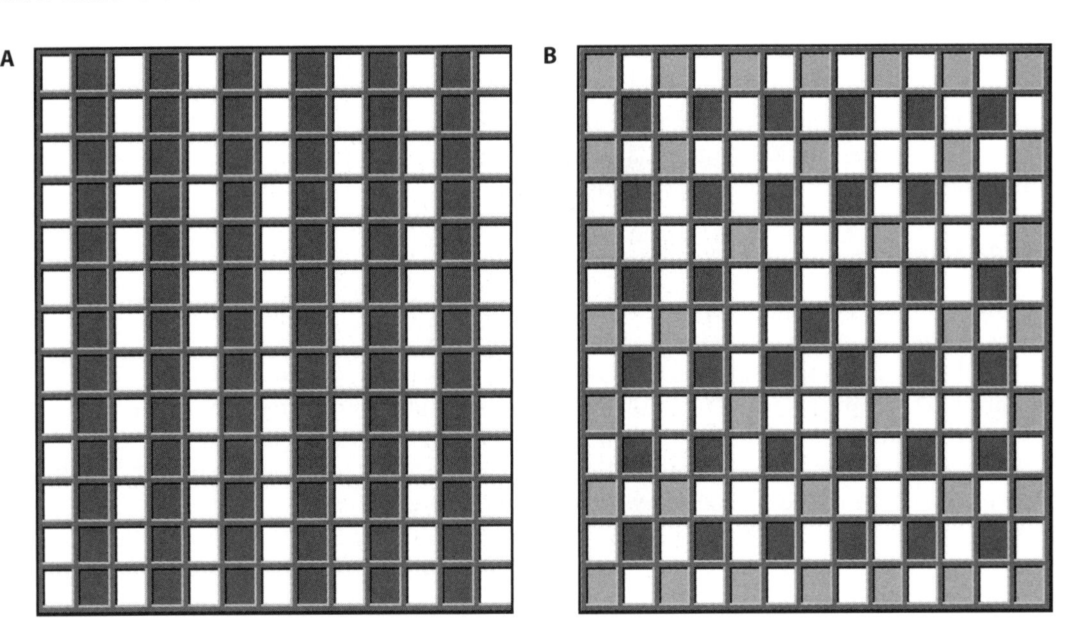

Figure 6-6. Pattern A is much easier to replicate than pattern B.

tiles face down, apply glue to mounting surface, place glued-covered mounting surface over tile backs, apply pressure until dry) is less time consuming and requires less precision handling but is perceptually more challenging. Thorough cleaning of tile surfaces while the grout is still moist will decrease the amount of resistive scraping required later. Simple designs that eliminate the need for cutting tiles also decrease task demand. Some materials are more difficult to handle than others, for example, precise placement of a small bead is more challenging than placing a 3/4-inch tile. The therapist needs to be observant of pinch requirements and adjust projects accordingly.

Mosaic work can also be graded to increase or decrease the cognitive or process demands. Following a pattern is simpler than creating one. The complexity of the pattern also dictates the cognitive and visual/perceptual challenge. Duplicating pictorial designs is more difficult than copying geometric ones. Most clients are able to repeat the sequence of gluing and placing, but for those with severe organizational or attention deficits, minimal color variation is recommended (Figure 6-6). Depending on the project, the therapist could color code areas on the backing prior to tiling to give the client even more visual cues.

Glass etching and painting are both fairly simple processes. In painting, less detailed designs with larger spaces are easier to do. The therapist can draw the design and fill in the artificial leading if needed to further reduce task demand. Etching is already only a two-step process; the primary concern is the caustic property of the etching cream

Main Therapeutic Applications

Physical Dysfunction

Mosaic work is a craft commonly selected to improve various types of pinch and other fine motor function. Picking up and placing the tiles is a repetitive activity using tip to tip pinch, and tile size can be altered to grade the pinch required. Using tweezers will provide added resistance and squeezing the tile cutters can be used to strengthen cylindrical grasp. Minimal proximal movement is needed for this activity, so a client with shoulder range of motion limitations can still be successful. Mosaic projects can also be structured to eliminate resistive forces—especially if grout is thoroughly cleaned while still wet—so it is appropriate for clients with weakness and/or fragile joints. Most steps can be done one-handed as well, especially if glue is spread over the entire backing surface rather than applied to one tile at a time. For this method, it may be helpful to have the design pre-drawn directly onto the substrate material. The cognitive aspects of planning and arranging the design can be beneficial for those clients with neurological impairment, but the therapist will need to provide structure and guidance to minimize frustration. A simple geometric design, or one with only two or three colors, may be best for a client with self-organization deficits (Department of the Army, 1971; Early, 2009; Overs, O'Conner, & Demarco, 1974). Mosaics could be done by bed-bound patients and those in isolation, up to the point of mixing and applying grout; at that point, the therapist can take the project to the clinic and do the grouting for them.

Mental Health

Making a mosaic project is a good way to assess or work on cognitive problems that often accompany psychiatric diagnoses such as decreased attention span and concentration, inability to plan or sequence, and poor awareness of spatial relationships. This may explain the prevalence of mosaic use in traditional psychiatric occupational therapy assessments and treatment (see Table 2-1). For example, the Perkins Tile Task, developed by Vicki Perkins for use in psychiatry, was presented at the 1986 Great Southern Occupational Therapy Conference in Charleston, SC. Quantitative research results, such as number of tiles used, amount of board surface covered, and tile placement were related to diagnostic groups (Perkins, 1986).

With skilled activity analysis on the part of the therapist, even very low-functioning clients can achieve a successful outcome. Thoughtful set up and instructions are necessary for clients with perseverative behavior or poor decision-making skills in order to minimize cueing or assistance needed from the therapist. It may be advisable not to use mosaics with a client who cannot tolerate frustration or attend to detail well. For such individuals, a painted glass project with the tangible boundaries of the tube leading may be preferable due to the imposed structure. In general, though, mosaic work is easily graded, which makes it a useful option for client populations with a wide range of cognitive abilities.

Pediatrics

Improved fine motor performance is a common therapeutic goal for pediatric clients. Mosaics provide an excellent opportunity to practice this skill, and the therapist can grade the size of the tiles to ensure the "just right challenge." The time required to glue all the tiles frequently exceeds the attention span of many children; gluing may need to be done in several sessions or using an alternative method. Seeds and beans are inexpensive alternatives to tiles that are satisfactory for children. Another advantage is that they can be applied in mass rather than individually, reducing the fine motor demand. Simply cover each section with glue, scatter the pieces over the glue, then shake off the excess onto a newspaper or other surface that can be folded into a funnel for pouring back into the container. Although this speeds up the process to accommodate shorter attention spans, it also changes the task demands, so the therapist should be certain that it accomplishes the therapeutic aim. Paper squares are another low cost alternative to tiles; simply cut or tear a variety of shapes, sizes, and colors of construction paper and glue them to a cardboard or paper background. In a large format, this makes an excellent multi-step group activity. Due to its sedentary nature, girls may enjoy mosaic craft more than boys. For hyperactive children, this craft may prove too challenging for both client and therapist (Rogers, 2010).

Adolescents

Older children and teenagers may enjoy making decorative mosaic projects such as flower pots, picture frames, or candleholders, but they are apt to find the traditional metal-framed tile trivet dated and unappealing. Adolescent clients can express their individuality by creating personalized designs or by using different materials as tesserae. This craft offers a therapeutic combination of both structured and unstructured components; for example, the designs, spacing, and colors can be changed to suit the maker, but the grout consistency and drying times are specific. This provides a useful analogy for life: some factors are open to change based on personal preference, but others have rules that must be followed for a successful outcome. Patience permitting, adolescents may like doing small projects such as inexpensive plain pins, bracelets, or pendants with glass seed beads. For this variation, glue beads immediately next to one another and omit grouting. The slow, detail-oriented nature of this process may be absorbing and soothing for someone in emotional turmoil (Brown & Stoffel, 2011).

Older Adults

A simple adaptation of mosaic craft for the elderly is to use larger tiles; bulk ceramic tile can be purchased in 3/4-inch size, rather than the 3/8-inch size. This increases both the visibility and the ease with which the tiles are handled. Since it also decreases the number of tiles needed to fill the space, the project can be completed more quickly. The therapist may want to choose highly contrasting colors to further improve visibility; if light-colored tiles are placed on a dark background, it is easier to discern appropriate spacing (Bonder & Bello-Haas, 2009). Because of their small size, mosaic materials are usually not breakable. This is particularly useful with elderly individuals because their reduced grip strength, coordination, and balance make it more probable they will drop things. Use of the tile cutters may be too difficult, or even contraindicated, but many projects do not call for cutting tiles. Making mosaics has low strength requirements, so it is a good craft choice for clients with upper extremity weakness. A typical project usually takes no more than two or three sessions, so it can be completed before the client loses interest or is discharged. Clients with organizational or memory problems will do best with a sample to copy. This simple, yet attractive craft can be appealing to the elderly because of its rich history and ageless quality.

Groups

Simple tile projects, especially those following a specified pattern, can be done as parallel activities in small groups. The therapist needs to be able to supervise for placement and spacing of tiles, but safety precautions are few. Group members could share glue and/or a common container for tiles, thus increasing opportunity for sharing and interaction. Group members could also work together to create a mosaic mural; this is more feasible in the clinic if using inexpensive and lightweight materials such as seeds or paper. If mosaic constructions will be hung, the background needs to be of sufficient thickness to support this. In most therapy settings, it is impractical to hang large mosaics made from ceramic tile due to their weight. Mosaic design is popular in outdoor applications; group members could collaborate to make items such as stepping stones or bird baths for a facility courtyard or garden spot. A 2005 article in a therapy publication describes the implementation of a mosaic project on a hospital cancer ward. Several patients designed and completed the wall hanging, largely with donated materials. The project, a depiction of a phoenix, proved to be an emotionally healing process for the participants, as well as a symbol of the hope of recovery for all patients (Taussig, 2005).

Case Study

Michael is a 77-year-old first generation immigrant whose family fled Bonn, Germany at the beginning of World War II. He later returned to Europe to study architecture in France but eventually rejoined his family in the United States. His father had started a successful retail business and his parents decided to make the United States their permanent home. Michael joined an architectural company and developed a name for himself as a restoration specialist for old buildings. At age 31, he married a young administrative assistant at the firm; over the next 10 years, they had four children.

All four children were well educated and all but the youngest followed their careers to different parts of the country. Michael continued to work on restoration projects and his wife returned to work after their last child left home. They enjoyed traveling to see their children but otherwise spent little leisure time together. His preferred pastimes were working on his computer and doing crossword puzzles, while she liked gardening and social activities. Michael retired at age 72 after suffering a light stroke. Five years later, he had a more severe cerebrovascular accident (CVA), requiring hospitalization and rehabilitation.

On admission to the rehab facility, Michael was thoroughly evaluated by the rehab team including an occupational therapist. Through a comprehensive evaluation, she found that Michael's left hemiparesis made ambulation unsafe and rendered his left upper extremity essentially nonfunctional. He had a left visual neglect and demonstrated impulsivity and perseveration when attempting tasks. His memory was intact but perceptual problems caused him significant frustration and mild paranoia, and he lacked insight into the scope of his functional limitations. Michael became increasingly depressed and noncompliant and was discharged from rehab due to poor participation. He was referred to home health, the therapist reasoning that he might perform better at home. The new therapist tried to interest Michael in previously enjoyed activities but to no avail. He was resistant to doing anything in which he could not be completely independent and was discharged from treatment after 2 weeks. His wife wanted to continue to work and began to have difficulty coping with his dependence, negative attitude, and distortion of reality. Lacking readily available support from her children, she finally elected to place him in a nursing home.

Michael adapted surprisingly well to the nursing home environment. The routine and structure seemed to calm his mind. He was cooperative and pleasant with the staff, but disinterested in social activities. He remained nonambulatory, inactive, and dependent for his self-care. In spite of his limitations, the nursing home occupational therapist believed that Michael had potential and requested a referral to her service on a trial basis. She attempted to evaluate his self-care ability, but he became frustrated and refused to complete the process. She assessed his motor function and found no tonal or other changes when compared to the home health records. The therapist then had Michael complete a tile trivet to assess his visual and cognitive skills, and general task behavior. Although he needed cueing for organizational deficits and left visual field scanning, he completed the trivet, then asked to do another to give to one of his direct care workers. She allowed him to do this at the next treatment session but still could not interest him in other activities. Michael was seen for five more visits in occupational therapy, but made only incremental improvements in mobility and self-care. He ultimately had to be discharged from therapy due to lack of sufficient progress toward self-care goals, but he began to voluntarily propel himself to the clinic and ask to work on crafts. He gradually began to participate in other nursing home activities and even took an interest in socializing and was more cooperative with the nursing home staff. Although his wife remained unwilling to take him home, she expressed to the therapist how much more pleasant their visits had become.

Discussion Questions

1. Michael wanted to continue making mosaics and doing other crafts, but the therapist was concerned about the cost of supplies. What compromises could be made in this situation?
2. Describe how this case study illustrates the value (and limitations) of a client-centered approach.
3. Why do you think this particular craft satisfied Michael's occupational needs/desires?

Resources

The Complete Book of Mosaics
By Emma Biggs and Tessa Hunkin
The Reader's Digest Association, 2006

The New Mosaics
By D. T. Dawson
Lark Books, 2001

The Mosaic Idea Book
By Rosalind Wates
Quarto Books, 2000
Project ideas, plus good introductory information about tools and materials.

Making Bits & Pieces: Mosaics
By Marlene Hurley Marshall
Storey Books, 1998.
Creative projects for the home and garden. Shows how to use broken pottery, glass, buttons, and jewelry in constructing mosaics. Colored photographs of artists' work as well as how to do the projects. Good index.

Decorative Mosaics
By Elaine Goodwin
New Holland, 2005
Well-illustrated history of the craft. Clear colored photographs of materials, tools, and techniques. Includes 14 projects, an index, and a short list of suppliers.

Mosaic Basics: Everything You Need to Know to Start Making Beautiful Mosaics
By Teresa Mills
Barron's Educational Series, 2006
Basic techniques and projects, graded for skill level

The Art of Making Mosaics
By Louisa Jenkins and Barbara Mills
D. Van Nostrand Company, Inc., 1957
Discusses materials. Has a chapter on children's mosaics and church art.

References

Better Homes and Gardens. (1966). *Stitchery and crafts.* New York, NY: Meredith Press.

Biggs, E. (1999). *The encyclopedia of mosaic techniques: A step-by-step visual directory with an inspirational gallery of finished works.* London, UK: Quarto Publishing.

Brown, C., & Stoffel, V. C. (Eds.). (2011). *Occupational therapy in mental health: A vision for participation.* Philadelphia, PA: F. A. Davis.

Cheek, M. (1998). *Mosaics: Inspirational ideas and practical projects to make in a weekend.* New York, NY: Lark Books, Incorporated.

Department of the Army. (1971). *Craft techniques in occupational therapy.* Washington DC: US Government Printing Office.

Earhart, C. A., Allen, C. K., & Blue, T. (1993). *Allen diagnostic module.* Colchester, CT: S & S Worldwide.

Early, M. B. (2009). *Mental health concepts and techniques for the occupational therapy assistant* (4th ed.). Philadelphia, PA: Lippincott Williams & Wilkins.

Gillette, N. (July 2, 1989). *Personal communication—telephone interview and letter regarding Nedra Gillette's Battery.* Birmingham, AL.

Hemphill, B. J. (1982a). *The evaluative process in psychiatric occupational therapy.* Thorofare, NJ: SLACK Incorporated.

Hemphill, B. J. (1982b). *Training manual for the BH battery.* Thorofare, NJ: SLACK Incorporated.

Hemphill, B. J. (1988). *Mental health assessment.* Thorofare, NJ: SLACK Incorporated.

Hooper, C. R., & Bello-Haas, V. D. (2009). Sensory function. In B. R. Bonder, & V. D. Bello-Haas (Eds.), *Functional performance in older adults* (3rd ed.). Philadelphia, PA: F. A. Davis Co.

Jacobs, K. (1991). *Occupational therapy: Work-related programs and assessments* (2nd ed.). Boston, MA: Little, Brown, and Company.

Janitch, V. (1973). *Country crafts.* New York, NY: Viking Press.

Lapidus, S. (Ed.). (1977). *Ceramics, mosaics, and stained glass: A creative introduction to methods and materials.* New York, NY: David McKay Company, Incorporated.

Matsutsuya, J. S. (1969). The interest checklist. *American Journal of Occupational Therapy, 23*(4), 323-328.

Moseley, S., Johnson, P., & Koenig, H. (1962). *Crafts design.* Belmont, CA: Wadsworth.

Overs, R. P., O'Conner, E., & Demarco, B. (1974). *Avocational activities for the handicapped.* Springfield, IL: Charles C. Thomas.

Perkins, V. J. (1986). *Quantitative assessment of a mosaic tile task.* Abstracts of the Fourth Annual Meeting. The Great Southern Occupational Therapy Conference, Charleston, SC.

Reader's Digest. (1979). *Crafts and hobbies.* Pleasantville, NY: Reader's Digest Association, Inc.

Roger, S. (2010). Common conditions that influence children's participation. In J. Case-Smith, & J. C. O'Brien (Eds.), *Occupational therapy for children,* (6th ed., pp. 146-192). Maryland Heights, MO: Mosby Elsevier.

Taussig, V. (2005). Healing through creative mosaics. *Advance for Occupational Therapy Practitioners 21*(21), 17.

Taylor, J. B. (2008) *My stroke of insight* (p. 114). New York, NY: Viking Penguin.

VanZandt, V. (1973). *Crafts for fun and profit.* London, UK: Aldus Books.

Wasinger, S. (2009). *Eco-craft: Recycle, recraft, restyle.* New York, NY: Sterling Publishing Co./Lark Books.

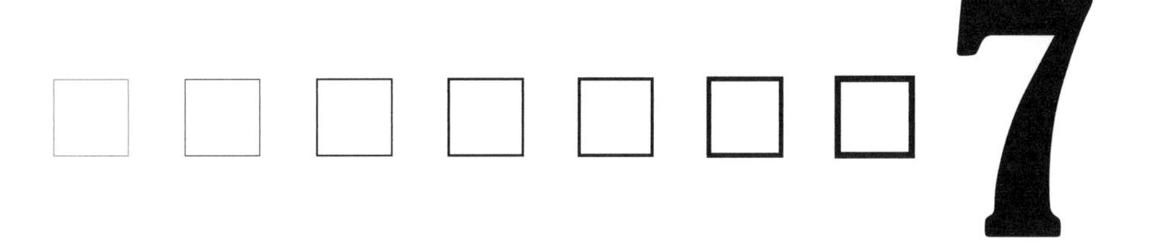

Woodworking

Objectives

The student should be able to:

- Discuss historical/cultural examples of woodwork
- List basic supplies and materials needed to do woodwork and know how to complete and grade a basic project
- Explain advantages and limitations of woodworking activities in therapy
- List precautions of woodworking activities
- Describe how woodworking activities can be used therapeutically with various client populations

Man has made functional articles from wood, including furniture and various types of containers, for thousands of years; and woodcarving may have been one of his earliest artistic endeavors. (Griswold, 1969). Wood has helped meet some of our most basic human needs: in heating for warmth and cooking; as material in sports equipment and musical instruments to meet recreational needs; as sculptures used in religious ceremonies and for decoration; and in creating structures for transportation such as bridges and railroad ties (Douglass, 1960; Scharff, 1952). Woodworking encompasses a number of crafts beyond construction, including making small furniture, chip carving, wooden block printing, whittling, toy manufacturing, and wood sculpting (*Reader's Digest*, 1979).

Cabinet and furniture making, and other woodcrafts are routinely employed in therapy programs to address vocational skills (Cottrell, 1996). Wooden kits are common projects in mental health treatment and used to a lesser extent in rehabilitation for physical dysfunction as well (Blundon & Smits, 2000; Specht, King, Brown, & Foris, 2002). Adapted equipment, largely unknown today, such as the bicycle saw, treadle lathe, and treadle sander were standard equipment in early occupational therapy clinics. Although these machines are more likely to be seen in museums today, some modern occupational therapy clinics and educational programs still have woodworking shops that contain large power tools like the drill press, table saw, jig saw, and band saw. Other clinics use projects that require only hand tools or hand-held power tools. In the following applications, only hand tools will be described since they are widely available, of relatively low cost, and are less dangerous than power tools. Most woodworking tools and supplies can be purchased at hardware or home improvement stores in the community.

Tubbs, C., & Drake, M. *Crafts and Creative Media in Therapy, Fourth Edition (pp. 75-86).*

Because occupational therapists are expected to be experts in equipment adaptation, they should make an effort to gain at least rudimentary skills with carpentry tools. Even though many commercial devices are available, cost may be an issue, or a client may need an item customized for a particular purpose. In addition, woodworking is a popular hobby, especially among men, and the therapist will need basic knowledge of the tools and processes involved in order to problem solve with clients whose goal is to resume this leisure occupation. Some therapists may even find themselves providing therapy services in developing countries, where a majority of the assistive devices will have to be fabricated (Werner, 2009).

Special Considerations and Precautions

Woodworking has broad appeal because articles made of wood are ubiquitous in our environment. Even those individuals with little or no artistic interest may value woodcraft because of its many functional applications. Wood projects, especially kits, are easy enough for even low-functioning clients to complete successfully; they are also easily graded up for clients needing more of a challenge. Several factors will influence how woodcrafts might be incorporated in a therapy setting. Power tools are expensive, dangerous, and take up a great deal of space, so many clinics will opt to use kits exclusively. Some therapists may have the ability to supply "homemade" kits for simple projects; having a friend or family member involved in woodworking is ideal for access to scraps and tools, since kits purchased in hobby stores or from craft catalogs can be cost-prohibitive for some clinics.

Hand tools for woodworking can pose hazards such as sharp edges or pointed ends. This is a consideration for all clients, but especially for those with decreased strength, coordination, or sensation, or with compromised immune systems. Supervision is a must when clients are using any woodworking tools. The woods pieces themselves may also cause splinters, and clients with diminished sensation, or those who are impulsive, for example, may warrant extra caution during handling and sanding of wood. Finishes such as paints and stains that are often used with wood projects can be messy and require special solvents for cleaning, and some may have toxic fumes. The therapist should guard against spills on clothing or work areas by using adequate newspaper, gloves, drapes, and so on. Fumes are inevitable with some substances and those should be used only outside or in well-ventilated areas. Paint or stain fumes, as well as sawdust from cutting or sanding, may be detrimental for clients with respiratory illnesses, and necessary precautions, such as the use of masks, should be observed. Noisy hammering may also be disruptive for some settings and/or clients.

A finished product is only as good as the care taken in its construction. Inadequately sanded surfaces will stand out when a finish is applied. Glue, which may be used in assembly, will resist most finishes, so any visible excess should be wiped clean immediately. Sanding with the grain and applying paint or stain in a single direction will result in the most professional appearance. Wood is somewhat forgiving in that it can sometimes be trimmed or re-sanded to improve fit, form, or look. Brushes (and all tools) should be thoroughly cleaned after use to keep them serviceable and extend their life; good quality implements can be expensive to replace.

Project—Small Pilgrim Stool

Plan It

This small stool has five pieces (Figure 7-1) that will have to be cut from board lumber, increasing the complexity over that of a kit. Softwood such as pine or fir is recommended rather than a hardwood such as oak, but either will work. Scrap wood is also a possibility if it is of sufficient size and thickness. Beware of splinters with any wood. This stool has a simple rabbet joint and is assembled with screws and wood glue, but could also be nailed together. Remember that any visible glue should be wiped off after application at the joints; screws or nails should be used before the glue dries to increase the strength of the finished product. Remember that sanding or use of products with fumes may be contraindicated for clients with respiratory issues.

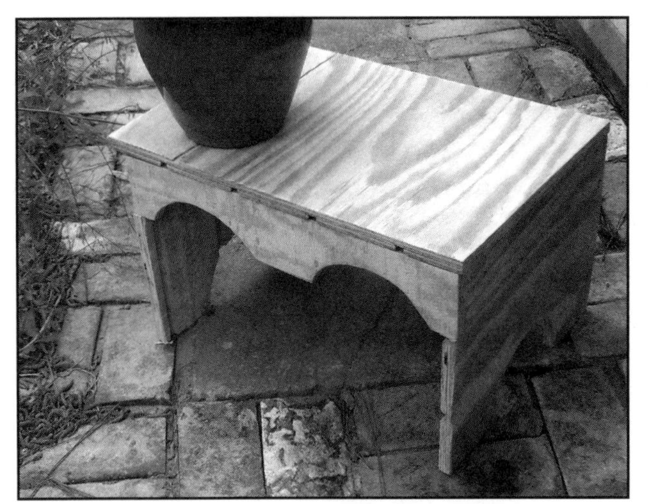

Figure 7-1. Pilgrim stool made from scrap lumber.

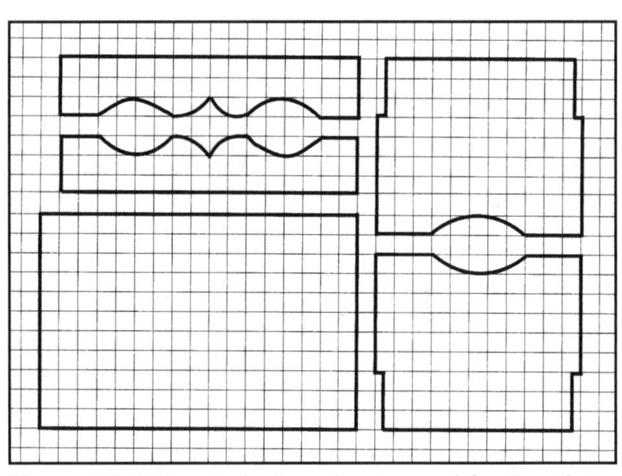

Figure 7-2. Pattern to be traced onto wood for the pilgrim stool (1 square = 1 inch).

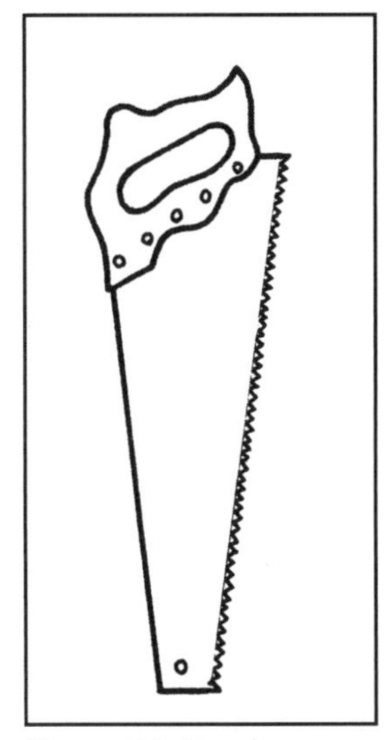

Figure 7-3. Hand saw.

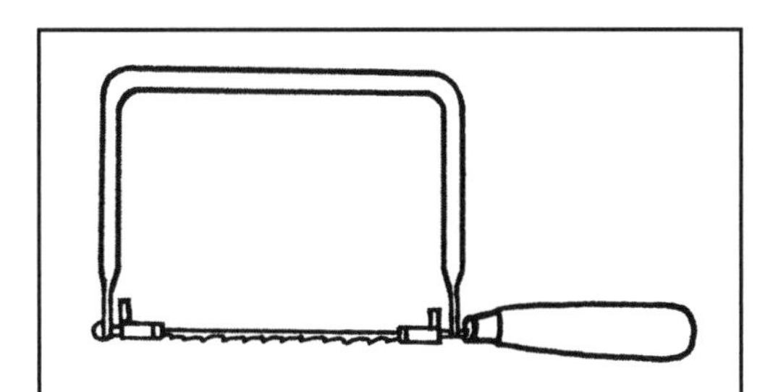

Figure 7-4. Coping saw.

Get Ready

Supplies

- 3/4-inch thick wood, cut into pieces according to pattern (Figure 7-2) using the grid to enlarge
- Sandpaper
- Wood glue
- Screws
- Wood putty or wooden plugs
- Stain or paint, as desired

Tools

- Carpenter's square
- Pencil
- Hand saw (Figure 7-3)
- Coping saw (Figure 7-4), optional
- Drill (hand-operated or power)

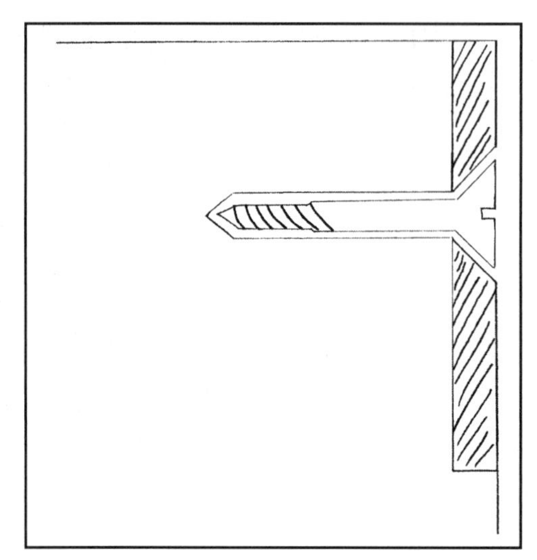

Figure 7-5. Countersunk screw in rabbet joint.

- Paint brushes, rags, etc. as needed for application and clean up of selected finish. Be sure to read finish label for application and clean-up instructions.

Time required: 1 to 2 hours, depending on how much the wood is prepared in advance

Approximate cost: $4 to $5 (can also be done more cheaply with scrap)

Do It

Process

1. Use a carpenter's square and pencil to transfer the enlarged pattern (see Figure 7-2) to the wood.
2. Cut out pieces using the hand saw (see Figure 7-3) and coping saw (see Figure 7-4). If the curved design is too difficult, simply cut the pieces straight across.
3. Assemble the pieces to see if they fit; adjust as necessary.
4. Sand each piece.
5. Mark and drill the holes as shown on pattern.
6. Glue the pieces together, making sure to thoroughly wipe away any visible glue.
7. If desired, counter-sink the screw in the rabbet joint (Figure 7-5).
8. Fill the holes with wood putty, let dry, and re-sand. The holes can also be filled with wooden plugs, which can be purchased or cut from doweling of the corresponding diameter.
9. To finish, use stain or paint as desired, remembering to read label directions first.

Change It

This stool could be varied by changing the pattern for the side pieces, or by staining or painting it. To grade the activity down, use a simple kit, in which all the parts are precut and require only a minimal amount of sanding. Kits typically contain sandpaper, all parts—pieces are usually made of pressed wood with a hardwood veneer—and nails if necessary. It is probably a good idea to have extra nails and sandpaper on hand. To grade the activity up, the template can be modified to include more curves in the side or leg pieces, or rounded corners on the top piece. The pieces could be nailed together instead of screwed, which alters grip and strength demands. The stool can also be embellished using a woodburning tool or by painting with stencils.

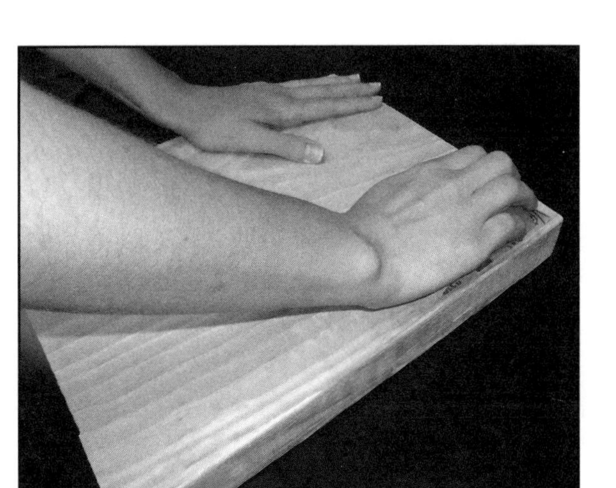

Figure 7-6. Sanding with a plastic sanding block to accommodate decreased grasp and facilitate weight bearing.

Document It

Woodcrafts are excellent for strengthening, endurance, and weight bearing and could be documented as such, as in the examples below:

- "The client was able to sand for 15 minutes without taking a rest break, demonstrating an increase in upper extremity endurance."
- "The therapist provided the client with an adapted sanding block to allow him to incorporate the affected upper extremity in spite of decreased grasp."
- "When sanding pieces of the project on an incline, the client was able to achieve > 90 degrees of shoulder flexion without complaint of pain." (Figure 7-6)

Woodcarving

Woodcarving—cutting a design into a wooden surface to create a sculpture—usually requires skill and practice, but can be simplified for use in therapy by using board scraps or prepared beveled wooden plaques. Balsawood, a very soft, lightweight wood, works well and can be purchased in various size blocks. Pine and basswood are other softwood options (Marshall, 1975). Hardwood should be avoided as it is too resistant and therefore dangerous for clinic use. If a more prominent relief appearance is desired, a stain or dye can be rubbed on the wood prior to carving (Hall, 2001). Carving, because it is a constructive/destructive craft requiring physical force, may facilitate emotional expression. Some carvers have even said that this process "frees" the wood as well (Fidler & Velde, 1999). For remediation of physical dysfunction, it may be most useful in working on strength, endurance, and coordination, but care should be taken that the client is safe to use the carving tool. This woodcraft requires few tools and the material is economical.

Other Ideas and Grading

A number of projects are possible using only some of the steps of woodworking. For example, various sizes and shapes of wooden plaques are available that require only sanding; they can then be decorated as desired. Other small wooden shapes (e.g., craft sticks or clothespin halves) are common items in craft catalogs and stores. These can be assembled and finished in multiple ways and they require no sanding. Wooden boxes are widely available from craft suppliers and can be decorated in different ways after sanding. Some have recessed tops that can be filled with a mosaic design after the wood is finished. Assorted wood scraps could be turned into picture frames or rustic plaques for mounting pictures or objects using only a simple pattern and a few tools. Woodcarving, described earlier, could be used to embellish features

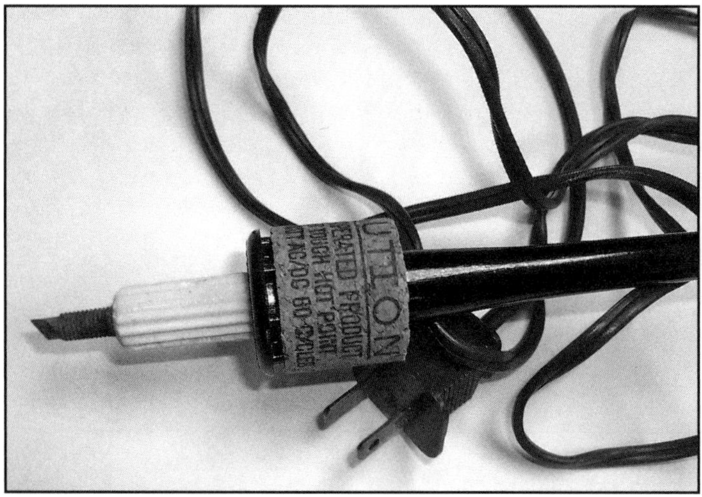

Figure 7-7. Woodburning tool.

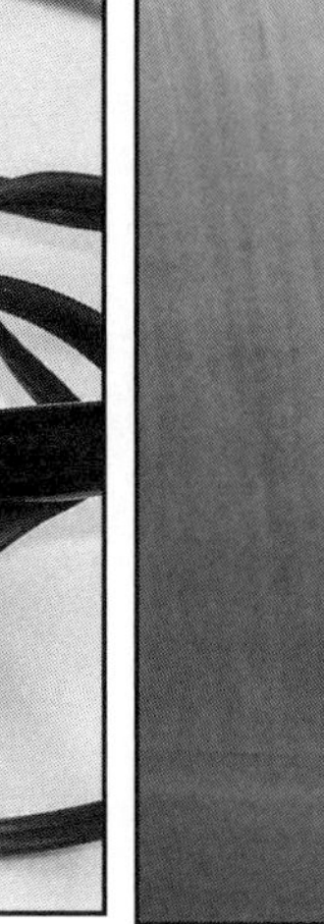

Figure 7-8. Woodburned picture.

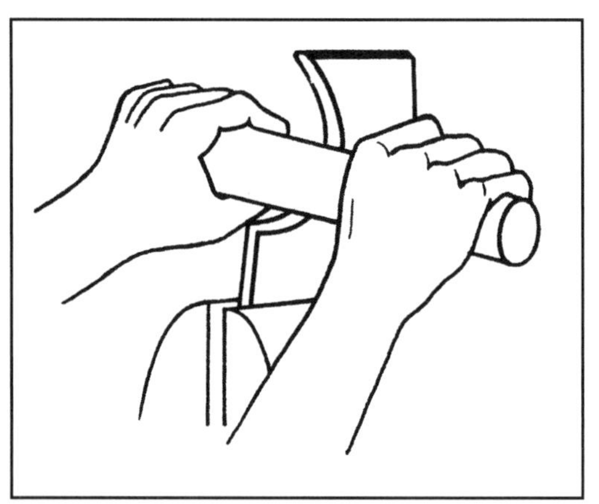

Figure 7-9. Cylindrical sanding block.

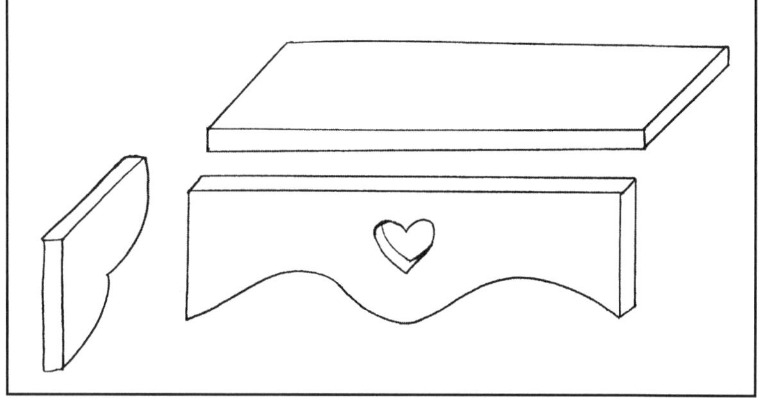

Figure 7-10. A common wood kit project.

of wooden objects, allowing individual design variations while retaining simplicity in tool and space requirements. Stick-on or pressure-sensitive veneer, available at many home improvement stores, can be used as decorative additions similar to appliqué. This material is thin enough to cut with scissors and an unfinished version will accept many coloring media such as stains or paints (Hall, 2001). Woodburning is a somewhat forgotten craft, but some clients may enjoy it. Skillful use of a woodburning tool (Figure 7-7) can result in intricate designs using less strength than necessary needed for carving (Figure 7-8). The tool tip is very hot, necessitating the appropriate precautions including careful attention to manufacturer's directions for use.

Sanding has been an important tool in the occupational therapist's treatment armamentarium for many years. In the past, there were many different designs for sanding blocks, which were simply blocks of wood or plastic to which sandpaper was attached with tacks or staples. Some had handles on top or had cut-out holes for the thumb or fingers, and each was planned to place a client's hand in the desired position. Cylindrical sanding blocks had sandpaper affixed to doweling (Figure 7-9) in order to facilitate wrist extension and flexion in all finger joints. Another aid was the sanding table, similar to an incline table, which could be raised or lowered to achieve range of motion of different upper extremity joints. These adaptations, along with other listed below, are still useful in structuring woodwork to achieve quite specific goals.

To grade woodworking down, choose a simple project with just a few large pieces; these can usually be completed in one or two sessions (Figure 7-10). Numerous kits are available on the market, and ideally, the client would have several from which to choose. The activity demand can be controlled not only by reducing the number of pieces, but also by the means of assembly (e.g., those that require only glue, or glue and nails). For a one-piece project, have the client sand and apply finish to a simple wooden plaque, then use it to mount a photograph or other picture.

Woodworking can be graded up by having the client wear wrist weights while sanding, or do the sanding with the pieces clamped on an incline. Wood pieces can be stabilized in a position such that specific motions are required, or so that more or less effort is needed. The therapist is encouraged to personally try each movement to make the most accurate activity analysis (Department of the Army, 1971). For clients with decreased grip strength or poor precision grasp, hand tools can be adapted by adding foam padding to the handles. Sanding blocks of various sizes and shapes can accommodate differences in grasp as well. Smaller projects are not necessarily less complex; the therapist should consider the number of pieces, how they are to be assembled, and finishing required. Small parts are difficult to manipulate and clients with impaired coordination or dexterity will do better with projects with larger pieces and less detail.

Main Therapeutic Applications

Physical Dysfunction

Because woodworking is most traditionally identified with masculine interests, this can be a valuable activity/occupation for men who have lost some of their physical capacities. The use of power tools may be one way for some clients to compensate for lost strength, assuming all safety hazards have been considered and accounted for. As customary gender roles have become more blurred in some cultures, woodworking as a hobby has become more acceptable for women as well. Many women head single-parent families or live alone and can attain a real sense of independence and achievement by learning basic woodworking skills. Simple home repairs are part of the area of occupation of home maintenance and many of these involve competent use of basic tools associated with woodwork such as hammers and screwdrivers.

Woodworking is an ideal hobby for the client with a chronic condition who may be unable to return to regular employment after discharge. Community craft centers, vocational schools, or even the shops of individual woodworkers may be potential sites for shared workshop space and tools for the client wishing to pursue or resume this pastime after discharge. The Jacobs Prevocational Skills Assessment contains components of woodworking tasks such as hand tool use (Jacobs, 1991). Considering other factors such as vision, judgment, and physical limitations, the therapist should use professional judgment in advising a client to pursue this hobby or line of work on an independent basis.

Improved upper extremity range of motion, strength, and dexterity in the hand can be achieved through carpentry. Hammering, carving, hand drilling, sawing, sanding, and painting all require combinations of upper extremity movement and, in general, the larger the project, the greater the movement required. By changing the height or position of the wood and the type of tools used, a therapist can structure the task for almost any upper extremity joint motion and muscle activation. Many wood projects do not require precision work and could therefore be accomplished by visually impaired clients. Clients with the use of only one hand can utilize clamps or other stabilizing devices and sanding is an excellent weight-bearing activity. Although a deviation from the standard protocol, sanding may be an acceptable variation of the compressive activity (scrubbing) used in treating some chronic pain conditions such as complex regional pain syndrome (Cooper, 2002).

Mental Health

Woodworking is a familiar and respected craft and objects made from wood may hold symbolic meaning. For example, a piece of furniture may conjure memories of home or family, or a carved walking stick may have connotations of respect and authority (Fidler & Velde, 1999). Because of these associations, completion of a wood project supplies a genuine feeling of accomplishment, one means of bolstering self-esteem, and helps establish a sense of normalcy. Woodworking is easily graded for the wide range of functional levels found in mental health clients. Graded appropriately, it can be used just as well for the client with moderate mental retardation as with the cognitively intact client with a substance use disorder. Woodworking may help illuminate, or remediate, deficits in sensory processing, motor control, praxis, attention span, sequencing, spatial operations, and problem solving. For example, woodwork is a component of several crafts in the Allen Diagnostic Module (Earhart, Allen, & Blue, 1992). Most steps are straightforward and can be stopped and started at any point, making it useful for clients with decreased attention or memory (Brown, 2011).

Pediatrics

For children as young as toddlers, elements of woodworking are part of play, for example, the popular hammer-and-peg toys. They help develop hand-eye coordination, motor control, and object manipulation. By the age of 3 years, many children enjoy constructing with wooden blocks, and building activities, often associated with masculinity, may be activities in which fathers can be encouraged to participate with their sons. As they mature, children begin to envision ideas too complicated for them to execute, but by around age 5, a child may start a project and want to continue to work on it day after day. As the child begins to count and discriminate sizes and shapes, woodworking is a natural way to learn shapes and use numbers in measurement (Kaluger & Kaluger, 1984). Small, odd shapes and sizes of wood can be gathered at most lumber yards or cabinet-making shops. As with all clients, but especially with children, wood should be checked for splinters before using. Children may enjoy gluing these odd pieces for sculpture; surfaces can be sanded, painted, collaged, or decoupaged.

Children like to make both useful objects as well as those that are imaginative and symbolic and may do well using prepared wood pieces such as craft sticks or clothespins. Children may be able to complete simple kits, but woodworking from plans and raw materials is too difficult for most. Due to the relatively short attention span of children, projects that can reignite their interest over multiple sessions are best.

Adolescents

Teenagers are more likely than younger children to be able to draw and follow plans. This increases their options for woodworking projects and allows for creativity, which is sometimes the key to adolescent participation. Carved wooden sculptures may appeal to adolescents for the same reasons (Gaitskell & Hurwitz, 1975). As mentioned earlier, woodworking may help adolescent boys with male identification and may be perceived as a step toward adult occupation and responsibility. Traditionally, occupational therapists used activities such as sanding, sawing, and hammering to sublimate negative emotions; some authors now believe they may exacerbate those feelings in some clients (Early, 2009). In any case, teenagers can experience a sense of self-efficacy by making items they can personalize for use in their rooms or for gifts to friends. Woodworking may also spark vocational interests in adolescents that they may not have otherwise considered.

Older Adults

Client factor problems common to geriatric clients are diminished memory, vision, and hearing, as well as decreased mobility and increased pain (Bonder & Bello-Haas, 2009). Deficits in these areas may affect their ability to do complex woodworking, but simplified projects can be equally beneficial. Precut kits are structured and often have only a few steps. The client can spend as much time as needed on steps that are repetitious, such as sanding or rubbing with stain, and each step can be taught separately, reducing demand for short-term memory. When selecting finishes, consider using dark paint or stain to create more contrast, allowing clients with low vision to more easily critique their work (Bonder & Bello-Haas, 2009). Since the elderly have reduced sensation, more vulnerable skin, and heal more slowly than younger people, the therapist needs to take extra precautions to avoid injury. For some clients, painful joints or diminished sensation may be a contraindication for this craft.

In a nursing home setting, some clients may enjoy woodworking as part of an ongoing leisure or activity program, and older women tend to be more willing to do traditionally masculine projects like woodworking than are men to do feminine crafts such as needlework. Those with furniture-building experience may enjoy miniature reproduction using softwood, simple hand tools, and glue (*Better Homes and Gardens*, 1966). Woodburning is another simple alternative woodcraft, but the therapist must decide if the safety concerns outweigh the potential benefits.

Groups

Aside from large projects such as furniture, woodworking does not lend itself well to collaborative group efforts. It is useful, however, for parallel group activity. Working on simple kits seldom requires constant supervision and may give clients opportunities to help one another and share materials. Elderly men working side by side may create an atmosphere that facilitates motivation and even friendly competition. Adult groups could participate in making items for philanthropic purposes, such as making simple wooden toys for hospitalized children. Group work will of course necessitate that the therapist pay special attention to any potential dangers.

Case Study

Paul, a 30-year-old sign painter was involved in a work-related accident in which he became unconscious after touching a boom that was in contact with live power lines. He fell from a 20-foot scaffolding, with a tree breaking his fall about halfway down. He remained alone and unconscious for several minutes. Men working nearby noticed him just as he was regaining consciousness and took him to the hospital emergency room. He spent 3 days in the hospital while they tried to locate the source of his severe neck and back pain. Paul also experienced periods of mild confusion and mood swings. The physicians were unable to find any structural or physiological reason for his pain, and he returned to work 1 week after discharge. The pain persisted and Paul was eventually referred to a chronic pain treatment program. Paul participated in the program on and off for 2 years. During this time, his relationships both at work and at home deteriorated. He both enjoyed and needed his job and was afraid of losing it if he took time off. Instead he took pain medications in ever-increasing amounts but achieved only minor relief. His temper became a problem, and he often got into arguments and fights with his coworkers.

At home, Paul and his wife argued about their young children and her wish to return to work. Their 3-year-old was diagnosed with cerebral palsy with mental retardation and was completely dependent. Although Paul's wife had not worked since the child's birth, she found being at home with the children much more stressful since his injury and hoped to return to nursing work. Suitable childcare was problematic and the family physician recommended residential placement for the 3-year-old. Despite his wife's opposition to this idea, Paul remained suspicious of her motives and accused her of having an affair. She confronted him by calling him paranoid and selfish. As the conflicts escalated Paul's anxiety, he became unable to function at work. The pain center psychiatrist suggested more intensive treatment, referring him to the outpatient unit of a local rehabilitation hospital. A team that included an occupational therapist, physical therapist, psychologist, and vocational specialist evaluated him. The occupational therapist had Paul fill out an interest inventory and administered several work-related assessments. Woodworking, photography, and painting were the items Paul selected on the interest inventory. Although he scored within normal range in both gross motor and fine motor upper extremity testing, he was unable to tolerate sitting through the entire testing session and required redirection to complete the activities. During the team meeting, the physical therapist reported that Paul's walking tolerance was one-eighth of a mile, and the entire team noted his depressive symptoms.

Referencing the Person-Environment-Occupation (PEO) Model, the occupational therapist and Paul agreed on the following goals: to improve communication and stress management skills to reduce conflicts with his wife; to increase his sitting and standing tolerance, along with overall strength and endurance; and to explore and capitalize on avocational interests to increase his activity level. The therapist reasoned that Paul's functional difficulties were due to a combination of psychological, physical, and contextual factors, and each area was appropriate for intervention. As one component of his treatment, the therapist had Paul participate in a woodworking program, beginning with constructing a small wooden stool using just hand tools. Although it took him extra time, he was able to complete each step independently, including drawing the plans, cutting the wood, and assembling the pieces. While he was working, the occupational therapist and Paul talked about his situation at home and discussed ideas for better managing his anxiety.

One Saturday, after he had been in the program 3 weeks, Paul and his wife attended a craft fair together. The woodcrafts that he saw inspired him to be more ambitious with his woodworking in therapy, so the following week, he designed and made a small bookcase. Several other clients liked his design and asked if they could copy it for their projects. This positive feedback from his peers, along with satisfaction he gained from completing a project start to finish, increased his confidence and sense of contribution. In his weekly progress note, the occupational therapist was able to objectively document his improved self-concept and increased activity level. Paul wanted to work on more difficult projects and asked if he could be discharged from physical therapy to increase his time in the woodshop. The treatment team soon decided that it was time to discharge him from the rehabilitation program altogether.

Paul returned to work, and he began to use his father-in-law's garage workshop to continue doing woodcraft. He and his wife continued weekly visits to a psychologist for several more months and eventually he found that he was able to work without pain medication and was able to cope with problems at home more effectively. He no longer felt like a burden to his wife, but felt confident in his ability to be a productive family member. By the time the psychologist discharged him, Paul felt that he was almost back to normal.

Discussion Questions

1. What precautions were necessary during Paul's involvement with woodworking, especially early in his treatment?
2. List client factors and performance skills required for woodworking that the therapist may have focused on in documenting Paul's progress.
3. If this client had been a female (instead of a male) with the same diagnosis, would this have been an appropriate craft choice? Why or why not?
4. If you wanted to start using this craft in your clinic, what are some obstacles/problems you might encounter? How would you respond to them?

Resources

The Big Book of Weekend Woodworking: 150 Easy Projects
By John and Joyce Nelson
Sterling Publishing/Lark Books, 2005

The Art of Woodburning—30 Useful and Decorative Projects
By Betty Auth
Sterling Publishing Co., 2001

The Complete Manual of Woodworking
By Albert Jackson, David Day and Simon Jennings
Alfred A. Knopf, 1997
A detailed guide to design techniques and tools for the beginner and expert. Has a glossary, index, and excellent photos, drawings and explanations. Shows photos of various woods and describes their properties.

Shop-Tested Small Furniture You Can Make
By James E. Blume (Ed.)
Meredith Books, 1997, 2nd edition
Twenty-five projects for the skilled hobbiest. Accurate patterns.

Time-Life Books: The Art of Woodworking Series
Series Editor, Pierre Home-Douglas
Time-Life Educational

Chip Carving: Design and Pattern Sourcebook
By Wayne Barton
Sterling Publishing Co., Inc., 2007
Patterns, useful techniques, and information on tools.

Easy Carpentry Patterns for Children
By Jerome E. Leavitt
Dover Publications, 1986

How to Carve Wood: A Book of Projects and Techniques
By Richard Butz
The Taunton Press, 1984
Good book for the beginner.

Modern Woodworking
By Willis H. Wagner
The Goodheart-Willcox Co., Inc., 2006
A comprehensive basic text presenting power and hand tools with emphasis on safety.

Woodcraft
By Bernard S. Mason
A. S. Barnes and Co., Inc., 1973
Older volume but interesting wood crafts for the pioneer outdoorsman.

Amateur Craftman's Cyclopedia
By Popular Science Monthly
Popular Science Publishing Company, Inc., 1937
While most of this nostalgic how-to book is on woodcrafts, there are sections on electricity, radio, metal craft, photography, and weather measurement tools.

References

Better Homes and Gardens. (1966). *Stitchery and crafts*. New York, NY: Meredith Press.

Blundon, G., & Smits, E. (2000). Cognitive rehabilitation: A pilot survey of therapeutic modalities used by Canadian occupational therapists with survivors of traumatic brain injury. *Canadian Journal of Occupational Therapy, 67*(3), 184-196.

Bonder, B. R. & Bello-Haas, V. D. (2009). *Functional performance in older adults* (3rd ed.). Philadelphia, PA: F. A. Davis Co.

Brown, C. (2011). Schizophrenia. In C. Brown, & V. C. Stoffel (Eds.), *Occupational therapy in mental health: A vision for participation*, (pp. 179-191). Philadelphia, PA: F. A. Davis Co.

Cooper, C. (2002) Hand impairments. In C. A. Trombly, & M. V. Radomski (Eds.), *Occupational therapy for physical dysfunction* (5th ed.). Philadelphia, PA: Lippincott Williams & Wilkins.

Cottrell, R. P. F. (1996). *Perspectives on purposeful activity: Foundations & future of occupational therapy*. Bethesda, MD: American Occupational Therapy Association.

Department of the Army. (1971). *Craft techniques in occupational therapy*. Washington, DC: US Government Printing Office.

Douglass, J. H. (1960). *Woodworking with machines*. Bloomington, IL: McKnight & McKnight Publishing Company.

Earhart, C. A., Allen, C. K., & Blue, T. (1993). *Allen diagnostic module: Instruction manual*. Colchester, CT: S & S Worldwide.

Early, M. B. (2009). *Mental health concepts and techniques for the occupational therapy assistant* (4th ed.). Philadelphia, PA: Lippincott Williams & Wilkins.

Fidler, G., & Velde, B. (1999). *Activities: Reality and symbol*. Thorofare, NJ: SLACK Incorporated.

Gaitskell, C. D., & Hurwitz, A. (1975). *Children and their art* (3rd ed.). New York, NY: Harcourt, Brace, Jovanovitch.

Griswold, L., & Griswold, K. (1969). *The new handicraft processes and projects* (10th ed.). New York, NY: Van Nostrand Reinhold Company.

Hall, M. A., Wrobel, J., & Salamony, S. (2001). *Decorative crafts sourcebook*. San Diego, CA: Thunder Bay Press.

Jacobs, K. (1991). *Occupational therapy: Work-related programs and assessments* (2nd ed.). Boston, MA: Little, Brown, and Company.

Kaluger, G., & Kaluger, M. F. (1984). *Human development—The span of life*. St. Louis, MO: Times Mirror/Mosby College Publishing.

Marshall, E. M. (1975). *Occupational therapy fundamentals of work*. Thorofare, NJ: SLACK Incorporated.

Matsutsuya, J. S. (1969). The interest checklist. *American Journal of Occupational Therapy, 24*(4), 323-328.

Reader's Digest. (1979). *Crafts and hobbies*. Pleasantville, NY: The Reader's Digest Association, Inc.

Scharff, R. (1952.) *Handbook of crafts*. Greenville, CT: Fawcett Publications.

Specht, J., King, G., Brown, E., & Foris, C. (2002). The importance of leisure in the lives of persons with congenital disabilities. *American Journal of Occupational Therapy, 56*(4), 436-445.

Werner, D. (2009). *Disabled village children*. Berkley, CA: Hesperian.

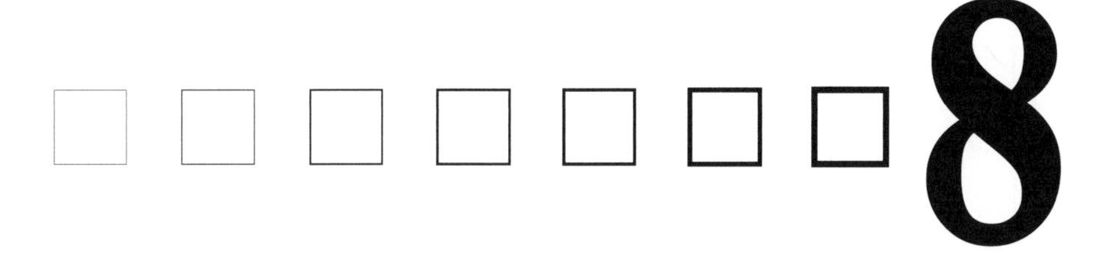

Metal Crafts

Objectives

The student should be able to:

- Discuss historical/cultural examples of metalwork
- List basic supplies and materials needed to do metalwork and know how to complete and grade a simple project
- Explain advantages and limitations of metalwork activities in therapy
- List precautions of metalwork activities
- Describe how metalwork activities may be used with various client populations

The word *metal* has its root in the Greek word *metallon*, which means "something diligently sought" (Griswold, 1969). Metalworking has existed for at least 12,000 years; metal was so important to the development of civilization that historic eras were named after it, namely the Iron and Bronze Ages. Copper and gold were probably discovered first, but all elemental metals are known to have been used in prehistoric times and, around 2000 B.C., metal workers discovered the process of making bronze, a hard metal alloy. Harder metals and alloys were used to make tools and weapons, while softer metals were used in ornamentation. Copper, a very malleable element, was often hammered into utilitarian and decorative objects, not far removed from the copper tooling we do today (*Reader's Digest*, 1979). Tin, also an elemental metal, tends to be most often used in practical rather than decorative applications. Other metals such as gold, silver, bronze, iron, pewter, and aluminum are still used today in craftwork, but in contemporary occupational therapy clinics, copper, tin, and aluminum are the most commonly used.

Types of Metal Crafts

Metal can be worked in numerous ways, including piercing or cutting, bending, soldering, hammering, or casting, and can be decorated by tooling, etching, or enameling. Metals can be purchased in sheets, discs or other shapes, or in the form of wire. Tooling, a method of making a design on a sheet of metal foil, is a common application of metal craft in therapeutic settings. Rolls of metal foil for tooling come in copper,

Tubbs, C., & Drake, M. *Crafts and Creative Media in Therapy, Fourth Edition (pp. 87-100).*

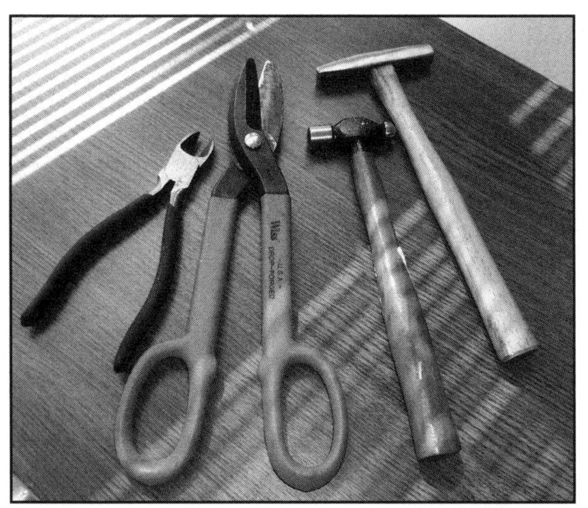

Figure 8-1. Common tools and supplies: side cutter, tin snips, ball peen hammer, planishing hammer.

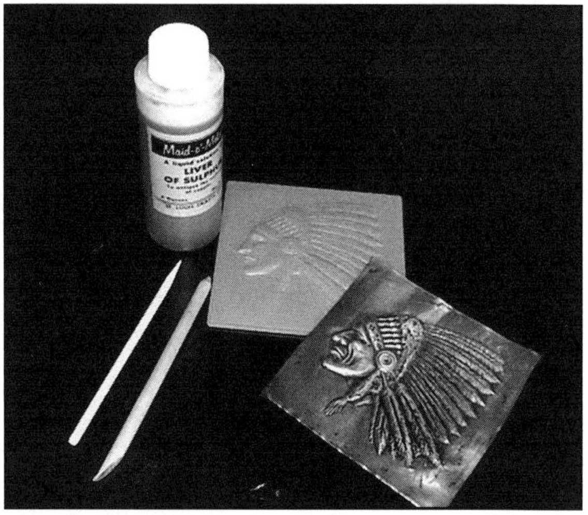

Figure 8-2. Copper tooling supplies: dowels, liver of sulfur, plastic template.

aluminum, and brass, with aluminum being significantly less expensive. Metal squares for tooling come in copper or aluminum and the aluminum is available in several different colors; however, the convenience of precut squares makes this option somewhat more expensive. The thickness of the metal foil or sheet is expressed in a numerical term known as gauge; the thicker the foil, the lower the number. Most tooling is done on 30- to 40-gauge metal. Copper has been most commonly used, probably because its malleability yields a more detailed design. Crafting metal for hammering, bending, or punching is also available as discs and other shapes in thicker gauge, or as wire for bending. Thickness and pliability of wire is also expressed in gauge; this is addressed in Chapter 16. For the most part, metals used in crafts are fairly easy to bend, cut, or pierce.

Embossing is a method of working the metal from the back of the foil to raise the design on the front, and chasing is the same process but done from the front of the foil. When both are combined to get a picture, it is called repoussé, which means "worked from both sides." The term *copper tooling* is inclusive of all three of these methods. (*Reader's Digest*, 1979). Hammering imparts a texture to the metal. Tin punch, another metal craft more commonly seen in therapeutic applications, involves piercing the metal with an awl, often following a pattern. Etching and enameling are methods of making designs on the surface of the metal. Etching is done using an acidic compound that erodes the metal surface, while enameling is the process of painting and firing glazes on the metal surface. Enameling is often used to produce beautiful jewelry and other decorative objects, but it requires skill and is often too costly and/or time consuming for most therapy clinics. Basic tools and supplies used in metal work are gloves, steel wool, tin snips, awls, blunt wooden instruments for tooling, various types of pliers, ball peen or planishing hammer (Hill, 2008), and liver of sulfur compound for "aging" copper (Figures 8-1 and 8-2).

Special Considerations and Precautions

Several factors should be kept in mind when considering the use of metal crafts in therapy. Since cost is almost always an issue, the price of metal supplies—copper in particular—must be considered. For most clinic use, though, after the initial expense of the copper, only a few basic tools are needed to complete most projects. Choosing small projects, or using more common materials, such as aluminum foil and steel wire, can be cheaper alternatives. Know the properties of the metals chosen; for example, some metals become brittle after excessive bending or hammering and this can ruin a project. Having knowledge of the materials beforehand will minimize waste. A facility should probably not make the investment in more expensive forms of metal work unless they are certain of using it frequently.

Since many clients are inexperienced in any type of metal work, some may find it less desirable as a craft choice. As with any craft, the therapist should offer project options based on analysis of the number of steps, the difficulty and timing of each step, and whether or not sharp tools or materials are involved; clients are more likely to value their creations when they have done most of the work on their own. Some forms of metal craft traditionally used in occupational therapy such as copper tooling or tin punch may be perceived as dated, and the therapist should try to choose projects and styles in keeping with current trends. Working with metal does present some dangers; the raw edges are sharp, as are many of the tools, and steel wool can cause splinters or skin irritation. The chemical compounds used in coloring, etching, or enameling metals may also pose respiratory or skin hazards, so working in a well-ventilated area and wearing gloves is recommended. Thus, for clients with certain medical diagnoses, such as emphysema or diabetes, some forms of metal work should be used with special caution. Noise, as well as odors, may also be problematic. Metal punch, for example, is a very loud process; the therapist should make sure that the client, and anyone else in the area, can tolerate this.

In spite of some of the challenging aspects of working with metal, it does offer broad therapeutic potential and many attractive, even beautiful, end products are possible.

Project—Template Tooling

Plan It

The process described here is for using templates; plastic picture templates are available for purchase or the maker can create one using any rigid raised design (Figure 8-2). Tooling custom designs can also be done by tracing, then chasing/embossing the picture. This method is more complex but could be used successfully with simpler designs. Aluminum is much cheaper than copper, but will not yield quite the detail possible with copper.

Get Ready

Supplies

- 36-gauge sheet copper (or aluminum), slightly larger than template to be used
- Plastic picture templates (or other suitable raised design templates)
- Modeling (oil-based) clay or sawdust paste
- Liver of sulfur (optional)
- Water (optional)
- Spray lacquer or acrylic sealer
- Masking tape
- Newspapers

Tools

- Small blunt hardwood dowels for tooling
- Small sharpened hardwood dowels for detailing (some tooling dowels have both a sharp end and a blunt end)
- Tongue depressor
- Brush for liver of sulfur (optional)
- Glass baking dish for liver of sulfur solution (optional)
- Gloves
- Steel wool
- Metal shears or scissors

Do It

Process

1. Cut the copper to the correct size, slightly larger than the template.

2. Clean one side of the copper thoroughly with steel wool. Avoid touching this surface with fingers from this point on.
3. Place the copper over the back (indented) side of the template* clean side down, fold edges over, and secure with masking tape, making sure there are no exposed sharp edges.
4. Place this on a stack of newspapers or other semifirm surface. Using the blunt wooden dowel, gently rub evenly over the design to create a beginning impression in the foil, working from the center out.
5. Continue to rub the design with the blunt dowel, gradually revealing more detail.
6. Refer to the front side of the template as needed to see where more work is needed. Use the sharpened dowel for detailed areas and lines, but do not press so hard as to puncture the copper.
7. Once the design is completely revealed, fill in the indention with modeling clay or sawdust paste, smoothing slowly and evenly to fill in the back of the indented surface. This step prevents the raised design from being pushed back in once the copper is removed from the template. This step may be safely omitted with small projects.
8. Remove the copper from the template. Remember to try not to touch the front with fingers, as body oil will resist the liver of sulfur (described in step 12). With a pointed tool, gently impress in the detailed lines of the design on the front if needed/desired.
9. Lightly but thoroughly rub over the front of the copper with fine steel wool to clean off any dirt or oil left from the tooling process.

The tooling can be considered complete at this point. If an antiqued look is desired, follow the remaining directions below.

10. Prepare a liver of sulfur solution in a shallow glass pan by following the label directions.
11. Dip the copper in this solution, or if the copper is too big to fit in the pan, it can be applied with a brush. As a word of warning, liver of sulfur fumes have a "rotten egg" odor which clients may find unpleasant. People with allergies or respiratory problems should avoid these fumes.
12. After the metal is dry, buff the front of the design with fine steel wool. This will allow the black oxidation from the liver of sulfur to remain in the crevices and provide contrast for the raised design.
13. After the desired polish and contrast is achieved, move to a well-ventilated area, or outside, and spray with a thin layer of clear lacquer or acrylic.
14. The finished tooling may be mounted on wood using copper escutcheon pins, or it can be placed in a picture frame.

**If the template is flat on the back, the copper will have to be tooled on the convex image. After removing the metal from the template, the filler for the back will need to be inserted carefully to avoid bending the foil. The front should then be thoroughly cleaned as described above.*

Change It

Using alternative methods to decorate the metal such as those described in the following section will vary the activity demands and one or another may be more appealing to a given client. In general, the activity can be graded down by using a thinner gauge metal and a smaller picture. It can be graded up by using a larger, more detailed picture or by having the client attach the finished piece to a mounting surface using small copper nails. Each of the other techniques described in the following section have different activity demands and may be considered graded up or down, depending on the individual client and the particular therapy goal.

Document It

Statements such as the ones below can be used to document the use of metal craft as a means of achieving an occupational goal.

- "The client was guided in using a pencil grip for holding the wooden dowel (during tooling) in order to facilitate ability to hold her pencil when doing writing activities."

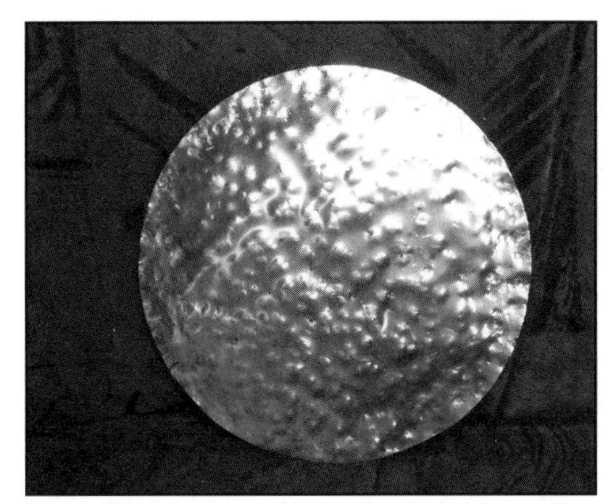

Figure 8-3. Hammered (planished) aluminum disc.

- "The client exhibited adequate grip strength and pressure to thoroughly reveal the template design."
- "In order to work on short term memory skills, the occupational therapist instructed the client in the first three steps of the metal craft activity."

Planishing/Hammering

Hammering requires fewer tools and supplies than tooling but imparts a texture rather than a design (Figure 8-3). This process toughens the metal and the planished piece(s) can be used in a more complex, multi-step project. This metalwork method requires less persistence and attention to detail, but has different motor demands (strong gross grasp instead of writing grasp) and can be noisy.

Supplies

- Sheet of 36-gauge copper slightly larger than the form over which it will be hammered (or a precut aluminum disc)
- Fine steel wool
- Liver of sulfur (optional)

Equipment

- Chasing hammer or small ball peen hammer
- Thin plastic or wooden square the desired size of finished piece (not needed if a disc is used)
- Scissors or metal shears (not needed if a disc is used)

Process

1. Cut the copper to size with scissors or snips. The length should be about 1 inch longer on each side than the form around which it will be shaped.
2. Place the copper over the form and bend the edges around and underneath.
3. Holding the piece still with one hand, hammer the metal using the planishing or ball peen hammer, taking care not to hit the stabilizing hand. A clamp or vise could be used to hold the piece if necessary.
4. Continue this process until the desired look is achieved.
5. Remove the metal from the form. Keep the edges folded so that the exposed border is smooth. Using small copped escutcheon pins or glue, attach the piece to a background such as a box lid or plaque.
6. If desired, the copper piece can be antiqued, before attaching it to the background, using the liver of sulfur method described previously.

Metal Punch

The copper piece can also be punched using a hammer and nail to create a design. For this method, the copper should be secured to a wooden or cardboard form that will allow for penetration of the nail. Simply transfer a design from paper onto the metal, then hammer the nail through at points 1/4- to 1/2-inches apart all along the outline. This can also be done with tin or aluminum, but copper requires the least amount of force.

For any of the above methods, experimenting on a scrap of metal is recommended before starting to work on the actual project. This will both save costly materials and minimize frustration on the part of the crafter.

Tooling With Aluminum Foil

This adaptation costs only pennies but can result in a nice-looking end product.

Supplies

- Wooden or cardboard form
- Thick cotton string, beans, or any other scrap items that can be used to create a raised surface design
- Spreadable glue
- Black acrylic or tempera paint
- Clear acrylic spray
- Heavy duty aluminum foil
- Metallic ribbon or metal foil tape (optional)
- Paper towels

Tools/Equipment

- Spoon
- Scissors
- Fine steel wool
- Gloves (optional)
- Paint brush (disposable foam brush is fine)

Process

1. Cut a piece of foil slightly larger than the form to be covered.
2. Gently crumple the foil into a ball. Straighten it back into flat sheet and smooth it with the back of the spoon to create a wrinkled effect. Try to avoid tearing the foil, but tears can be corrected after gluing.
3. Brush glue on the form and add objects to create a raised design. Once the glue is dry, cover with the (wrinkled and smoothed) piece of foil. The edges can be folded around and under the form, or the foil can simply be laid over the top, leaving the edges free to fold under or be secured with metallic tape later if desired.
4. Gently tool the foil down around the raised design using either end of a spoon or a small blunt end dowel, being careful not to puncture the foil. Once the design is satisfactory to the maker, the project can be considered finished. If a more antiqued look is desired, continue with steps 5 and 6.
5. If desired, brush a thin layer of black acrylic paint over the foil; allow it to dry.
6. Using steel wool (wearing gloves), gently rub the paint off until the desired look is achieved (Figure 8-4).
7. Once complete, the foil can be removed from the form, or left attached, depending on how it is to be used. Attach the embossed foil to a wooden plaque or box lid, for example, using either glue or metallic tape. Avoid getting glue on top of the foil, as it will dull the finish. If glue does get on the foil, wipe it off as soon as possible.

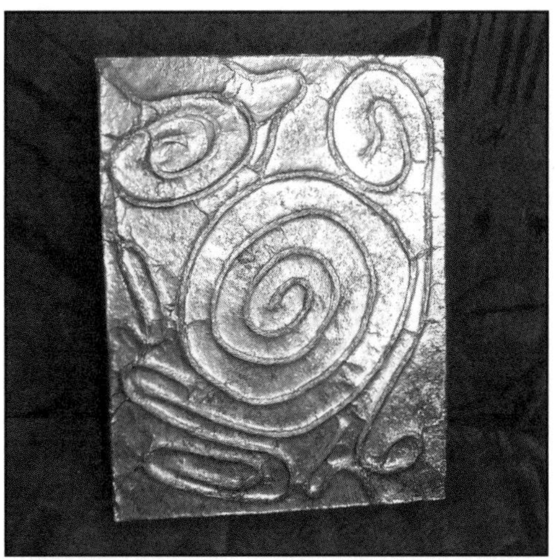

Figure 8-4. Tooled aluminum foil plaque.

Other Ideas and Grading

The differences in the properties of various metals, and the forms in which they are available, enable the therapist to incorporate metal crafts in working on a broad range of client goals. The following section describes additional creative possibilities while taking into account more pragmatic concerns such as cost and time constraints. Economical projects can incorporate aluminum foil, soda pop cans, or tin vegetable cans. For a simple children's activity, cut foil into small rectangles and have them twist them into tight cylinders, then into circles, to form a silver chain for a Christmas tree. Beverage and food cans can be cut with tin snips, and bent, punctured, or hammered into various shapes (Hill, 2008; Wasinger, 2009). For example, form a candleholder by cutting the top off a soda can, then cutting the sides into strips and curling them down—one at a time—with needle nose or round nose pliers. Once the top and bottom are removed, vegetable cans can be cut open and flattened out with a rubber mallet, then cut and/or molded as with other sheet metal blanks. Sharp edges are unavoidable, so either sturdy gloves or extra caution are recommended in handling. Wares at country flea markets also provide abundant inspiration for "yard art" or functional items made with various type metal cans.

Nail punching is in an old American craft used in making the panels on pie safes and other food storage cupboards. These panels were designed to let air in but keep mice and insects out. Today, some therapists call this technique nail art and provide clients with nail punching kits to create objects that look antique (Johnson, Lobdell, Nesbitt, & Clare, 1996). Again, simple projects such as hanging ornaments can be done with nothing more than recycled metal pieces and a common hammer and nail.

Plate metals can be cut using a jeweler's saw to create a silhouette effect, although the skill level required is beyond that of most clients. A simpler alternative is to etch designs onto metals using an acidic compound. Cover nonetched areas with a resist (a compound that seals off the metal surface), then place the piece in an etching bath to remove the shiny finish from the exposed areas. An etching project could easily be completed in one session. To achieve interesting patinas on metals, experiment with applying household chemicals, such as bleach, ammonia, or other cleaning liquid, to them (Hall, 2001). As seen in the projects section, copper can be darkened and given an antiqued look by using liver of sulfur; black tempera paint on aluminum foil will yield a similar effect. Then simply use steel wool to polish the metal to the desired finish.

Metal in its wire form lends itself to other types of crafting, especially jewelry making (see Chapter 16). Wire mesh of various gauges can be shaped and used in applications such as containers, candle holders, or as a decorative addition in mounting pictures or tooled metal. Form metal mesh into a cylinder, fasten, and cover with colorful paper and découpage medium to make attractive candle lanterns; gloves should always be worn when handling heavier wire mesh such as chicken wire. Or staple window screen to the back of an old wooden frame and attach dried flowers to the front to create a rustic wall hanging (Hall, 2001). Old screen or other lightweight metal mesh can also be cut into shapes with tin snips and painted. The paint will not completely cover the entire surface, creating an interesting mottled effect. Keep in mind that cutting mesh or sheet metal with tin snips will require hand strength and is not recommended for clients with unstable or painful joints.

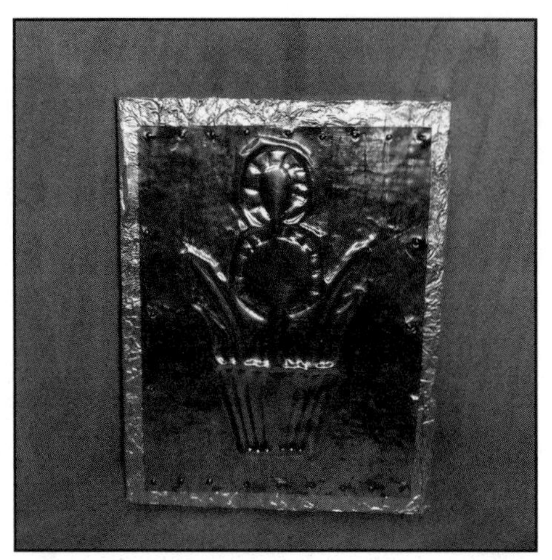

Figure 8-5. Tooled copper plaque, done from a line drawing without a template.

Some types of metal can be purchased as leaf, which comes in tissue paper thin sheets. It can be used on clear glass, picture frames, or boxes, or strategically placed in découpage-type applications. This form of metal crafting is less resistive than some other types, but the material is expensive, so the therapist should have experience with it before considering it for use in therapy. Enameling is another process that requires special skills, but it offers a wide array of possibilities in both color and design. While traditional enameling requires a kiln for firing pieces, special metal paints are now available that produce a similar appearance without heating. These may be useful for working with children, for example they could make one-of-a-kind buttons, pins, or refrigerator magnets from copper discs or other shapes. Another product, called metal clay, has the look of crafted silver jewelry after molding and firing (Kay, 2005).

Because metal work has so many variations, the innovative therapist can envision ways to grade a project to fit most any client's skill level. Copper tooling, the metal craft most well known in occupational therapy clinics, is simplified by using templates—the smaller the easier—or alternatively, made more difficult by using client-created designs (Figure 8-5). For those clients with weak upper extremities or inefficient grasp, higher gauge (thinner) foil and/or large-handled tools can be used. Hammering projects can be large or small; again, softer or thinner metals will offer less resistance. A pierced or nail punch project can be extremely simple, especially when the object is already formed and marked with the design, but it requires bilateral coordination when done in the traditional manner with hammer and nail. As with tooling, strength requirements can be decreased by using a lighter weight metal. If use of sharp objects is prohibited, blunt tools can be used in a similar way to chase or stipple the metal. Obviously, the use of a heating device in any part of the process (e.g., kilns, torches, or soldering irons) increases the task demand as well as its dangers. Considering the large range of possibilities, the therapist should actively assist the client in selecting the project based on resources, the activity demands of each step involved, and the amount of time available for completing it.

Main Therapeutic Applications

Physical Dysfunction

The tooling process is sometimes chosen to work on common motor goals such as strengthening of wrist and finger musculature or to facilitate a three-jaw chuck or other grasp. Nice results are possible even for clients with hand weakness or poor coordination and clients with the use of only one hand can also perform this craft successfully. Because a relatively strong and static pinch is needed to control the modeling tool, a client may need frequent rest periods, and this activity would be contraindicated for a client with a diagnosis such as rheumatoid arthritis, in which resistive and repetitive motions can exacerbate joint damage (Melvin & Jensen, 1998). Although a client with hemiplegia may need some assistance for taping edges, tracing designs, or other preparatory steps, he or she may be able to use the affected hand to stabilize the piece during tooling. Liver of sulfur, steel wool, and lacquer applications can also be done while the object is stabilized, either with the affected extremity or with dycem. Regardless of diagnosis, clients should wear gloves to protect their skin when using steel wool.

Copper tooling, either with a template or the client's own design, can be used with blind or partially sighted clients. They can feel the contours of the picture in the same way they feel the dots for reading Braille. Again, precautions need to be taken to cover all sharp edges with masking tape, as the blind person is unable to see this danger. Bed-bound patients can do copper tooling, but it is advisable to use the liver of sulfur and steel wool on a bedside table, in another room, or not at all. Tooling is a quiet activity that requires little space and a project can typically be completed in one or two sessions.

Hammering a metal sheet, as in planishing, involves strong grasp, elbow flexion and forceful elbow extension, ulnar and radial wrist deviation, and shoulder stability. The resistive forces in these processes need to be factored into their selection; weak or inflamed joints could be damaged by the repetitive motion or impact (Department of the Army, 1951, 1971; Deshaies, 2006; Dunton, 1945; McCann, 1978; Melvin & Jensen, 1998; Rich, 1960). In addition, hammering could pose difficulty and/or danger for a client with incoordination or proximal instability or weakness. Hammering can be beneficial, however, in improving endurance or grip strength and metal piercing is useful for working on bilateral and hand-eye coordination. Hammering as part of a piercing or nail punch project has essentially the same benefits and dangers as planishing; the safety issues in hammering a nail are obvious. As always, it is up to the therapist to analyze the activity, and structure it based on therapeutic goals.

Mental Health

Because copper tooling on templates is a success-assured activity, it is a traditional occupational therapy activity in psychiatric settings. Low self-esteem, a common problem among psychiatric clients, is often improved by doing a project with a successful outcome (Early, 2009). This craft is easily graded to match the abilities of the client and can be used to focus on attention span, sequencing, decision making, or self-control. The therapist might offer a variety of templates from which to choose, placing clients in a situation where they can make an independent choice and exert some control in an environment—usually the hospital—where they otherwise have very little. An angry client with destructive tendencies may find this controlled, repetitive craft to be a good way to sublimate harmful hostile urges and avoid frustration that may occur with more detail-oriented activities (Early, 2009). For depressed clients, who often have a low energy level, copper tooling can be accomplished with slow, rhythmic movements that they are able to do despite their fatigue. The sharp edges of the copper, however, may be a temptation for self-injurious or suicidal clients. Clients with memory or cognitive problems should also be successful with this simple craft (Ayers, 1949; Early, 2009).

For clients who are sometimes challenged in identifying the boundaries of reality, such as those with schizophrenia, the structure and well-defined limits offered by template tooling is helpful. The activity requires little concentration or cognitive processing, skills that are sometimes lacking in clients with psychotic disorders. The here-and-now quality of this activity enables the client to see immediate results and exercise reality testing to counter disordered thinking. Clients with dementia benefit from copper tooling for many of the same reasons as those with schizophrenia; a good outcome can be achieved in spite of low cognitive functioning and the lack of attention to environment cues sometimes seen in this population (Brown & Stoffel, 2011).

The inherent restrictions in using a template can provide control for a client experiencing mania or hypomania that has difficulty with boundaries, limits, and/or self-regulation. The resistance of the copper can provide an acceptable outlet for excess energy. Since the activity is relatively short-term, it is useful for those who are easily distracted or lose interest quickly. Hammering metal was traditionally used in mental health to externalize hostility and anger in a constructive process. In some cases, however, these negative emotions have escalated rather than decreased, so the therapist should be alert to this potential (Department of the Army, 1971; Fidler & Fidler, 1954; Wilkinson & Heater, 1979).

Pediatrics

As with other clients, copper tooling on templates ensures a successful outcome for children. Template use is less desirable, though, if the goal is creativity or self-expression and older children may prefer to design their own patterns. The gross motor aspect—and noise—of hammering often appeals to children, and the process is simple. If the copper sheets are thin enough, children can do tooling/chasing and piercing with alternative tools such as toothpicks, household implements, or pushpins. In some cases, the child may only be able to handle large-handled implements and/or may lack the coordination necessary to do a bilateral task such as the punching with a hammer and nail. The same precautions that apply to adult physically and mentally disabled clients should also be observed with children and adolescents.

Adolescents

Adolescents with a physical or mental disability are likely to have many of the same difficulties as adults with similar diagnoses, including decreased self-esteem and an external locus of control, but are also struggling developmentally with gaining independence. Teens may have a negative response to authority, or may come from backgrounds with little structure. Sequential metal crafts offer this needed structure and more complex projects provide opportunities for collaboration with the therapist or peers. Adolescents may be capable of formulating their own designs, which will foster decision-making skills and self-confidence (Early, 2009). Some, especially girls, may prefer making metal jewelry or decorative boxes more than pictures or home décor items, and creating and wearing handmade jewelry may boost the self-esteem of those dealing with body image distortions. Introduction to metal crafts may even spark an interest that develops into a lifelong hobby. In a general sense, metal crafting is gender neutral; the therapist can increase the appeal to both boys and girls by thoughtful project selection.

Older Adults

The no-fail nature of copper tooling using a template makes this craft appropriate for elderly clients, including the diverse nursing home population (Gould & Gould, 1971; Plautz & Camp, 2009). It is age appropriate and should appeal to both men and women, yet has few cognitive requirements and can be done by individuals with decreased coordination or use of only one upper extremity. With geriatric clients, it is advisable to start the activity with precut foil sheets, not only to reduce the number of steps, but to minimize their chances of getting cut. This population is especially vulnerable to injury due to their tender skin, decreased sensation, and a reduced rate of healing. Liver of sulfur may cause eye irritation for some clients and those with increased sensitivity to glare may have difficulty seeing the design on the shiny metal surface (Hooper & Bello-Haas, 2009). Older clients may also enjoy working on tin punch items that are reminiscent of earlier Americana.

Groups

Once set up, copper tooling could easily be done with several clients at once working in a parallel group. Doing original designs may prove too time consuming, but most clients can complete tooling on templates with little or no assistance. Other simple metal projects such as nail punch may be similarly feasible with multiple clients. This type craft is usually not conducive to having several clients work together on a single item. If working with a group, the therapist must have a heightened awareness of the previously noted precautions.

Case Study

Glen, a 78-year-old male client, was admitted to the geriatric psychiatric unit of a local hospital. His internist was concerned about his apparent depression and recommended hospitalization, to which he and his family agreed. He appeared clearly depressed, but the treating psychiatrist wanted to rule out dementia, as the two illnesses often look similar in the elderly. Because the occupational therapist used activities for determining whether functional deficits were truly cognitive or more emotional in origin, he had become a key member of the evaluation team. He and the certified occupational therapy assistant (COTA) utilized primarily the Learning/Cognitive Disabilities theories in evaluating and treating their clients.

On the afternoon of admission, the occupational therapist performed a screening interview with Glen and his daughter-in-law, yielding the following information. He was born and raised nearby and married his childhood sweetheart right after high school. They bought a small farm and had five children within 6 years. During their marriage, Glen always helped take care of the house and the children in addition to his farm work. Involvement in the church was also an important part of life in their rural community. He and his wife continued to farm the land after the children had all left home but were disappointed that none of them had chosen to take it over. Nonetheless, it never occurred to them to sell the farm and retire.

Just over a year ago, Glen's wife died after a long struggle with congestive heart failure. During her illness, he not only cared for her, but also continued to manage the farm with little assistance from their children. Following her death, his vitality gradually declined. He paid less attention to the operation of the farm, avoided community and church events, and became uncharacteristically dependent on his son and daughter-in-law. Most recently, he had begun to neglect his personal hygiene and stayed in bed or the recliner much of the day. Since one son and his wife were the only family members still living nearby, the siblings agreed that their father should move in with them. Despite the move and increased attention from family, his condition worsened and by the time he was admitted, he did little more than eat, sleep, and stare at the television.

The next morning, the occupational therapist completed Glen's evaluation, including assessment of his sensory and motor function and his self-care skills. He also evaluated his cognitive status using the large Allen Cognitive Level Screening test. During these assessments, Glen had repeatedly said, "I can't remember anything" and responded, "I don't know" to most questions. It appeared that he could not or would not make an effort to participate in conversation. Test results showed that motor function was within normal limits for a man his age, although motor retardation was evident. He was able to dress and groom himself independently but only with much prompting and encouragement. On the Allen Cognitive Level Screening, he scored level 5.0, spontaneously correcting an error he made, although he needed extra time and cueing to keep working. Glen seemed to have some hearing loss, but otherwise his sensory skills were essentially intact.

That afternoon, the occupational therapist and Glen agreed on the following long-term goals: to increase his self-esteem/improve mood through the use of satisfying activities, to increase his overall activity/occupation level and endurance, and to improve initiation and completion of self-care activities.

The occupational therapist asked the COTA to have Glen try a copper tooling activity. He reasoned that this craft would not require a great deal of energy or concentration and that Glen might find the repetitive rubbing motion soothing. In addition, the product he created might demonstrate to him that he was still capable and competent.

Initially, Glen tried to get the therapist to choose the template design for him, so the COTA narrowed the choices to three: praying hands, a horse head, and a deer. Glen eventually chose the praying hands, and the COTA helped him tape the precut copper foil on the back of the template. Glen began tooling and worked without stopping until the session was over. The next day the therapist took the first few minutes of the session to have him apply the liver of sulfur solution to the tooling. During the third session, he polished the piece and then nailed it onto the lid of a small wooden box. He seemed more pleased with his effort than was indicated by his statement, "I guess it turned out alright." He put the box on the bedside table in his hospital room and said he would keep his watch in it. Glen asked the COTA if he could do another tooling for his granddaughter.

The psychiatrist, along with the treatment team, ultimately determined that Glen was experiencing a major depressive episode but also had some beginning cognitive decline as well. The treatment team, client, and family all agreed that it would be best if Glen stayed with his son and daughter-in-law indefinitely. By the time he was discharged, however, Glen had fully resumed his self-care, was participating in all therapy activities, and was making plans to attend the senior center near his son's home. On a follow-up visit at the hospital, he stopped by the therapy department to tell the COTA that he had been attending craft classes at the senior center and was working at home on a "yard art" project for his daughter-in-law's flower garden.

Discussion Questions

1. Should the therapist have allowed Glen to do a second copper tooling project during remaining therapy sessions, or encouraged him to do other activities instead? Explain your answer.
2. Considering Glen's previous occupational history, was a craft an appropriate activity choice? If so, might another type of craft have been more appropriate? Explain.
3. Do you think the therapists should have had Glen work in a group instead of having individual treatment sessions? Why or why not?

Resources

Metalcraft
By Mary Maguire
Barrons Educational Series, 2005

Metalcraft for the Home: 20 Step-by-Step Projects
By Lisa Brown
David and Charles, 2001
Projects of varying difficulty. A nice section in the back on tools and techniques.

The Metal Craft Book
By Janice Eaton Kilby
Sterling Publishing/Lark Books, 2002
Variety of projects and information for the beginner

The Encyclopedia of Jewelry Making Techniques
By Jinks McGrath
Running Press, 2010 Reprint Edition
A comprehensive visual guide to traditional and contemporary techniques.

Excellent photos of 31 processes for making exquisite to playful jewelry. Shows shaping, forging, fusing, soldering, casting, and surface decorations for mostly metal jewelry and the tools required. Good index.

References

Ayers, A. J. (1949). An analysis of crafts in the treatment of electroshock patients. *American Journal of Occupational Therapy, 3*(4), 195-198.

Brown, C., & Stoffel, V. C. (Eds.). (2011). *Occupational therapy in mental health: A vision for participation.* Philadelphia, PA: F. A. Davis Co.

Department of the Army. (1951). *Occupational therapy.* Washington DC: US Government Printing Office.

Department of the Army. (1971). *Craft techniques in occupational therapy.* Washington DC: US Government Printing Office.

Deshaies, L. (2006). Arthritis. In L. W. Pendretti, H. M. Pendleton, & W. Schultz-Krohn (Eds.), *Pedretti's occupational therapy: Practice skills for physical dysfunction.* St. Louis, MO: Mosby.

Dunton, W. R. (1945). *Prescribing occupational therapy* (2nd ed.). Springfield, IL: Charles C. Thomas.

Early, M. B. (2009). *Mental health concepts and techniques for the occupational therapy assistant.* Baltimore, MD: Lippincott Williams & Wilkins.

Fidler, G. S., & Fidler, J. W. (1954). *Introduction to psychiatric occupational therapy.* New York, NY: The MacMillan Co.

Gould, E., & Gould, L. (1971). *Crafts for the elderly.* Springfield, IL: Charles C. Thomas Publisher.

Griswold, L. (1931). *Handicrafts.* Colorado Springs, CO: Outwest Printing and Stationary Company.

Griswold, L., & Griswold, K. (1969). *The new handicraft processes and projects.* New York, NY: VanNostrand Reinhold Company.

Hall, M. A., Wrobel, J., & Salamony, S. (2001). *Decorative crafts sourcebook.* San Diego, CA: Thunder Bay Press.

Hill, S. (2008). *The illustrated guide to crafting with tin, wire, and foil.* London, UK: Anness Publishing, Ltd.

Hooper, C. R., & Bello-Haas, V. D. (2009). Sensory function. In B. R. Bonder, & V. D. Bello-Haas (Eds.), *Functional performance in older adults* (3rd ed.). Philadelphia, PA: F. A. Davis Co.

Johnson, C., Lobdell, K., Nesbitt, J., & Clare, M. (1996). *Therapeutic crafts: A practical approach.* Thorofare, NJ: SLACK Incorporated.

Kay, A. (Ed.). (2005). *Create your own jewelry.* London, UK: Anness Publishing, Ltd.
McCann, M. (1978). *Health hazards manual for artists.* New York, NY: Foundation for the Community of Artists.
Melvin, J., & Jensen, G. (1998). *Rheumatologic rehabilitation series: Assessment and management.* Bethesda, MD: American Occupational Therapy Association.
Plautz, R. E., & Camp, C. J. (2009). Long-term care. In B. R. Bonder, & V. D. Bello-Haas (Eds.), *Functional performance in older adults* (3rd ed.). Philadelphia, PA: F. A. Davis Co.
Reader's Digest. (1979). *Crafts and hobbies.* Pleasantville, NY: The Reader's Digest Association Inc.
Rich, M. K. (1960). *Handicrafts for the homebound handicapped.* Springfield, IL: Charles C. Thomas.
Wasinger, S. (2009). *Eco-craft: Recycle, recraft, restyle.* New York, NY: Sterling Publishing Co./Lark Books.
Weisberg, N., & Wilder, R. (1985). *Creative arts with older adults: A sourcebook.* New York, NY: Human Sciences Press.
Wilkinson, V. C., & Heater, S. L. (1979). *Therapeutic media and techniques of application: A guide for activities therapists.* New York, NY: Van Nostrand Reinhold Company.

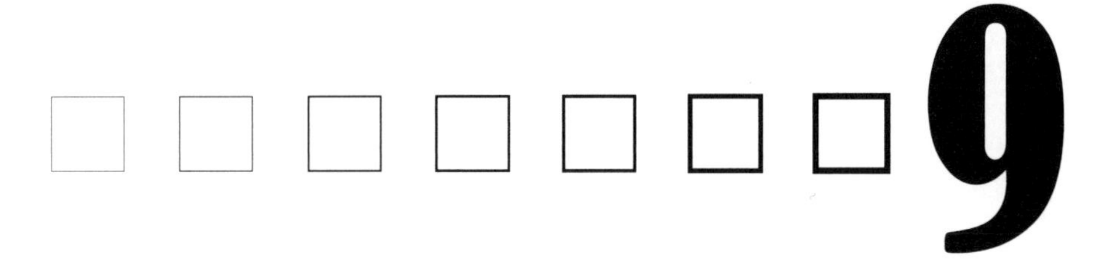

Ceramics

Objectives

The student should be able to:

- Discuss historical/cultural examples of clay/ceramic work
- Know basic supplies and materials needed to do ceramics and know how to complete a pinch pot, a coil pot, and a slip cast pot
- Understand advantages and limitations of clay activities in therapy
- List precautions of ceramic activities
- List ways to grade ceramic/clay activities
- Articulate the application of ceramics activities with various client populations

The ancient craft of pottery involves simply shaping clay—an especially plastic earth—allowing it to dry, and then baking it at a high temperature for a long period of time. Creating earthenware may be one of the oldest crafts, along with leather- and woodworking. We know humans have been shaping and baking clay for at least 10,000 years. In fact, the durability of pottery fragments has made it possible for archeologists to learn much about prehistoric humans. On the other hand, because pottery is breakable, intact ancient pieces are rare. Although technology has improved the durability of many materials, the characteristic properties of clay products, and the process of creating them, have changed little over the years (Budworth, 1970; Marmer, 1997).

The term *ceramics* encompasses pottery; ceramic sculpture; ceramic tiles used in kitchens and bathrooms; ceramic building blocks, roof tiles, and decorative facades for buildings; ceramic beads for jewelry; and even the ceramic tiles used to protect the bodies of space shuttles. Clearly, the full range of ceramics is beyond the scope of this book. The following pages, however, thoroughly explain the basic processes to make smaller pots and sculptures (Figure 9-1) most commonly used in occupational therapy interventions. In a rehab setting, the most frequently used ceramics forms are slip-molded or hand-built greenware and ceramic sculpture. Although few clinic schedules allow clients and therapists the time to do wheel-thrown pots, essentials of the procedure are also included in this text. Newer materials appear on the market with regularity, allowing for creative uses of clay-like materials without the inconvenience and expense of firing a kiln (Dierks, 1994). The basic shaping and sculpting are the same but the baking process will vary with the product; examples of these products are listed in the Other Ideas section.

Tubbs, C., & Drake, M. *Crafts and Creative Media in Therapy, Fourth Edition (pp. 101-118).*

The Value of Ceramics in Therapy

Looking back into the history of all cultures, from the most primitive to the most advanced, each used the earth to their advantage and fashioned useful articles from clay. Clay is a central part of our collective unconscious. Experiencing a bundle of clay in our hands connects us, throughout the ages, to one of the most central parts of being human. It relates to any gender, any age group, and any generation.

Pauline du Plessis, OTR/L

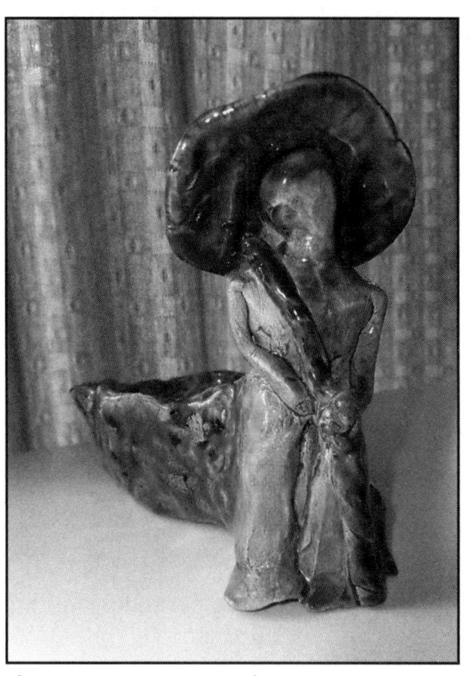

Figure 9-1. A ceramic sculpture.

Special Considerations

Ceramics or clay work has many advantages as a therapeutic medium. It offers plenty of room for creativity, self-expression, and variation of end product. It can be graded to accommodate diverse functional levels and involves a process familiar to most. It is a safe activity and can even be done without tools if necessary. Ceramics work can be structured such that it consists of only a few steps, or of many. There is a vast selection of clay types, building processes, and glazes.

Drawbacks of ceramics include cost, time, and space required, but all of these factors can be mitigated to some extent. Traditional clay work requires time for preparation, drying, firing, and cooling. Alternative clay products, such as those that air-dry or can be baked in an oven, speed up the process considerably, but are more expensive and may result in a less impressive end product. Space requirements for ceramics vary, but generally speaking, this craft requires more space than most due to the fact that pieces must be properly stored between each phase of the process, and equipment requirements. Cost, like the other factors, is highly variable but traditional clay is relatively cheap, usually less than $30 for a 50-pound block. For clinics that do their own firing, there is the considerable start-up expense of a kiln and the room containing the kiln must meet certain safety specifications regarding ventilation and fire codes. In addition, sinks used in this area will also need special clay traps installed.

Although a ceramics project can be structured such that it poses few risks, certain precautions should be considered. Working with clay is drying to the skin, so application of moisturizer after the session is recommended. Clients with delicate skin or peripheral neuropathies may or may be able to work with clay since even the smoothest clay has some abrasive quality. Polymer products may be preferable in this instance. Some greenware cleaning procedures can create dust, so clients with respiratory problems may need to

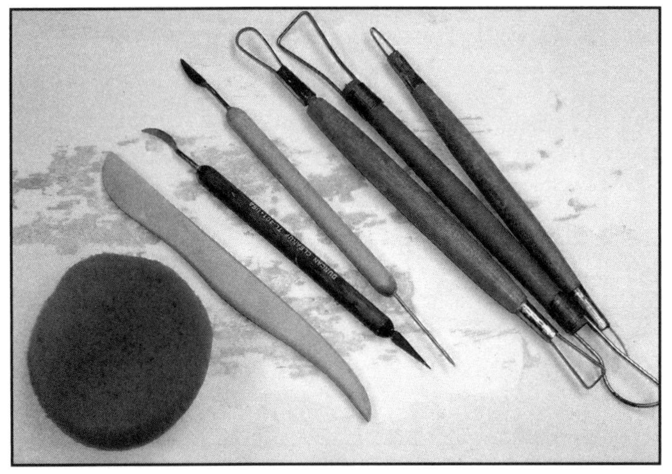

Figure 9-2. Ceramic tools: sponge, fettling knife, cleaning tool with needle tool, and wire loop tools.

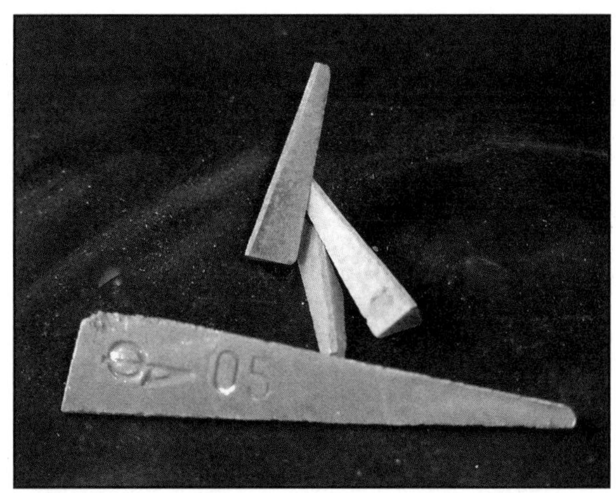

Figure 9-3. Pyrometric cones used to regulate temperature in kiln firing.

wear a mask or have someone else complete this step for them. Clients who may not differentiate edible from non-edible materials should be closely observed during ceramics work. This craft may be contraindicated for those with arthritic conditions due to the potential for joint damage during the application of force in shaping; the small joints of the hand are especially vulnerable. Working with this medium is also contraindicated for anyone with an open wound that might come in contact with the clay (Department of the Army, 1971; Hamill & Oliver, 1989; Turoff, 1949; Wilkinson & Heater, 1979). Similarly, an incompletely healed wound may not tolerate the stresses placed on it during the kneading or molding process (Kasch & Walsh, 2006).

Supplies

As long as safety guidelines for kiln wiring and venting are observed, it is possible to do ceramics in an area adjoining the occupational therapy clinic. The therapist should consult the facility safety officer or a local ceramics store for specific requirements. Clay sediment traps in the sink drains allows residue to be easily removed and thus avoid costly plumbing problems. Beyond this, the following supplies and equipment are sufficient for regular use of traditional ceramics in the clinic, including those techniques discussed in this book. Of course, more sophisticated materials and techniques are available.

- Ready-mixed clay (for hand-building or throwing)
- Ready-mixed slip (for using molds)
- Ready-mixed glazes and underglazes
- Bisque stains and sprays
- Fine-grain sponges (Figure 9-2)
- Pyrometric cones (Figure 9-3)
- Kiln wash

Tools/Equipment

- Covered plastic storage containers
- Storage shelves for finished pieces
- Kiln
- Kiln furniture: Stilts and shelves (Figure 9-4)
- Canvas-covered boards
- A wedging board (Figure 9-5)
- Clay pull (cutting wire) (Figure 9-6)
- Fettling knife (see Figure 9-2)

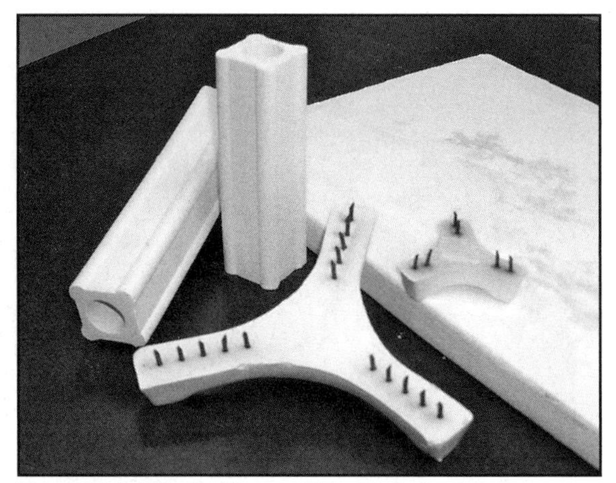

Figure 9-4. Kiln furniture: stilts and shelves.

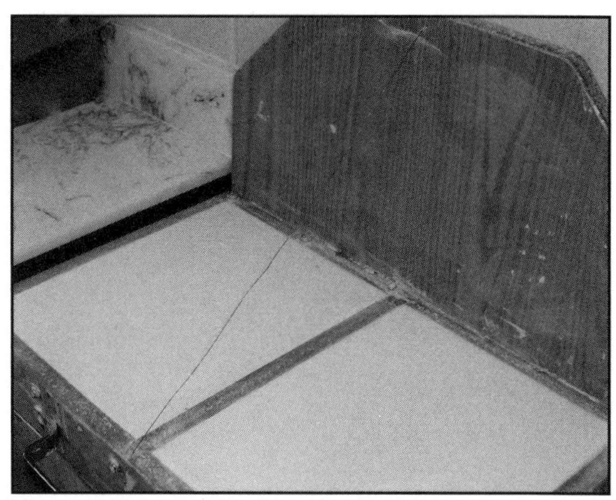

Figure 9-5. A wedging board.

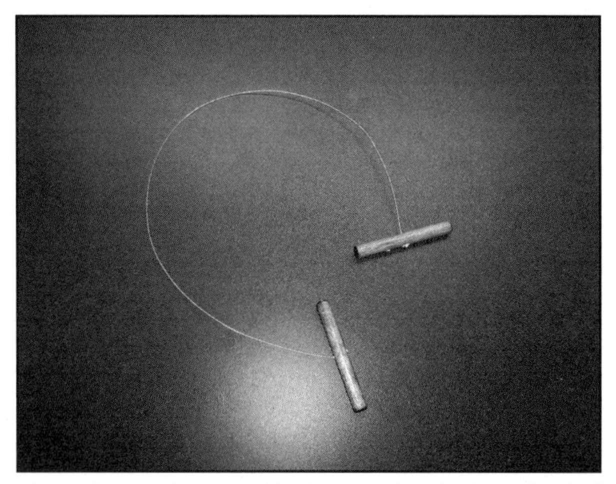

Figure 9-6. A clay pull—Used to cut cleanly through a ball of clay.

- Sgraffito/cleaning tool (see Figure 9-2)
- Needle tool (see Figure 9-2)
- Wire-loop tool (see Figure 9-2)
- Rolling pin
- Plaster or masonite bats
- Slip molds
- Slip strainer
- Mold straps (Figure 9-7)
- Sink
- Plastic water bowls
- Glaze brushes

Process

Most therapists buy ready-mixed clay; preparation of clay from powdered material is difficult and requires costly machinery. Clay is usually purchased in 25- to 50-pound plastic bags and the cost for 50 pounds is around $30. Clay comes in a variety of grays, browns, and reds and some have grog—previously fired with ground clay added. The grog adds strength to the clay but it can be abrasive to the hands, so this variety

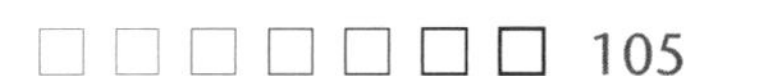

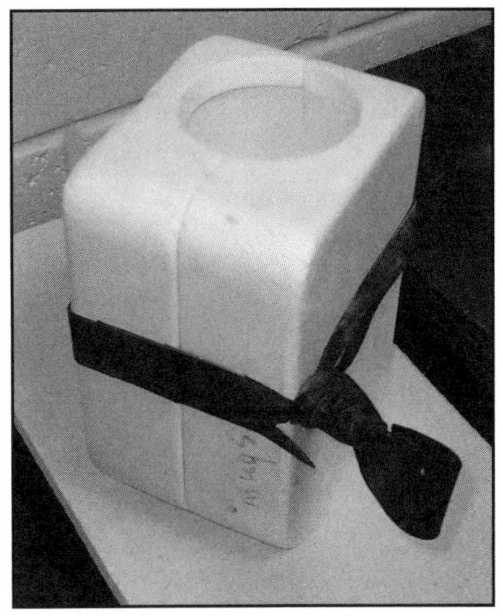

Figure 9-7. Mold straps on a slip-cast mold.

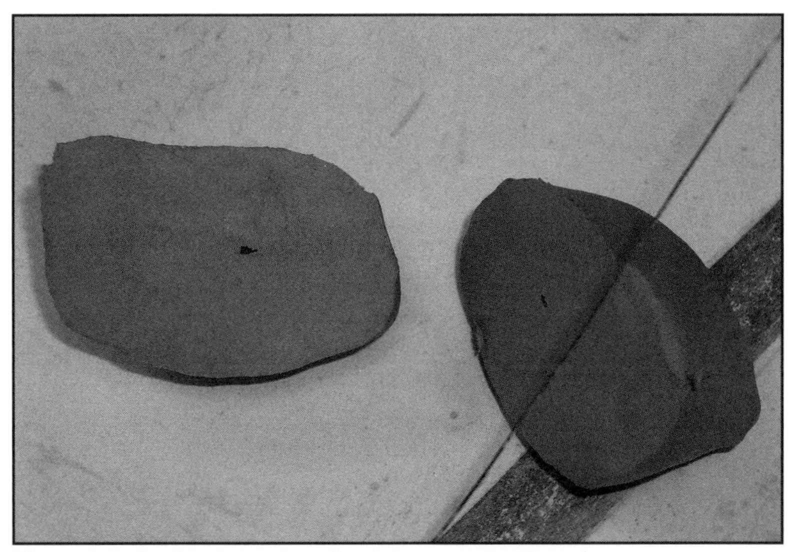

Figure 9-8. Cutting through wedged clay; note the air pocket.

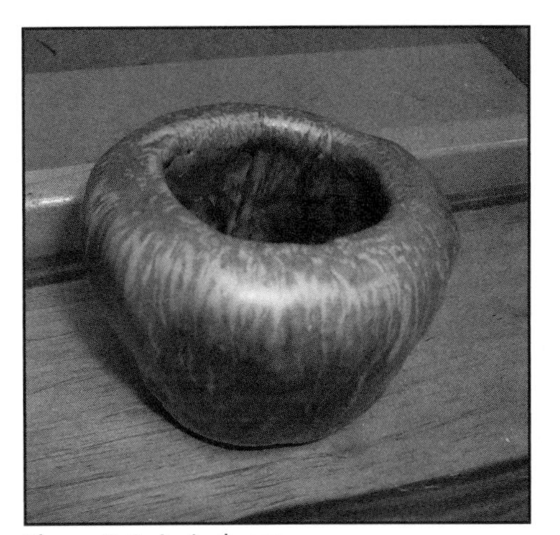

Figure 9-9. A pinch pot.

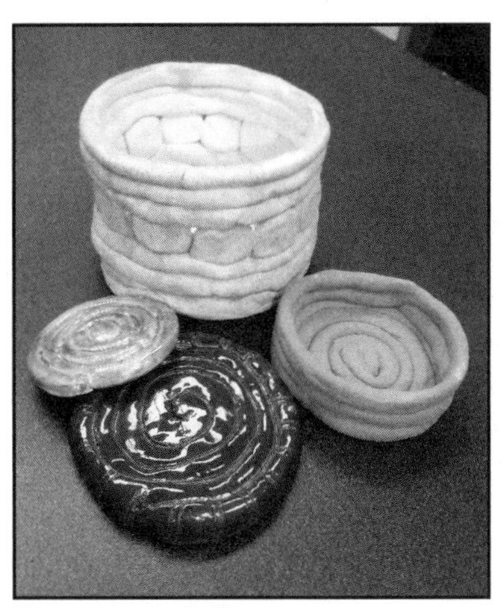

Figure 9-10. Coil pots.

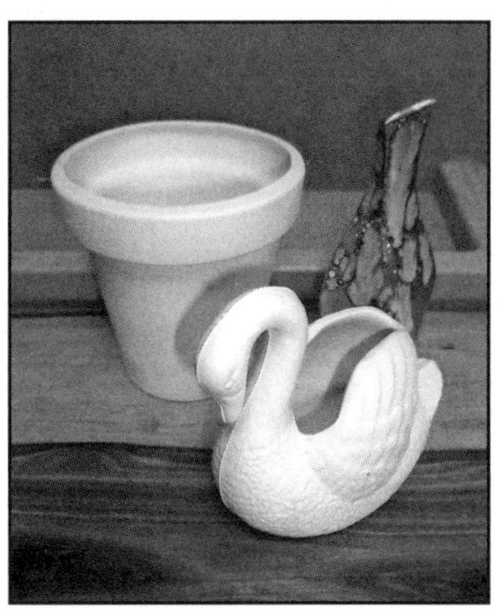

Figure 9-11. Slip-cast pieces, bisqueware, and glazed.

is contraindicated for some clients. Different clays can be fired at different temperatures; however, most occupational therapists simplify their ceramics operation by firing at only one or two temperatures, usually between 1800°F and 2000°F or between 980°C and 1100°C.

The first step in preparing the ready-mixed clay is to cut and form it into usable 3- to 4-inch diameter pieces. This is most easily accomplished by using the clay pull, which is a tool one can easily make by cutting a 20-inch length of thin wire or nylon fishing line and tying each end to a large button or bead. The clay pull (see Figure 9-6) is grasped at each end and wound around the fingers until taut. The line is then laid across the block and pressed straight down through the clay until the proper size piece can be pulled off. This piece is then wedged, a process necessary to equally distribute moisture in the clay. This makes the clay softer and easier to handle and gets rid of air pockets that could expand during firing, causing the piece to explode in the kiln. Professional potters wedge clay by kneading, but the most common method used in therapy is repeatedly throwing the clay onto a wedging board (see Figure 9-5). Before beginning to form an object, the clay should be checked for air pockets by cutting through the center of the lump with a wire or clay pull (Figure 9-8). If it will not be used immediately, it should be wedged again before using.

There are six basic methods of forming ceramics in occupational therapy. They are described and illustrated next sequentially from the easiest technique (pinch pots) to the most difficult and exacting (the potter's wheel). This chapter describes the most commonly used processes (Figures 9-9 through 9-11) in ceramics rather than a single project from beginning to end. The preparation, time required, cost, grading possibilities, and emphasis documentation will be highly variable depending on the method selected.

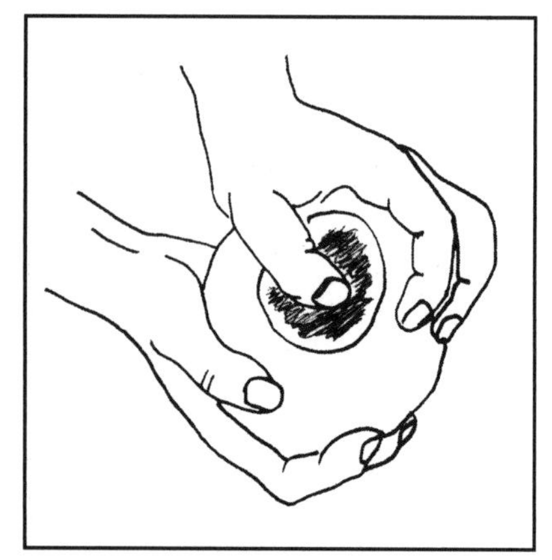

Figure 9-12. Forming a pinch pot.

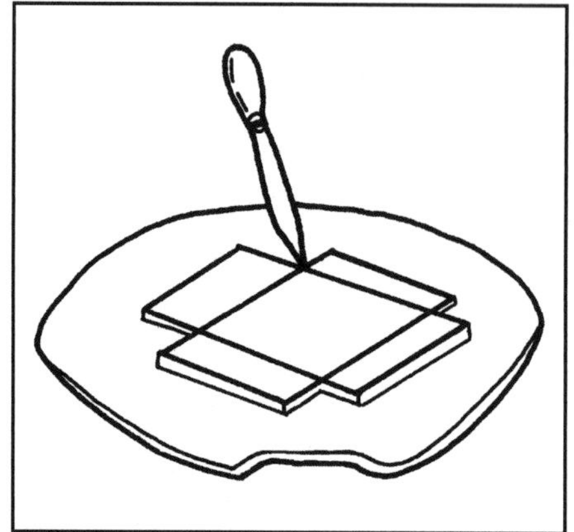

Figure 9-13. Cutting around a paper pattern with a fettling knife.

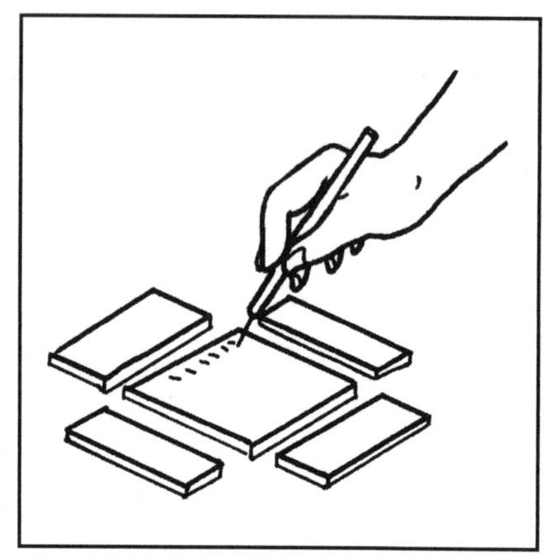

Figure 9-14. Crosshatching with a clay needle.

Pinch Pot

Process

1. Form the clay into a ball.
2. Stick the thumb into the top of the ball. This makes the first opening.
3. With the thumb of the dominant hand on the inside and fingers on the outside, begin to press gently out with the thumb, moving the form either clockwise or counter clockwise while keeping the piece supported with the nondominant hand (Figure 9-12). Continue to move the emerging vessel in this fashion until the walls and bottom are uniformly ½-inch thick or less. If small cracks appear on the edge near the opening, just pinch them together.
4. Set the pot on a canvas-covered board and, using both hands, smooth the walls. Do not use water to smooth the walls at this point, as it will weaken them.
5. Set the pot aside to dry on a mesh shelf or grate so air can reach all surfaces.
6. After it is leather hard (the hardness of good shoe leather), smooth the pot with a damp, fine-grain sponge. At this stage, carve or incise the surface for decoration if desired.
7. The length of the drying process depends on the temperature, humidity, and ventilation. The therapist will need a few trials to find how long it takes a piece to become bone dry—when the piece is no longer cool to the touch—but in a climate-controlled environment, this should become fairly predictable. Once bone-dry, the piece is ready to bisque fire—a process to be described later.

Slab Building

Process

1. On a canvas-covered board, roll the wedged clay with a rolling pin to an even thickness of ¼ to ½ inch.
2. Lay a previously made paper pattern on the clay. Cut around the pattern with a fettling knife (Figure 9-13), a special tool for cutting clay.
3. Allow the pieces to sit for a short time to stiffen slightly, then join the pieces in the manner described below.
4. Lift the base off the canvas and place it on a plaster bat.
5. In a crosshatch manner, incise or score all the edges that are to be joined using needle tool (Figure 9-14). Both edges of each seam should be prepared in this way.
6. Moisten both edges with a finger before pressing them together. This moisture goes into the incisions, forming slip, or liquid clay, which acts as a sealer. Be careful not to allow the clay to become too wet, however, since this may weaken the structure.

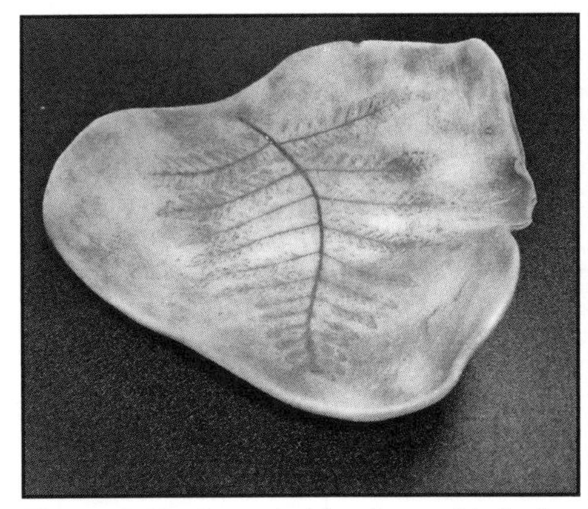

Figure 9-15. Curved slab piece with leaf imprint.

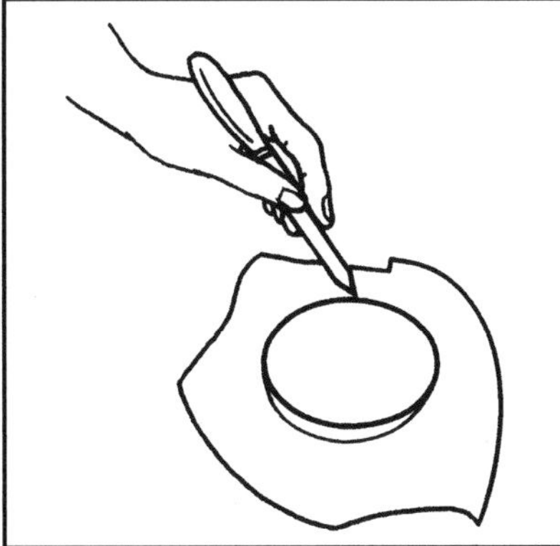

Figure 9-16. Cutting a round base for a coil pot.

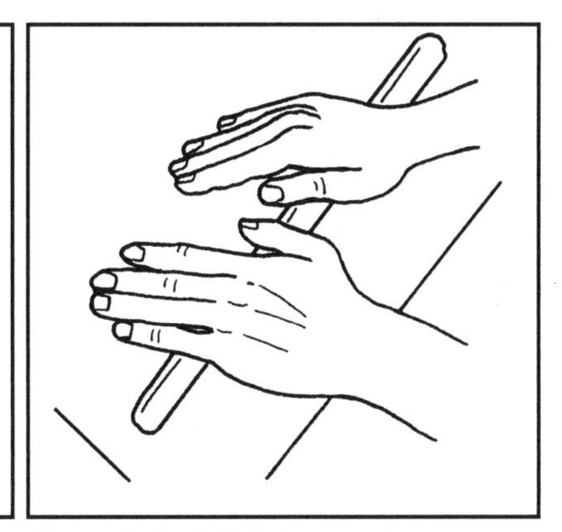

Figure 9-17. Coils being made.

7. Strengthen the joints by pressing a thin rope of clay along the seams on the interior surface and smoothing it into the walls.
8. Set the piece aside until it is leather-hard; it can then be decorated by sgraffito; textured with a comb; or imprinted with buttons, shells, or other small objects (Figure 9-15).

Of all forming techniques, slab building may offer the most opportunity for variety. Napkin rings or other small cylindrical objects can be constructed with one joint. A simple slab scored on the bottom to prevent warping and decorated with surface designs makes an attractive trivet. A free-form vase or other vessel can be made by draping a trimmed clay slab over another object to dry. Buttons, beads, or ornaments for suspending can all be cut from a plain slab and decorated as desired.

Coil Building

Coil building is a modification of the slab-building technique.

Process

1. Make a round or oval base slab (Figure 9-16).
2. Make coils with another piece of clay by rolling it back and forth with both hands on the canvas-covered board (Figure 9-17).
3. Score or incise around the entire edge of the slab, where the coil will be placed.
4. Wet the scored edge and lay the coil on it, pressing lightly to bond the two pieces.
5. Lightly moisten the top of the coil; lay another coil on this seam and lightly press.
6. Continue this process until the desired height is reached. If the pot is to curve outward, set each coil a little to the outside of the one below it. If it is to curve inward, place each coil a little toward the inside of the preceding coil. Make sure each coil is securely sealed to the one below all the way around.
7. When the desired shape and size are reached, smooth the sides. On the other hand, if you like the look of the coils, you need do nothing to the surface. It is possible to use coils in making the base, but it will not be as strong as a slab base. In each slip-bonded joint lies the potential for weakness and cracking.

Another easy coil method can be used, especially for wide, low bowls that have the potential to collapse from their own weight while damp. Select a ready-made bowl and line it as smoothly as possible with plastic wrap. Lay the slab for the base in the bottom of the bowl, and arrange the coils up the sides of the bowl. With this method, the coils can even be made into a design. After all coils are laid, smooth the inside of the bowl to fasten them together for strength and to allow easy cleaning later. The coiled bowl should be left inside the ready-made bowl until it is leather hard, then it can be lifted out. Any unwanted marks from the plastic wrap can be smoothed at this time.

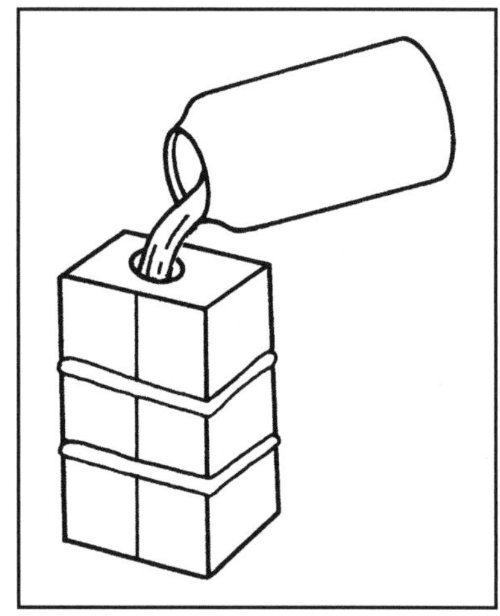

Figure 9-18. Pouring slip into a mold.

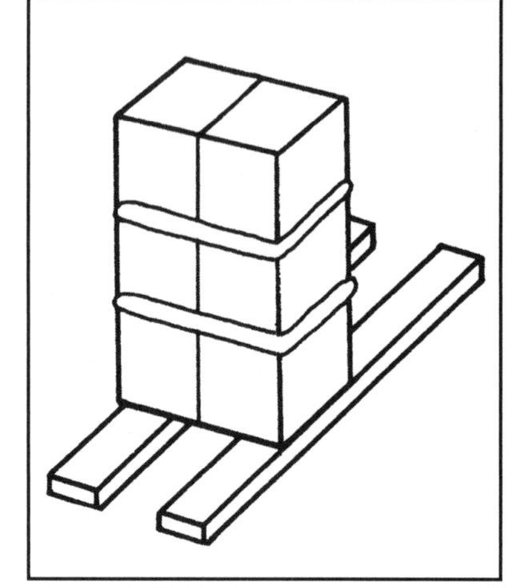

Figure 9-19. Draining the mold.

Sculpture

In occupational therapy, sculpture is an activity in which the therapist usually offers very little instruction or direction to the client. Sculpture often combines the techniques used to make pinch pots (see Figure 9-1), slab containers, and coil vessels. One such technique involves hollowing out the center of chunk of clay by using a wire loop tool. Systematically cutting away pieces of clay from the middle or inside of a bulky sculpture prevents an explosion, since pieces with thick walls are prone to explode in the kiln. Another technique is to use a paper core or substructure and form the clay sculpture around it. The paper-based core, which supports the sculpture's walls and keeps it from collapsing, will burn away in the kiln, leaving a hollow vessel. There are other more complex building techniques but many are too involved for most clinical situations. Attaching multiple parts to a sculpture can be problematic; they often break off in handling or firing. To minimize this, use the above scoring and moistening techniques for joining any added parts.

Slip Casting

Slip casting is the process of pouring liquid clay into a plaster mold, allowing the clay to accumulate as a layer on the plaster wall, and pouring out the remaining liquid clay. Slip casting is often used in therapy because chances of a successful product are good, pleasing the client and improving self-confidence. Molds are usually purchased rather than made; they are moderately priced and available at local ceramic or hobby stores. The therapist may choose to have the patient complete the entire process below, or simply clean and glaze the greenware after it has become leather-hard or fully dried (see below).

Process

1. First check the molds for cleanliness and gently wipe them out with a damp sponge or fine bristle paintbrush, if necessary, to remove old clay.
2. Fit the mold sections together and fasten them tightly with mold straps or giant rubber bands (see Figure 9-7).
3. Mix and strain the slip to remove any lumps.
4. Pour the slip into the mold pour spout (Figure 9-18), filling it to the top.
5. As the plaster absorbs moisture, the slip will sink down in the pour spout. It is necessary to check the mold every few minutes and continue to refill it to the top.
6. When the thickness of the solid clay near the plaster becomes approximately ¼ inch, pour out the remainder of the slip by turning the mold over to drain (Figure 9-19). This slip can be saved and reused if stored properly in an airtight container.
7. After approximately 30 minutes, turn the mold upright and carefully remove half of the mold.

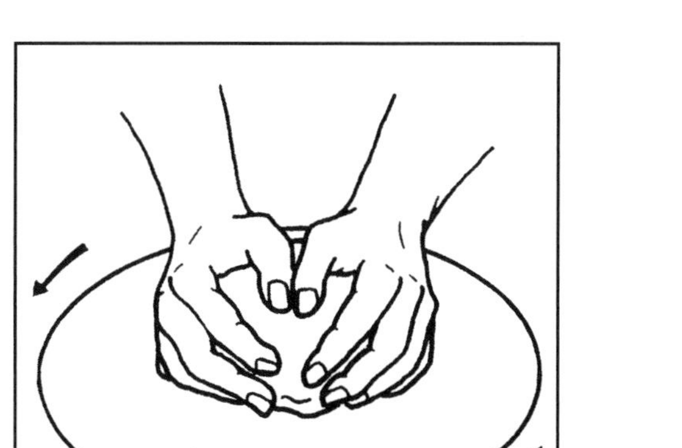

Figure 9-20. Centering the clay.

8. Cut off the excess clay in the pour spout. The piece can remain in the half mold until it becomes leather hard. It will then come out of the mold easily because it will shrink away from the plaster in drying.
9. If the slip casting has textured walls, allow it to dry before cleaning the seams with a sgraffito/cleaning tool. If the slip cast has no texture or detail, the seam can be removed at the leather-hard stage with a fine-grain sponge. There are a variety of other molds, including press molds and drape molds that can be used with regular clay instead of slip. These molds usually consist of one piece into which clay is pressed or draped and removed when leather hard.

Throwing on a Pottery Wheel

Throwing on the potter's wheel is one of the most sophisticated ceramic techniques. It requires skills and practice to create an attractive product; consequently, few therapy settings even have a wheel available. Only the most basic steps will be given here. Students wishing for more information will find a variety of sources, both written and video, on the Internet; and in many communities, local colleges or enrichment programs may offer classes. While pottery wheels themselves have become simpler to use, the basic throwing technique is timeless.

Process

1. Experiment with the foot pedal or switch to determine how much pressure or power is required to achieve the desired speed.
2. Affix a bat on the center of the wheel. Very slightly dampen the bat and keep a bowl of water and a sponge nearby.
3. Place a ball of wedged clay the size of an orange onto the center of the bat.
4. Start the wheel slowly and check to be sure the ball is in the center of the wheel. If it is not, stop the wheel and reposition the clay. Repeat this until the ball is as close as possible to the center. Then with the wheel stopped, press it down to secure it to the bat.
5. The clay must be kept "slippery" wet to slip through the hands, so the potter needs to constantly reapply water to the surface. The wheel should always be moving before the hands touch the clay and be kept moving after the hands have been gently removed from the clay. Begin to spin the wheel and press the palms of both hands down and around the base of the clay to center it (Figure 9-20). Keep the forearms braced on the thighs to help stabilize the hands and wrists. The force to the clay should be transmitted through pressure from the large bones of the arm and wrist and not directly from the hands. This will minimize muscle fatigue and help keep the pressure even.
6. Coning is the next step; first press the clay to raise it into a cone shape, then steadily press down on the top of the cone with the right hand while supporting the clay from the side with the left hand

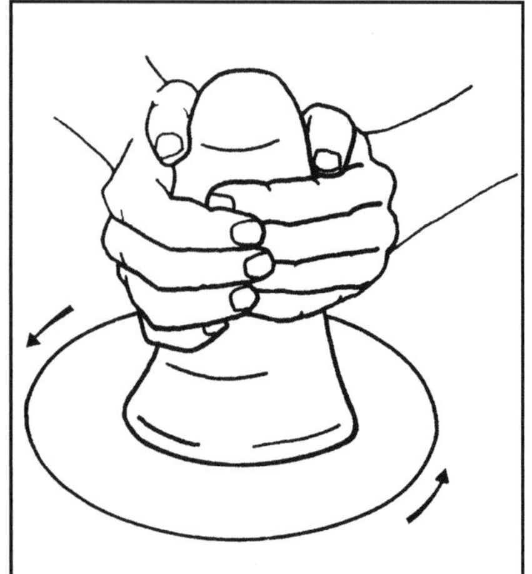

Figure 9-21. Coning the clay.

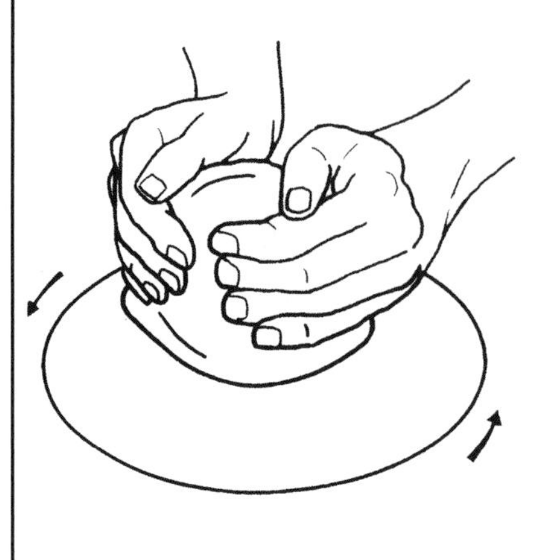

Figure 9-22. Pressing down on the clay in preparation for reconing.

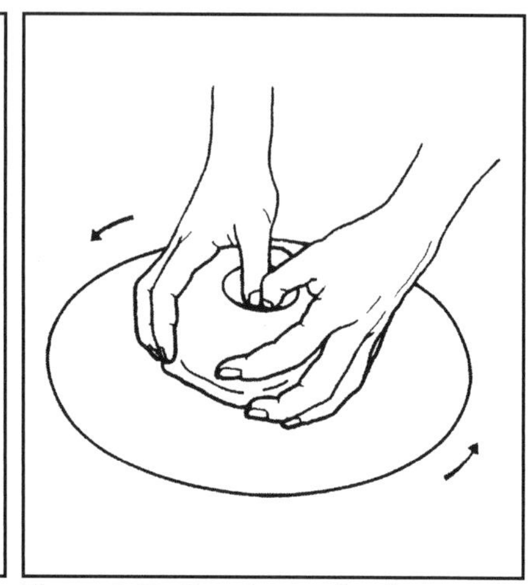

Figure 9-23. Opening up the clay.

(Figures 9-21 and 9-22). This is all done with the palms of the hands, not the fingers. This not only protects smaller, more vulnerable joints and their supporting structures but keeps the clay shape more uniform. Beginners can omit coning altogether and move immediately to step 7; advanced potters usually repeat the coning process several times.

7. The next step is to "open" the clay by pressing the right thumb into the middle of the centered clay as the wheel continues to move (Figure 9-23). Press the thumb to a depth that leaves about 1 inch of clay between the thumb and bat. Then place both thumbs in the hole and begin to slowly and gently widen it until the floor of the pot is the desired width.
8. Next, raise the walls by interlocking the thumbs and placing the fingers of one hand inside the hole and the fingers of the other on the outside. As the wheel spins, apply gentle pressure while pulling up at the same time; keeping the elbows in at the sides or on the thighs improves control. Continue until the desired height is reached. Beginners should attempt only smaller objects, about 6 inches tall and 4 inches in diameter. Simple cylinders or bowls are adequate to satisfy most beginners; forming the clay into more complex shapes takes skill and practice.
9. When the pot is fully formed, use a damp sponge to smooth and slightly dry the inside of the pot; excess water could weaken the walls.
10. Level the top of the vessel by placing the needle tool through the wall ¼ to ½ inch below the top while the wheel is slowly turning; trim away this clay until the top edge is even. Smooth the new rim with wet fingers or a sponge while the wheel is turning.
11. Release the vessel by sliding the pulling tool along the surface between the pot and the masonite bat one time. This is not necessary with plaster bats.
12. Set the pot aside on the bat until it is leather hard.
13. Lift the pot off the bat. Turn it upside down, center it on the wheel, and stabilize it at the bottom with three pieces of fresh clay. This process, called turning, involves trimming off the excess clay at the base.
14. While the wheel turns, hold the needle tool against the vessel to make concentric circles (Figure 9-24). This shows the potter where the clay is too thick so it may be trimmed, making the walls of the pot equally thick throughout.
15. Pare away the excess clay using cutting tools. Take the pot off the bat.
16. If desired, texture or score the walls for decoration and allow the pot to dry before firing. The beginner should not be discouraged if he or she fails more than once to obtain a satisfactory result; throwing on a wheel is a very difficult skill to master.

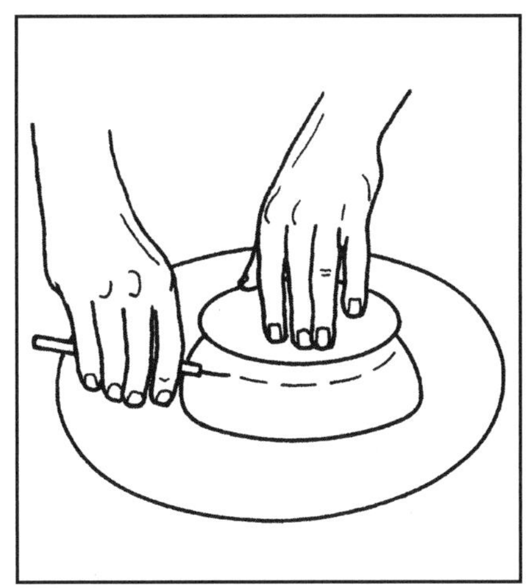

Figure 9-24. Trimming the pot with the needle tool.

Firing the Kiln

Pots should air dry at least 1 week before firing; the clay should not feel cool to the cheek. Kiln furniture, consisting of posts and shelves (see Figure 9-4), is used to allow for stacking several levels of items. The kiln should be loaded evenly, with pots at least 1 inch from the heating elements. In a bisque firing, pots can touch, but in glaze firing, pots should be on stilts and at least 1/2 inch apart to allow air to circulate. The kiln bottom and shelves should be brushed with several coats of kiln wash prior to loading to prevent glazed pieces from sticking; it is safest to avoid putting glaze on the bottom of pieces when possible.

The first firing is called the bisque firing, which causes the clay to harden enough so that it will not disintegrate if it becomes wet. For clients, all clay should be bisque fired to make the piece more durable before glaze is applied. Glaze firing is the second firing and done at a higher temperature. Bisque firing usually takes 4 to 10 hours, glaze firing takes longer (*Reader's Digest*, 1979). Each kiln comes with its own firing manual that provides a timing guide and specific loading directions. At either stage, it is important to increase the kiln temperature slowly to prevent the water in the clay from evaporating too quickly, causing the pieces to explode. Pyrometric cones (see Figure 9-3) are used to indicate kiln temperature; they bend at specific temperatures and are more accurate indicators than a thermometer. Although different clays and/or surface coatings require different temperatures, most therapists fire between the pyrometric cone range of 07 to 03.

Gas kilns have the potential to emit carbon monoxide, which can cause brain injury or death, so precautions for ventilation are particularly important with this kiln type (Anonymous, 1986).

Glazing

The dried but unfired pot is called greenware; after the first firing, it is called bisqueware. Glazes can be applied after a first or a second firing, or both. The type of glazing process used will depend on how the final product is to be used. Ceramic glazes used in clinics or other therapy settings are almost always ready-mixed, since some of the dry ingredients can be toxic. Commercial glazes have specific directions for application and firing temperature on the label. Glazes should dry at least 6 hours before firing.

Underglazes

Underglaze is one type of surface decoration. It can be brushed, sponged, spattered, or sprayed onto bisqueware; the label will provide specific instructions for application and firing. If the piece is also to receive an overglaze, it must be fired again. Overglazes are transparent or semitransparent and provide a water-impermeable surface. This necessitates a third firing but makes the article safe to use in applications such as vases or food containers. Underglaze offers opportunities for experimentation, such as brushing it into incisions on the surface to highlight them, or brushing it over a textured surface and then rubbing some of it away the glaze to emphasize the texture. Ceramic hobbyists often apply underglaze to greenware, but greenware is usually too fragile for most clients to handle with the delicacy required. In the therapeutic setting, it is best to bisque fire everything before underglazing or glazing.

Glaze firing is the last firing. Glazed pieces should be set on stilts and placed with at least ½ inch between each piece and the walls. This allows air to circulate, avoiding a spotty finish. It is sometimes difficult, but necessary, to wait the length of time required for proper kiln cooling. A rule of thumb is to let the kiln cool twice as long as it took to fire it to full temperature; this will prevent the glaze crackling from cooling too fast. Many newer glazes produce interesting and dramatic effects with little or no extra effort; see Appendix I for glaze retailers.

Bisque Stains

For purely decorative pieces such as figurines and some kinds of jewelry, bisque stains can be painted on the surface of bisqueware. These stains, which are unfired, are not moisture resistant and cannot be used in any container that may hold liquids. They have some qualities, however, that make them useful in the clinic. For example, they do not require as much time/as many steps as traditional glazes. They are best applied over gray clay, which becomes white after firing, as the color will be clearer than over red or brown clay (Marmer, 1997). Stains are applied in much the same way as liquid tempera paints, and like tempera colors, they need to have a protective finish over them. A basic spray lacquer sealer can be used but must be applied in an area with adequate ventilation, preferably outdoors. The therapist must decide whether or not to let the client perform this step of the process. The therapist should also take care to keep the sprayed pieces clearly separated from those to be fired; it is not always possible to tell them apart just by looking.

Other Ideas and Grading

Once the basic processes of building, throwing, or slip casting are mastered, the creator can try out numerous additional techniques to further decorate the pieces. As alluded to in above sections, ornamentation can be added to the leather-hard clay surface by scratching or incising with a pointed tool. Impressing and stamping (see Figure 9-15) are alternative ways of imprinting the surface with shapes or other recessed designs. A plain ceramic exterior can also be embellished with relief or appliqué techniques, accomplished by adhering small portions of coiled, rolled, or molded clay directly onto the surface (see joining method above in slab building techniques) or perforated by completely cutting out sections of the clay wall. Tools to form clay embellishments might include a rolling pin, cookie cutters, and a garlic or clay press. Children's craft dough accessories may also offer ideas for shapes and molding. Lastly, clay can be colored by the addition of oxides or dyes. The amount of pigment used will affect the final color after drying or firing (Ros, 2002).

As an alternative to kiln-fired clay work, there is a large selection of non-clay modeling products, from polymers to paper-based compounds. Some are air-dry, others are oven-baked. Brand-name products include Crayola Air-Dry Clay (Crayola, Easton, Pennsylvania), Craft Porcelain and Sculptamold (AMACO, Indianapolis, Indiana), Claystone and Boneware (Sculpture House, Inc., Skillman, NJ), Fimo (Staedtler Fimo, Neurnberg, Germany), Sculpey (Polyfoam Products Company, Elk Grove Villiage, IL). AMACO Magic Mud can be baked or air-dried, and air-dried items can be reconstituted and the material used again. These products are most frequently used to make relatively small objects and cost may be a limitation. When working with children, homemade—and inexpensive—salt dough is a useful option. After baking, salt dough articles can be painted with basic acrylic paints and sealed with a spray or brush-on lacquer.

Pinch and coil pots, slab building, and sculpture are simpler than slip casting and throwing on a wheel. Decorating options add complexity, as do multi-step glazing techniques. Non-clay modeling is the simplest option, but it definitely limits what can be created and increases costs. See the previous Projects sections as well as the information on client populations below for more suggestions regarding the grading process.

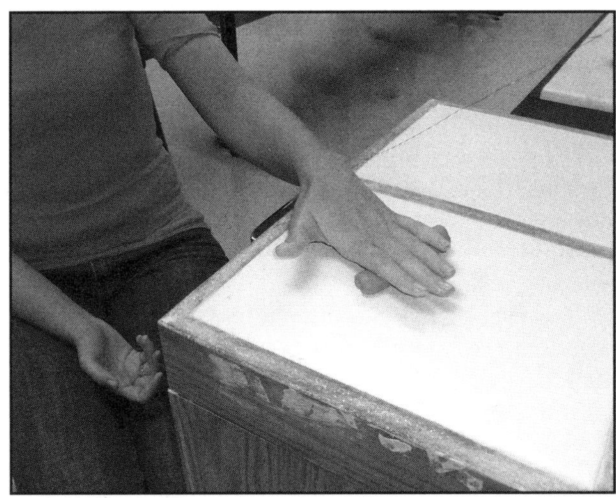

Figure 9-25. Rolling clay facilitates finger extension or graded weight bearing.

Main Therapeutic Applications

Physical Dysfunction

In years past, the clay manipulation in "ceramics class" was used to achieve many of the motor benefits for which therapy putty is now commonly used. Squeezing, pushing, pinching, patting, rolling, smoothing, and manipulating clay can strengthen or refine almost any desired wrist or hand movement. Working with clay strengthens the upper extremities and can be easily graded, from delicate manipulations such as carving, to larger, more resistive actions such as those needed for wedging. Correctly structured, clay work can involve the entire body (Fidler & Velde, 1999). Wedging, rolling, or pressing activates muscles in both the trunk and upper extremity and provides a way to stretch tight soft tissues (Figure 9-25). The therapist can adjust the table and chair to facilitate upper extremity movement patterns, biomechanically correct postures, or can even have the patient stand to work on balance or weight bearing. Positioning will dictate muscle demand; the therapist must call on activity analysis skills for the best placement of the work and selection of tools to be used. More distal muscles can be strengthened by making pinch pots; or coils can be made with minimal grasp ability. Rolling out a slab facilitates bilateral upper extremity movements; bilateral coordination is needed to put the slab pieces together. In the first case, the less cortical, more automatic nature of the activity may facilitate the incorporation of a hand that is weak or dominated by pattern movement (Zoltan, 2007). For clients with ataxia or tremors, the draped slab method may achieve the best results.

The therapist can grade for fine motor skill demand by having the patient use surface decoration tools, adding small hand-molded clay embellishments or complete either monochrome or detailed glazing. Prewedged clay or clay alternatives can be used bedside with clients; they are nontoxic, easily washable, and the building or sculpting process is quiet. It may be possible to use this medium for patients on isolation; it is less expensive than therapy putty and can be left in the client's room. A masonite square covered with paper can be used as a work surface and the whole project—the ceramic piece atop the working surface—can be put into a plastic bag to be carried to the kiln. Any contagions on the clay will be killed in firing; the paper should be bagged like any other infectious material and the masonite can be sterilized by washing with antibacterial soap. Clay is particularly suitable for low vision or blind clients because of its tactile qualities. The person can actually feel the shape being created and be more certain of the appearance of the end product.

Mental Health

For consumers in mental health settings, the opportunity for expression of mood and thought is perhaps the most beneficial aspect of working with clay. As evidenced by the number of traditional psychiatric occupational therapy evaluations that use clay (see Table 2-1), this medium provides an opportunity for the client to project feelings and their perspective of reality (Bruce & Borg, 2002). Clay sculpting is viewed as the least structured of all projective assessments because of the effort required in controlling it (Hemphill, 1982). A structured task may illuminate cognitive deficits such as the inability to follow instructions; a non-structured task may show depressed mood or bizarre thoughts. For clients with cognitive deficits such as difficulty with abstraction, having a variety of samples assists in conceptualizing the process. Structured slab and coil construction can help with sensory integration for adult psychiatric clients, since both wedging and rolling provide range of motion and proprioceptive input to the upper extremities (King, 1974). The nature of the material is also useful in that it allows clients to make mistakes but then be able to reverse them (Hemphill, 1982).

Some individuals believe that wedging or pounding clay helps release aggressive hostility; however, for some clients, it may cause emotional escalation and the therapist should be observant of the effects of this activity. The therapist must also be vigilant when clients are using clay tools because they can easily become weapons (Early, 2009).

Pediatrics

Clay is a natural medium for children. They play in their food—squeezing and manipulating it—or make mud pies in the same way they handle clay. Clay allows this same unstructured exploration of materials. Therapists can provide clay activities to facilitate intrinsic hand strength, which is a prerequisite for in-hand manipulation skills (Henderson & Pehoski, 2006), but children who have had little experience in working with art materials or tools will usually not work as long or as independently with clay. They may produce an unrecognizable form and want to move on to more familiar activities. The reverse can also be true; the novelty of the material may encourage play and experimentation (Kuhaneck, Spitzer, & Miller, 2010). Children at a more mature stage may name the form even though it may still be unrecognizable. As they advance developmentally, they will begin to make the head separate from the body, and add facial features, progressing in the same stages as they do in drawing. Pre-adolescent children try to make realistic-looking items but younger children may be less intentional about making a permanent object. They are usually more willing to put their clay back into the container after they have satisfied their curiosity. While sometimes even young children may want the piece fired, they may not care about glazing it (Gaitskell & Hurwitz, 1975). Clay is a common ingredient in implementing play therapy as it fits well with the exploratory and self-initiated nature of this treatment approach. It is also suitable for the destructive and messy tendencies of children (Axline, 1947). Children who have never been allowed to be messy or who have been punished for getting dirty or soiling themselves may have difficulty initially but eventually most children overcome this anxiety and enjoy the freedom of working with clay.

The main precaution in using clay or similar substances with the pediatric population is ingestion of the materials. Even though clay is usually not toxic, glazes are very dangerous and it is best to avoid using them with small children unless constant supervision is provided. The therapist can allow children to paint their bisque-fired clay objects with tempera paints rather than glazes. Children tend to make small objects with many appendages, such as legs for animals, which almost always break off either before or during firing. In some cases the pieces can be glued together after firing but the object will lack durability. Making small hand-built objects is a good choice for pediatric bedside therapy, since clay is easily washed off the hands.

Adolescents

Adolescents may see ceramics as a functional craft and may be drawn by the professional appearance of the end product. Teens will benefit from the manipulative nature of this medium as they search for self-identity and outlets for expressing it. As a rule, they are mature enough to participate in all steps of the process and in some situations may even be allowed to assist in setting up and firing the kiln. Older children and adolescents are more likely to want their objects fired and glazed. The structured nature of the glazing and firing processes are instructive in prevocational lessons such as following procedures/rules and having to wait for results.

Older Adults

Many of the same indicators for use of ceramics in rehabilitation for physical dysfunction apply to the geriatric population as well. Project selection will vary according to cognitive and physical ability. For example, although slip molding leaves little room for creativity, it may the preferred means of enticing a regressed client to participate. Simple hand-built projects, on the other hand, are a better option for working on hand strength, attention to task, or self-expression. Clients can be reminded that the process of making something is just as important as a beautiful end product (Weisberg & Wilder, 1985).

Orthopedic limitations and/or pain are common in the elderly, so the therapist must grade the activity based on range of motion and hand function requirements, and the client's tolerance of resistance. Sensory loss, such as low vision, decreased hearing, and reduced tactile perception, is also likely in this population (Bonder, 2009), but these deficits should not prevent participation in ceramics work. In fact, this craft choice may be more suitable than many others. For the visually impaired, for example, clay may provide a creative experience they could not have with something more exacting like needlework. Although diminished sensation increases the risk of an unnoticed injury, working with clay can be beneficial in sensory re-education or desensitization. To facilitate memory and other cognitive function, the completed ceramic objects can be incorporated into a reminiscence group and used as a springboard for discussion.

Groups

Clay is a good medium to use when working with groups of clients. Hand building and coiling are unstructured enough that a therapist can supervise several clients at once. While it is unlikely that a group of clients would create a single group project, the expressive quality of this medium is excellent for fostering self-revelation and discussion during the shaping of individual pieces. Clients can glaze their pieces in a group setting as well. In fact, some sheltered workshop programs are based largely on ceramics production.

Case Study

A 26-year-old married female, Jean, was admitted to a 20-bed inpatient psychiatric unit in a small private community hospital with a diagnosis of Major Depressive Disorder, first episode (American Psychiatric Association, 2000). Jean and her husband had recently moved to the city from a smaller town where her parents lived. She had left her elementary teaching job to follow her engineer husband, whose company had transferred him to a nearby plant. Her symptoms upon admission were loss of appetite and weight loss, insomnia or early morning awakening and fatigue, decreased attention span, delusional thinking related to contamination of canned and frozen foods, agoraphobia, and suicidal thoughts without concrete plan for accomplishment. The facility's occupational therapist used an eclectic approach, relying on the theory that best fit the client, but had often realized good results with the psychoanalytic approach. She used the observation-based Comprehensive Occupational Therapy Evaluation for assessment; she considered it efficient for obtaining a great deal of information in a relatively short amount of time. On this occasion, she included the client in a paper craft group for observation. Jean showed mild to moderate dysfunction in all areas except appearance and reality orientation, which were normal.

The therapist also had Jean complete a magazine collage; she noted that Jean chose very few pictures and many of them were dark in color or theme. In collaboration with Jean, the therapist subsequently set goals to increase client activity level, attention span and concentration, and self-esteem—along with learning practical strategies for coping with stress—through craft and educational group involvement. Although Jean lacked insight for in-depth future planning, she was amenable to the goals suggested.

The next day, Jean and one other client attended the craft group. The therapist presented several options; since Jean was unable to make a decision, she was simply given a grapefruit-sized ball of clay. At first she seemed unsure of how to start, but she did mention having used clay with her elementary students. After several self-deprecatory statements, she began to smooth and manipulate the clay. Jean spoke little during the 90-minute session, but by its conclusion she had formed a representation of a seal on a rock. The therapist helped her cover it with plastic so it would not dry out and told her she could continue to work on it the next day. At the next session, she used a wire loop tool to hollow out the rock and give it more definition. Two days later it was dry enough to fire along with the projects of several other clients.

The kiln was fired on Friday and allowed to cool over the weekend. Jean seemed to be waiting her therapist on Monday, anxious to open the kiln. The nursing staff reported that Jean had been much more animated over the weekend and attributed her improvement to both medication and therapy. As they opened the kiln, the therapist warned Jean that her sculpture could have exploded because the seal body was so thick, but fortunately, the piece fired well. Jean smiled when she saw her white bisque-fired seal. She immediately began to select glazes; she chose a glossy black for the seal and a matte green for the rock. That same day, the physician, along with the treatment team, decided that Jean was well enough to be discharged home. The therapist told her that she could come back by the hospital on Thursday to pick up her refired sculpture. When Jean appeared on Thursday, she was dressed for an interview for a teaching job.

At this time, she felt more comfortable sharing personal information with the occupational therapist. She told her that when she made the sculpture, she had felt like a seal stuck out on a rock, alone and away from her family and friends. She now felt like she could climb down off the rock and swim again. The therapist knew the pending job interview indicated that she was ready to re-engage in life. Jean thanked her and said she might visit again, but never did. Later, the therapist heard that she had indeed taken the teaching job in a suburban school and was doing well.

Discussion Questions

1. Would you have done anything differently with Jean? If so, what and why?
2. Do you associate ceramic work more with males or females? Why? How might you convince a client that it was not only for men (or women)?
3. How does/could ceramic work improve a client's self-esteem?
4. What are some questions you might ask clients to draw them out in a discussion of their ceramic sculpture or pot?
5. Of the models of practice discussed in this text, which one do you think would be most appropriate for this setting?

Resources

AMACO—A selection of book and video resources, including clay work with children and how to throw on a potter's wheel videos
At www.amaco.com/shop/
Resource materials tab

Safety Manual: Ceramics
By AMACO
American Art Clay Co., Inc., 1988
Covers all aspects of hazards in ceramics from clay, to glazes, to firing, to kiln wash (AMACO brand specific)

Polymer Clay Kids' Crafts: 30 Terrific Projects to Roll, Mold and Squish
By Irene Semanchuk Dean
Lark Books, 2003

Ceramics for Kids
By Mary Ellis
Lark Kids Crafts, 2002

Ceramics for Beginners: Surfaces, Glazes and Firing (A Lark Ceramics Book)
By Angelica Pozo
Lark Books, 2010

Instructional videos on glazing from Dick Blick Art Materials
http://www.dickblick.com/brands/amaco/

The Art of Metal Clay, Revised and Expanded Edition (with DVD)
By Sherri Haab
Watson-Guptill Publications, 2010
Techniques and projects for jewelry and small decorative objects with fired metal clay

Decorating Techniques (Ceramics Class)
By Joaquim Chavarria
Watson-Guptill, 1st Edition, 2000

Handbuilt Pottery Techniques Revealed: The Secrets of Handbuilding Shown in Unique Cutaway Photography
By Jacqui Atkin
Barron's Educational Series; First Edition edition, 2005
Handbuilding techniques explained, including coil, slab, and pinch pots

The Potter's Primer
By Morgen Hall
Krause Publications, 1997
Excellent photos of wedging, making slip, making molds, pouring molds, combining clay of different colors, glazing, making tiles, and the processes of coil, slab, sgraffito, sculpture, and firing

Step-By-Step Crafts: Painting Ceramics
By Caroline Green
Creative Publishing International, First Edition, 2000
Includes patterns for a range of skill levels and projects with helpful photos

References

American Psychiatric Association. (2000). *DSM-IV-TR*. Arlington, VA: Author.
Anonymous. (1986). Hazards in arts and crafts. *Emergency Medicine, 18*(18), 60-81.
Axline, V. (1947). *Play therapy*. New York, NY: Ballantine Books.
Bruce, M. A. G., & Borg, B. (2002). *Psychosocial frames of reference: Core for occupation-based practice*. Thorofare, NJ: SLACK Incorporated.
Budworth, D. W. (1970). *An introduction to ceramic science*. New York, NY: Pergamon Press.
Department of the Army. (1971). *Craft techniques in occupational therapy*. Washington, DC: US Government Printing Office.
Dierks, L. (1994). *Creative clay jewelry: Designs to make from polymer clay*. Asheville, NC: Lark Books.
Early, M. B. (2009). *Mental health concepts and techniques for the occupational therapy assistant* (4th ed.). Baltimore, MD: Lippincott Williams & Wilkins.
Fidler, G., & Velde, B. (1999). *Activities: Reality and symbol*. Thorofare, NJ: SLACK Incorporated.
Gaitskell, C. D., & Hurwitz, A. (1975). *Children and their art* (3rd ed.). New York, NY: Harcourt, Brace, Jovanovitch.
Hamill, C. M., & Oliver, R. C. (1989). *Therapeutic activity for the handicapped elderly*. Gaithersburg, MD: Aspen Publishers.
Hamilton, D. (1974). *The Thames and Hudson manual of pottery and ceramics*. London, UK: Thames and Hudson, Ltd.
Hemphill, B. J. (1982). *The evaluative process in psychiatric occupational therapy*. Thorofare, NJ: SLACK Incorporated.
Henderson, A., & Pehoski, C. (2006). *Hand function in the child: Foundations for remediation* (2nd ed.). St. Louis, MO: Mosby/Elsevier.
Hooper, C. R., & Bello-Haas, V. D. (2009). Sensory function. In B. R. Bonder, & V. D. Bello-Haas (Eds.), *Functional performance in older adults* (3rd ed.). Philadelphia, PA: F. A. Davis Co.
Kasch, M. C., & Walsh, J. M. (2006). Hand and upper extremity injuries. In L. W. Pendretti, H. M. Pendleton, & W. Schultz-Krohn (Eds.), *Pedretti's occupational therapy: Practice skills for physical dysfunction*. St. Louis, MO: Mosby.
King, L. J. (1974). A sensory integrative approach to schizophrenia. *American Journal of Occupational Therapy, 28*(9), 529-536.
Kuhaneck, H. M., Spitzer, S. L., & Miller, E. *Activity analysis, creativity, and playfulness in pediatric occupational therapy: Making play just right*. Sudbury, MA: Jones and Bartlett Publishers.
Marmer, L. (1997). Ceramics for business and pleasure: Why John Q. Public is embracing an art of antiquity. *Advance for Occupational Therapists, 13*(28), 14-15.
Reader's Digest. (1979). *Crafts and hobbies*. Pleasantville, NY: The Reader's Digest Association Inc.
Ros, D. (2002). *Ceramics: Decorative techniques*. Hauppauge, NY: Barron's.
Turoff, M. P. (1949). *How to make pottery and other ceramic ware*. New York, NY: Crown Publishers.
Weisberg, N., & Wilder, R. (1985). *Creative arts with older adults: A sourcebook*. New York, NY: Human Sciences Center.
Wettlaufer, G., & Wettlaufer, N. (1976). *Getting into pots: A basic pottery manual*. Englewood Cliffs, NJ: Prentice Hall.

Wilkinson, V. C., & Heater, S. L. (1979). *Therapeutic media and techniques of application: A guide for activities therapists*. New York, NY: Van Nostrand Reinhold Company.

Zoltan, B. (2007). *Vision, perception, and cognition: A manual for the evaluation and treatment of the adult with acquired brain injury* (4th ed.). Thorofare, NJ: SLACK Incorporated.

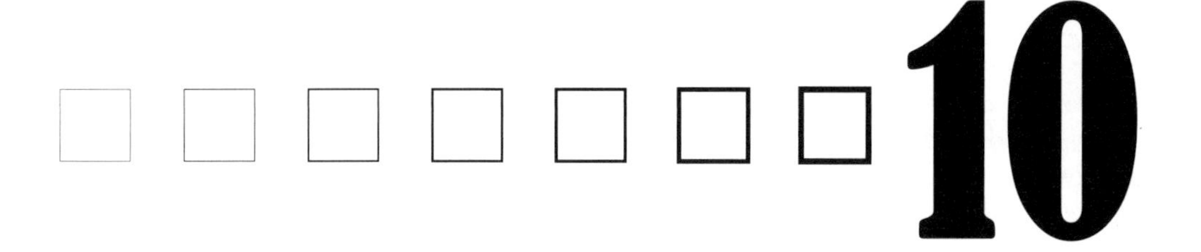

Leatherwork

Objectives

The student should be able to:

- Discuss historical/cultural examples of leatherwork
- List basic supplies and materials needed to do leatherwork and know how to complete and grade a simple project
- Explain advantages and limitations of leatherwork activities in therapy
- List precautions of leatherwork activities
- Describe how leatherwork activities can be used with various client populations

It would be difficult to find a person who has not used or worn leather or an imitation leather product. Common uses are countless and include shoes, belts, clothing, wallets, purses, upholstery, saddles, and animal leashes and harnesses, to name just a few. Leather is our most ancient fabric (*Reader's Digest*, 1979). Archeological work confirms that prehistoric humans used leather (Stohlman, Patten, & Wilson, 1969), and use of leather has been documented in Chinese, ancient Hebrew, Roman, American Indian, Eskimo, and early European cultures (*Reader's Digest*, 1979; Stohlman, Patten, & Wilson, 1969). During the Egyptian dynastic period, leather articles were considered gifts fit for royalty and the gods. Ancient Arabians tanned leather; they traded with the Moors, through whom leatherworking skills were passed to the Spanish and ultimately to the New World. Prior to European influence, Native Americans invented their own tanning method and used leather for clothing, tents, and canoes. During the Middle Ages, European leatherworkers formed craft guilds. In Russia and Poland, the value of leather was evident in its use as form of currency. Over time, modern synthetic materials and processes gradually reduced the demand for handcrafted leather, but it remains a popular art medium of both ancient and modern influence (Maguire, 2004).

Although its use in therapy is declining, some occupational therapists still use leatherwork with their clients. Early in the profession, leather was used to make adaptive devices such as slings and splints for clients, but, for the most part, commercial products have made this obsolete. A therapist's familiarity with leather craft, however, could provide the know-how to change or adapt commercial products if necessary.

Tubbs, C., & Drake, M. *Crafts and Creative Media in Therapy, Fourth Edition (pp. 119-130).*

Choosing Leather

Leather comes from fur- and wool-bearing mammals; from scaly creatures like snakes, alligators, and lizards; and from birds such as the ostrich. Leather is classified according to its animal source and the process by which it was tanned (Griswold, 1969). Cowhide is most common in therapeutic applications, as it is versatile and less expensive than other leathers. The unit by which it is sold is the square foot and its thickness is expressed by weight in ounces, for example: 2 to 3-ounce weight leather is approximately 1/16-inches thick and 7- to 8-ounce leather is approximately 1/8-inches thick. Weights are given in a range because leather varies in thickness even on the same piece. In occupational therapy settings where leather is used, it is usually stocked in 4- to 5-ounce weight for wallets and small projects, and 8- to 9-ounce weight for belts and purses. Used suede clothing and chamois leather (used in automobile cleaning) are economical sources of leather pieces as well (Maguire, 2004). For the contemporary clinic, these choices plus a variety of pre-cut, prepunched kits provide a sufficient selection.

Kits offer advantages that may outweigh their creative limitations. They not only save the therapist preparation time, but may also save their sanity when working in a busy clinic. In addition, since most clients are not experienced in leatherwork, they may prefer the structure of a kit. If a therapist does decide to include projects made from raw materials, the facility should stock the weights of leather described above—as well as lining leather, which is a different weight and texture—in addition to a range of laces, snaps, and fasteners. Kits should also be available, since the functional level and/or interest of clients will likely vary. Kits contain pre-cut pieces—some with a pre-embossed design—and the required needles and lace. The variety available in project kits allows the therapist to easily grade leatherwork for a client's functional level without stocking all the raw materials.

Special Considerations

Leatherwork is a relatively safe craft. Although sharp tools may be needed for parts of some projects, most of the process is done without them. Hammering during tooling and stamping may pose hazards if the client has decreased strength, coordination, or vision. Lacing needles are blunt and danger of a puncture injury is minimal. Since many leather projects can be easily transported, completed with few tools, and done without noise or fumes, they are suitable for most any setting.

Cost is an important factor to consider in leather crafting. Small economy kits can be purchased for about a dollar, but stocking a variety of kits, bulk leather, and tools can turn into a large expense. Some suppliers sell scrap leather in bulk; this is economical on the front end, but will require more of the therapist's time for preparation. If the clients are satisfied with small, simple projects, however, leatherwork is no more costly than many other crafts.

The fact that leather crafts are less familiar to most individuals than many other crafts may reduce their desirability. Some leather projects may be perceived by the client to be dated and/or too "western." The occupational therapist should be observant of trends and styles in selecting kits or patterns, especially if trying to appeal to younger clients. Traditionally, leatherwork has been a male-oriented craft, although many female clients enjoy it too.

Tools

The variety of leather tools available makes it difficult to decide which ones to acquire. The following tools will make it possible to complete most any therapeutic project:

- Rotary punch with replaceable cutting tubes (Figure 10-1)
- Rawhide mallet (see Figure 10-1)
- 3/4-inch oblong slotting punch
- Strap cutter
- Snap setter

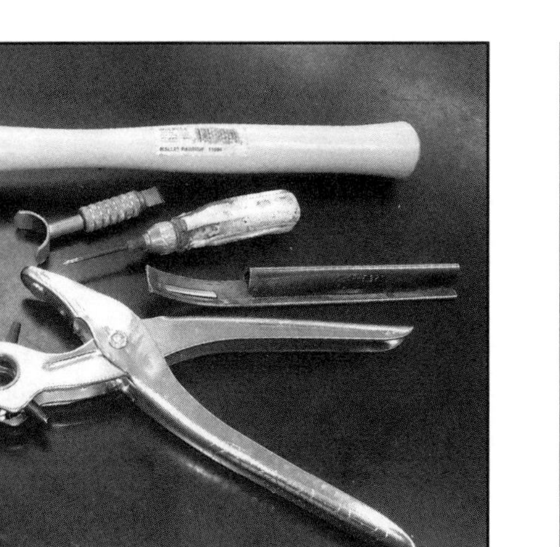

Figure 10-1. Common leatherwork tools: rotary punch, skiving knife, awl, swivel knife, and rawhide mallet.

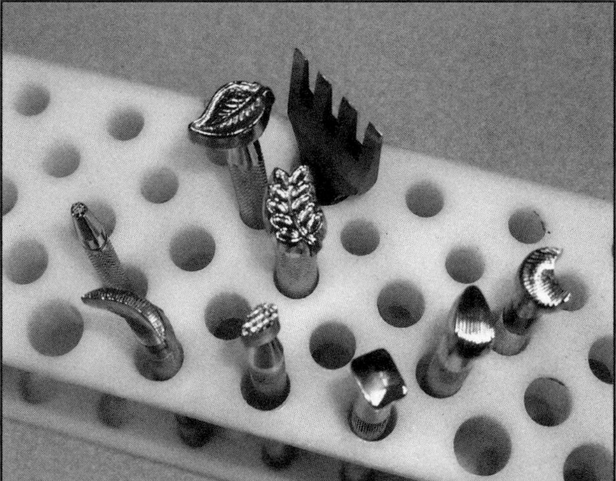

Figure 10-2. Left: a seeder, veiner, and background tool. Middle: A thronging chisel and leaf stamps. Right: a pear shader, camouflage tool, and beveler.

- Awl (see Figure 10-1)
- Leather shears
- Utility knife
- Skiving knife (see Figure 10-1)
- Ruler
- Thonging chisel or awl (Figure 10-2)
- Round drive punches
- Edge creaser
- Swivel knife (see Figure 10-1)
- Sponge and water dish
- Tracing modeler
- Lacing needles

The six basic tools for leather stamping are:

- The veiner (see Figure 10-2)
- The seeder (see Figure 10-2)
- The camouflage (see Figure 10-2)
- The beveler (see Figure 10-2)
- The pear shader (see Figure 10-2)
- The background tool (see Figure 10-2)

These six stamping tools used in combination can achieve many interesting and decorative effects. Other techniques may use plastic templates; these offer an inexpensive option for attractive designs that are quick, easy, and reusable. Alphabet stamps are handy for personalizing the project, and other pictorial stamps (see Figure 10-2) can be used to simplify design making.

Tooling and stamping are done on the smooth (grain) side of the leather piece (Figure 10-3).

Tooling Process

1. Select the design. If it is copied from a book rather than from a template, trace it with a pencil.
2. Cut the leather to the proper size.

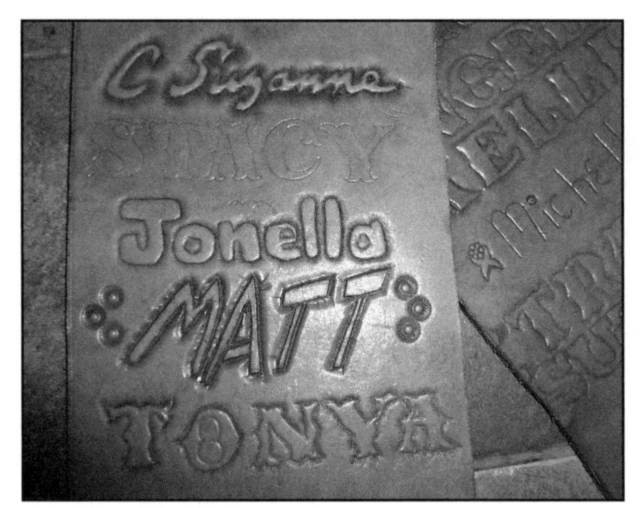

Figure 10-3. Stamping and tooling samples.

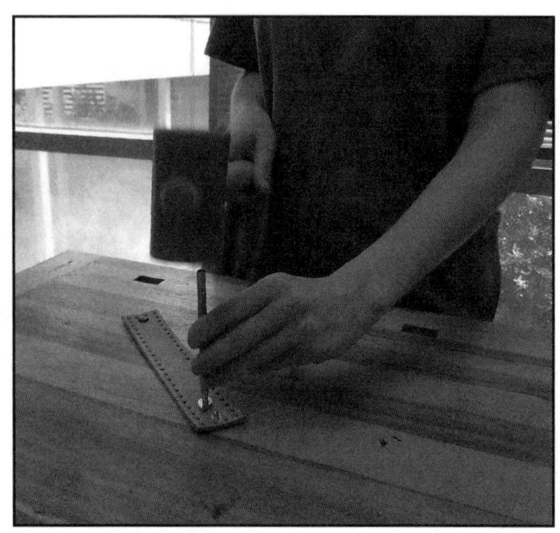

Figure 10-4. Striking the stamping tool requires a strong grasp and hand-eye coordination.

3. Moisten the leather on the flesh (rough) side first and then on the grain (smooth) side with a damp (not wet) sponge. Wait until the grain side of the leather returns to its original color; this will take a minute or less.
4. Place the traced design on the leather, writing side up, so that the pencil lead does not stain the leather.
5. With the pointed end of the tracing modeler, lightly press the design into the leather so that it is clearly visible.
6. Next score the traced design with the swivel knife. Allow the leather to dry somewhat, as wet leather tends to catch on the swivel knife and cause small tears and unevenness in the line. Using a swivel knife requires practice, so while the leather is drying, encourage the client to practice carving with a swivel knife on a piece of scrap leather. The leather should be just slightly damp so the knife can glide more smoothly.
7. After all lines are carved, moisten the leather again with a damp sponge in preparation for tooling the design.
8. Holding the stamping tools upright, strike the flat top with a rawhide mallet (Figure 10-4). The beveler (see Figure 10-2) is usually used first. The pointed end or toe of the beveling surface is placed in the cut made by the swivel knife facing toward the center of the design. Wrist and arm movements are used, rather than fingers, to manipulate the mallet in tapping the beveler as it moves along the carved line.
9. Use of the camouflage tool's half-moon shape (see Figure 10-2) is usually the next step in a tooled design.
10. Next, use the pear shader (see Figure 10-2) to create contours and shading.
11. The veiner is commonly used in nature designs, as its name comes from its similarity to leaf veins (see Figure 10-2) and the seeder is a small round design (see Figure 10-2) used for putting centers in flowers or similar motifs.
12. Use the background tool (see Figure 10-2) to impress the area around the design, causing it to stand out more dramatically. Each of these tools is held upright and tapped with the rawhide mallet. A steel-headed hammer will damage the chrome finish on the leatherworking tools and can also cause the tool to puncture the leather.

The creator can use stamping tools to either copy or create unique designs (see Figure 10-3). In either case, he or she should practice stamping on a piece of scrap leather before beginning the project. A wide variety of stamping tools other than those mentioned here are available. Some are just shapes; others are realistic pictures of objects and animals that will not require the skill and concentration of leather tooling, allowing a lower-functioning client the opportunity to successfully choose and create pleasing designs.

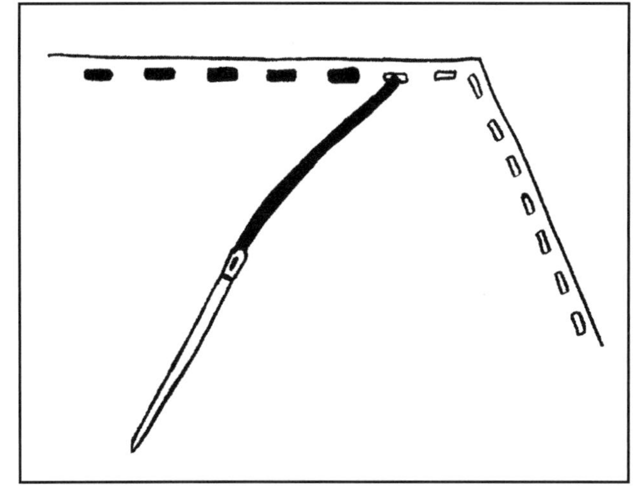

Figure 10-5. Running stitch.

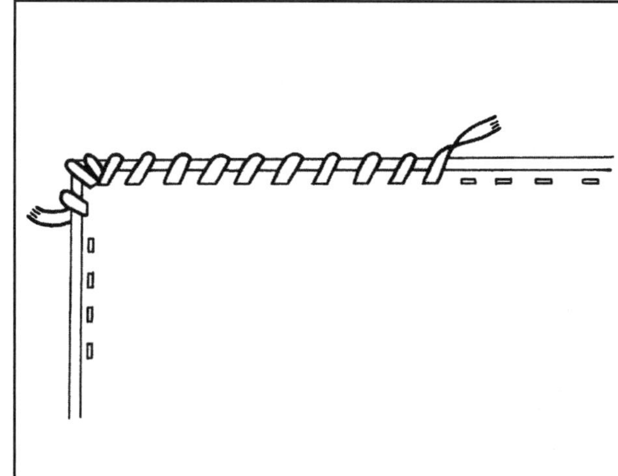

Figure 10-6. Whip stitch.

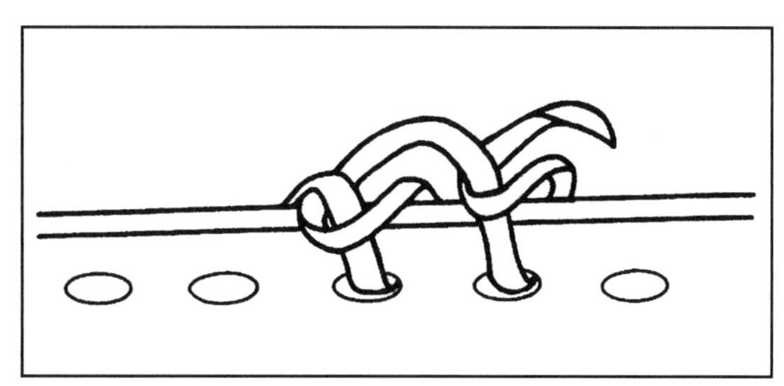

Figure 10-7. Single cordovan lacing.

Coloring Leather

The natural color of leather is one of its attractions. Nonetheless, clients frequently desire to add color to their work, and there are a number of coloring agents, dyes, and acrylic paints suitable for this. As with tooling and stamping, clients should be encouraged to practice on scrap leather before attempting it on their project. This can even segue into a life lesson—being sure of abilities and choices before making an irreversible commitment. Since each coloring agent has unique properties, it is important for both the therapist and client to read the label directions prior to using. A brush, a felt or wool dauber, or a fine-grained sponge is used to apply color. Vegetable stains will give an antique appearance. Moisture-resistant finishes include lacquers and waxes; treatment with neat's-foot or mink oil will waterproof leather but will also slightly darken the color. All finishes should be applied before pieces are assembled or laced.

Lacing

Due to the popularity of the Allen Cognitive Levels Screening Test (Earhart, Allen, & Blue, 1992) in assessment, lacing has become a particularly important leatherwork skill for the occupational therapist. Performance in lacing reveals information about tactile awareness, strength, motor planning, dexterity, visual perception, sequencing, frustration tolerance, and ability to learn and to recognize errors. Because of the variety of stitches—running stitch (Figure 10-5), whip stitch (Figure 10-6), single cordovan lacing (Figure 10-7), and other, more complex variations—it is easy to grade lacing up or down. For some leather projects, lacing the is primary operation, with little or no tooling/stamping involved.

Lacing Process

1. Glue the pieces together with a thin layer of rubber cement applied just to the edges of the surfaces to be joined. Avoid getting cement on anything but those surfaces; glue adheres quickly and can also stain the smooth (visible) side of the leather.

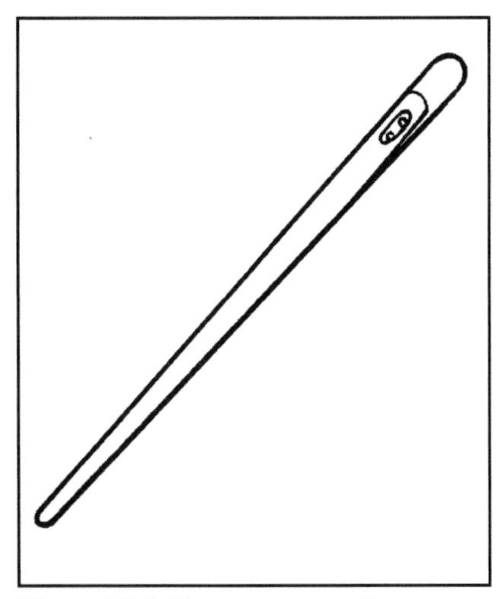

Figure 10-8. Two-prong needle.

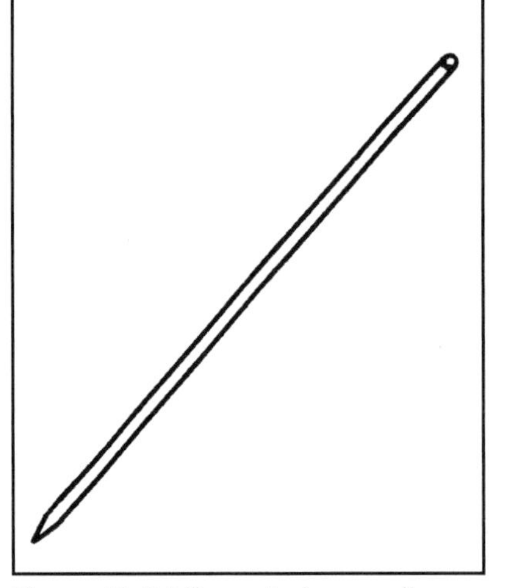

Figure 10-9. Life-eye lacing needle.

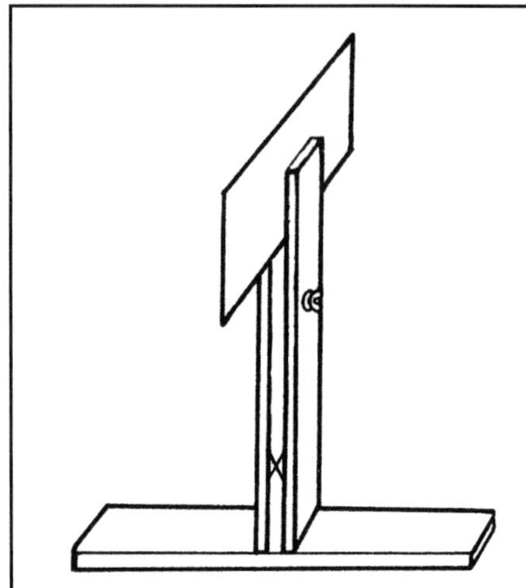

Figure 10-10. Lacing pony.

2. Mark a line 1/8 to 1/4 of an inch from the edge with a ruler and the pointed end of the tracing modeler to indicate where lacing holes will be.
3. Use scrap wood under the leather and place the thonging chisel (see Figure 10-2) 1/8 to 1/4 of an inch from the corner on the line.
4. Holding the chisel perpendicular to the leather, hit the chisel head with a rawhide mallet until the cutting blades go through to the wood and can be seen on the other side. Care must be taken to hit the chisel hard enough to make the lacing slots without cutting the leather in between the slots.
5. Continue making these slots wherever lacing will be used. A rotary leather punch (see Figure 10-1) can also be used to make the holes for lacing.
6. The two types of needles most commonly used for lacing are the two-prong needle (Figure 10-8) and the life-eye (Figure 10-9), neither of which have a traditional eye. To use the life-eye needle, cut the leather lace into a point and twist it into the hollow end of the needle. Regular large-eye needles can also be used, usually with waxed linen or nylon thread. The type of stitch will determine the difficulty of the actual lacing; see illustrations (see Figures 10-5 through 10-7) for basic stitch options. The running stitch and whip stitch are done as illustrated. The process for the single cordovan is similar to the whip stitch, but the lace is inserted back under the loop, from front to back, before it is tightened down. More specific instructions for lacing can be found in the references and the Resources section. There are several tips for lacing that will ensure a more attractive end product: keep the lace from becoming twisted; avoid pulling the lace too tight; and to finish off, trim the lace to a narrow point and tuck back through several stitches under the leather. Also keep in mind that the longer the working piece, the harder it will be to keep flat (Griswold, 1969). The lacing pony (Figure 10-10) is a tool for stabilizing a project for one-handed lacing. The pony is placed between the client's legs, with the leather held in the clamp at a comfortable working height.

Project—Whimsical Luggage Tag

Plan It

This project requires only a small amount of leather and can do done with or without tooling. The lacing can be done with leather thronging or with plastic lace. Plastic lace comes in assorted colors, and could be color-coordinated with dyed leather if desired. In making this tag, make sure the strap is long enough to go around a luggage handle and that a large enough opening is left to insert a name card.

Get Ready

Supplies

- Leather piece, 4- to 5-ounce weight, approximately 6 x 12 inches
- 3 feet of leather thronging or other lace
- Glue
- 1 to 2 snaps
- Paper

Tools

- Leather needle
- Scissors
- Ruler
- Marking pen
- Leather punch
- Thronging chisel, optional
- Rawhide mallet
- Snap setter

Time required: 45 minutes to 1 hour

Cost: Approximately $1

Do It

Process

1. Draw the desired pattern on a sheet of paper. The shape can be changed as desired as long as there is room to cut a window and a way to insert the identification card. Dampen and mark the edges of all pieces (except the top of the front piece) using the stitch marker. Using the leather punch or the thronging chisel and mallet, make lacing holes evenly around all marked edges.
2. Cut the picture out, then trace around it on the back (rough side) of the leather piece. Do this as close to the edge as possible to avoid wasting the material.
3. Cut out the shape from the leather. Then place it, rough side down, on the back of the remaining piece of leather. Draw around it and cut it out as well. Do not trace and cut both pieces at the same time because they will not fit together correctly when placed back to back.
4. From the remaining leather, cut a strip about 6 inches long and 1/2-inch wide to make a strap.
5. On the back of one piece, run a thin bead of glue around the outer edge, but leave unglued one section large enough to accommodate insertion of the identification card later. Let the glue dry for a few minutes.
6. Using the thronging chisel or the rotary punch, make lacing holes around the outer edge of the shape, except where the card is to be inserted.
7. Lace the piece using a whip stitch as illustrated (see Figure 10-6) and described in the previous section (Figure 10-11).
8. Use the slot punch and mallet to make a slot for the insertion of a strap. This can correspond with the opening for the name card or anywhere close to the edge of the piece.
9. Use the snap setter and mallet to add a snap to the strap, and to the opening for the name card if necessary.

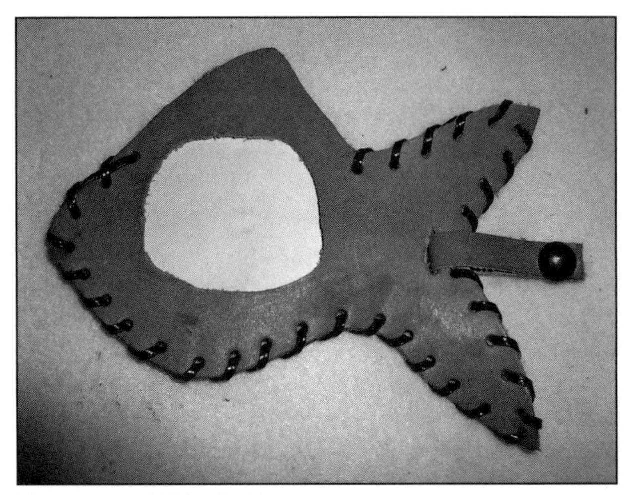

Figure 10-11. Whimsical luggage tag.

Change It

This project can be varied by making a different shape, or several different shapes, and by dyeing the leather or using colorful plastic lacing. To grade it down, make the shape a simple square, pre-punch the lacing holes, or have the client do just selected steps such as the lacing. To grade it up, have the client tool the leather to make distinguishing features on their shape of choice. Or use the double cordovan stitch for a greater fine motor and perceptual challenge.

Document It

Below are some suggestions for documenting the use of this activity to illustrate performance skills utilized.

- "The client was able to follow demonstrated instructions for stitching the leather project with only occasional cues to correct twisting."
- "The client was able to grasp the mallet but did not have enough hand strength to maintain grasp during resisted use of the tool. This indicates a likely inability to return to previous work tasks at this time."
- "The client was able to consistently flex and extend elbow during lacing activity for up to 10 minutes with no complaint of pain."

Other Ideas and Grading

Many simple yet attractive leather projects are possible using only cut suede, lacing and minimal tools, for example coin purses, napkin rings, picture frames, or toys (Maguire, 2004). One substitute material that can serve as a more affordable option in some projects is chamois cloth, available in auto parts stores, or the auto section of large discount stores This very soft, thin leather is perfect for decorative pillow appliqués or making children's stuffed toys (Maguire, 2004). Leather scraps left over from other projects, or purchased in scrap packs, can be used to make small items such as key rings, luggage tags, tassels, napkin rings, or hair barrettes. Leather thonging can be used in several ways besides lacing, for example braided to make bracelets or anklets, wrapped around purse handles or used to make knotted fasteners or decorative embellishments, or woven into coasters or trivets. Tooled leather pieces can be used as framed pictures or as fancy covers for boxes or journals. Leather picture frames can be made with simple patterns and minimal stitching. Leather can be colored with dyes but also with everyday items such as felt markers. Moccasins, slippers, or baby booties—while somewhat more complex and costly to make—may be popular choices for some clients. Both kits and patterns are available for these and other items. Link belt kits were once a staple therapy craft and are still available. The kit usually contains pre-cut pieces, a buckle, and the buckle connector and keeper, and assembly is simple and repetitive. Other items frequently made from kits include small coin purses, luggage tags, and wallets.

Leatherwork has many variations and likewise offers many grading possibilities. For any given project, a kit is simpler than starting from a pattern and raw materials. The therapist should not assume, however, that all kits are easy. Very simple "scratch" projects may require fewer skills than complex kits. Another way of grading is by choosing stitch difficulty; the running stitch and whip stitch are much easier to reproduce than the cordovan or double cordovan. Any project that calls for tooling or stamping necessarily has added steps, requiring more tools, time, and skills. The therapist can advise the client in simplifying, or even eliminating, the tooled design if necessary. In general, the more pieces a project has, the more complex its assembly. The addition of decorative stitching, color, or appliqué increases the demands of the activity. Most basic leather projects lend themselves well to grading by the therapist, and to modification by the client for individual taste and design preference.

Main Therapeutic Applications

Physical Dysfunction

Leatherwork is easily graded for use with clients with physical limitations. Lacing projects are ideal for use with bed-bound patients. They are quiet, do not require the use of water or other liquid, and do not create dust or fumes. In the event the client becomes fatigued or is interrupted, the project can be stopped at almost any point and resumed later without compromising the finished product. Leather tools can be disinfected, but steel rotary punches may rust if not completely dried after immersion in liquid. Leather itself is difficult to sterilize; chemicals in disinfectants may affect color and suppleness of tanned leather, and soaked leather will shrink. Simple projects that require few tools, such as link belts or pre-stamped kits ready for lacing, are the best alternative for isolated clients.

Leatherwork can be a good treatment activity for clients with goals of upper extremity strengthening and increased endurance. Cutting or punching leather utilizes resisted grasp, which also activates wrist musculature for stabilization. Resistive pad-to-pad pinch is used to hold the implements in tooling and stamping. Using the swivel knife requires static pinch as well, along with wrist ulnar and radial deviation. For safe and accurate tooling or stamping, proximal stability is necessary in the extremity used for holding the tool. Mallet use with the other extremity requires resisted cylindrical grasp, shoulder stability, and forceful elbow extension. Lacing involves intermittent activation of many upper extremity muscle groups and is good for working on range of motion, but the work can be positioned to compensate for poor proximal stability or inability to use one hand. Leatherwork can be a good method of achieving upper extremity strengthening, endurance or coordination goals using an activity more purposeful than exercise. The type and complexity of design can be graded to target strengthening or dexterity goals. For clients with fragile or inflamed joints, the therapist is cautioned against using resistive activities such as cutting with the swivel knife and hammering (Melvin, 1998).

Individuals with visual impairment can use leather craft to increase tactile awareness, an important compensatory skill. As the client works on the design, the impressions and contours can be felt with the fingers. The skills learned in leatherwork can be transferred to other activities such as handling coins and identifying textures in putting clothes on right side out.

Mental Health

Leather crafts were once commonly used in the treatment of mental health clients but leatherwork is now most closely associated with this population due to the popularity of the Allen Cognitive Level Screening in assessment of cognitive function. Low-functioning clients can be successful with easy projects such as link-belt kits or those requiring only simple lacing, and the ability to advance to more complex projects demonstrates functional improvement to the client in a very concrete way. Leatherwork can be used to address diverse mental health needs such as task persistence, problem solving, visual attention and processing, self-awareness, and the ability to follow directions. As commercial manufacturers rely increasingly on synthetics, natural leather products become more appreciated for their authenticity. Consequently, when a client completes a leather item, it may be perceived as something of value and permanence, enhancing a sense of self-worth. Leather projects are useful for clients experiencing mania because they can be highly structured, the material is controllable, and they can be frequently stopped and started without consequence (Early, 2009). Clients diagnosed with mental retardation may benefit from those aspects of leatherwork requiring motor coordination/dexterity skills and concentration for repetitive actions, such as stamping and lacing. Accuracy in lacing and time spent on the task without redirection are both objective ways of measuring and documenting improved performance.

Pediatrics

Leatherwork has been used only infrequently with younger clients in acute settings. Often, by the time acutely ill children were well enough to do leatherwork, they were discharged from the hospital. Leather projects were—and still are—more appropriate for children in longer-term settings, such as cancer hospitals or psychiatric facilities. Children should enjoy making items that they can use and boys in particular may like the "cowboy" look. Use of leatherwork is indicated in a school system setting only if the occupational therapist can relate it directly to an educational function such as use of scissors or handwriting. Kits offer the most satisfactory results for children and some are designed especially to appeal to children. For older children, hammering and tooling may be good outlets for excess energy (Early, 2009) and they provide strong proprioceptive input, but should be avoided for any child who is hypersensitive to the noise.

Adolescents

Older children and teenagers are more likely to use and enjoy making leather objects such as chokers, armbands, wallets, or coin purses. Leather tooling and stamping offer opportunities for expression of identity and some leather objects (e.g., wallets) are associated with adult responsibilities. Completion of a leather project, especially one with multiple steps, will offer a sense of accomplishment and competence.

Geriatrics

Stamping or tooling leather should be done with caution with the elderly because of the strength required to accomplish it safely. Some of the tools could cause cuts or bruises that will be slower to heal; older people are at higher risk for injury due diminished coordination, tactile sensation, and visual skills (Bonder & Bello-Haas, 2009). Osteoarthritis is also more common in older people and resistive gripping of tools may aggravate the pain or deformities symptomatic of this condition (Melvin & Jensen, 1998). Leather is considered by some to be a male-identified craft and the majority of elders are women, which may explain why leather crafts are used less often in therapy with older adults.

Groups

Leatherwork is not typically used as a group activity. Clients may work on simple projects in parallel groups, but few leather items are large enough to make teamwork appropriate or meaningful. Groups of higher-functioning clients, however, may be able to assist one another in planning and executing tooled designs.

Case Study

Rafael, a 23-year-old from East Los Angeles, was arrested outside a bar where he had been fighting, and later admitted to the county's alcohol and drug treatment unit as part of a jail diversion program. Due to his frequent and excessive alcohol use that had resulted in many encounters with the law, he was deemed substance dependent, qualifying him for a 28-day inpatient treatment program.

During the initial interview, the occupational therapist learned about Rafael's background. His mother's parents were migrant workers in the fruit orchards of California and his father had illegally come across the Mexican border to find work. Rafael was the youngest of their eight children and stated that his parents were too busy to pay much attention to him growing up. He had dropped out of high school when he was in tenth grade "because it was boring," and since that time had worked at a variety of unskilled day labor jobs. Rafael had always associated alcohol with machismo and had never considered his drinking abnormal, in spite of negative consequences. He was engaged at one time, but the wedding was called off after he hit his fiancé in the face during a drunken rage. Following this incident, his family asked him to leave their home, as they were both fearful of and embarrassed by his behavior. Although he had been arrested for public intoxication before, this was the first time he had ever undergone treatment.

The occupational therapy department had a variety of assessments available, and Rafael's therapist chose an Interest Checklist, the daily activities time chart, and the Allen Cognitive Levels Screening Test, based on interview results that suggested maladaptive leisure choices, impaired problem solving and judgment, poor self-control, and lack of time management skills. On the Interest Checklist, he indicated a strong interest in leatherwork and sports. He told the therapist he had once watched an uncle in Mexico doing leather tooling and had wanted to work with leather ever since. The completed daily activities chart demonstrated little variety and few productive pursuits during a week's worth of activities, along with a low sense of autonomy in those that he did do. During the follow-up discussion, he told his therapist that he had always been passive in groups and allowed others to make decisions for him. Rafael scored a 5.4 on the Allen Cognitive Levels Screening Test; the therapist also documented observation of decreased dexterity in manipulating the needle and lace.

As Rafael and the occupational therapist worked together to devise a treatment plan, he told her he would like to learn skills that would help him get a stable job. After discussing the more comprehensive role of occupational therapy in his treatment program, they set the following goals: to develop a daily activity plan/schedule and carry it out during the 28-day treatment program, to list at least three realistic options for employment, to consistently exhibit self-control and incorporate problem solving and positive coping strategies during group and individual activities, and to increase the strength and dexterity of his upper extremities.

During the first week of treatment, Rafael was able to complete a tooled leather belt that he planned to keep and wear. He was clearly pleased with the outcome and wanted to do something more complicated. For his second project, he decided to make a shoulder bag for his mother in preparation for her upcoming visit. During this same time, he began a weight-lifting program with the recreation therapist and his strength and endurance began to show improvement. During his last week, he decided to try to make something for his estranged father as a peace offering. With minimal guidance from the therapist, he designed and completed a tool belt for his father, who worked in construction. During the process, he demonstrated the ability to problem solve, and dealt with frustrations and setbacks in a positive way. During the last group session he proudly displayed the finished project and engaged in the discussion about present accomplishments and future plans and strategies for remaining sober.

Discussion Questions

1. What questions might you ask Rafael at the time of his discharge to help him assess whether he had achieved his goals?
2. How is this occupation relevant to Rafael's vocational needs?
3. For what cultural/age/gender groups might leatherwork especially meaningful? Explain your answer.
4. What leather project materials or kits (if any) do you think might be best to stock in an occupational therapy clinic? Why?

Resources

Leather Jewelry: 30 Contemporary Projects
By Nathalie Mornu
Sterling Publishing/Lark Books, 2010
Small projects with explanation basic techniques suitable for the beginner

Making Stylish Belts: Do-it-yourself Projects to Craft and Sew at Home
By Ellen Goldstein-Lynch
Quarry Books, 2007
Belt projects from a variety of materials, including leather

The Leatherworking Handbook: A Practical Illustrated Sourcebook of Techniques and Projects
By Valerie Michael
Cassell, 2006
Describes techniques, tools, and equipment needed for all the basic processes involved in leatherwork. Projects are diverse in level of difficulty

Gorgeous Leather Crafts: 30 Projects to Stamp, Stencil, Weave, and Tool
By Kari Lee
Sterling Publishing/Lark Books, 2003

Leathercraft
By Chris H. Groneman
Sayani Press, 2010
A reprint of a classic leather how-to book.

References

Allen, C. K., Earhart, C. A., & Blue, T. (1992). *Occupational therapy treatment goals for the physically and cognitively disabled.* Bethesda, MD: American Occupational Therapy Association.
Bonder, B. R., & Bello-Haas, V. D. (2009). *Functional performance in older adults* (3rd ed.). Philadelphia, PA: F. A. Davis Co.
Early, M. B. (2009). *Mental health concepts and techniques for the occupational therapy assistant* (4th ed.). Philadelphia, PA: Lippincott Williams & Wilkins.
Griswold, L., & Griswold, K. (1969). *The new handicraft orocesses and projects* (10th ed.). New York, NY: Van Nostrand Reinhold Company.
Maguire, M. (2004). *Craft workshop: Leatherwork.* London, UK: Southwater, Anness Publishing, Ltd.
Melvin, J., & Jensen, G. (1998). *Rheumatologic rehabilitation series: Assessment and management.* Bethesda, MD: American Occupational Therapy Association
Reader's Digest. (1979). *Crafts and hobbies.* Pleasantville, NY: The Reader's Digest Association Inc.
Stohlman, A., Patten, A. D., & Wilson, J. A. (1969). *Leatherwork manual.* Fort Worth, TX: Tandy Leather Company.

11

Needlework

Objectives

The student should be able to:

- Discuss historical/cultural examples of needlework
- List basic supplies and materials needed to do various types of needlework and know how to complete and grade a basic project
- Explain advantages and limitations of needlework activities in therapy
- List precautions of needlework activities
- Describe how needlework activities might be used in therapy with various client populations

The term *needlework* is quite broad, including everything from sewing clothing, to making boat sails or repairing fishing nets, to creating intricate tapestries that may hang in an art museum. In 18th and 19th century America, needlecraft was often the measure of a woman's worth. Young women did needlework samplers with the same dedication and expectation of judgment that today's young women complete term papers or work-related projects. Sewing clothing for the family, along with quilting and mending, were constant female occupations (Banks, 1979). Quilting dates at least as far back as the Crusades; the process was found useful in adding warmth to clothing and bedding. Patchwork quilting resulted from a need for frugality among pioneer women who could not afford to waste even scraps. Appliqué, a technique sometimes incorporated in quilting, also developed out of economy; it was used as a substitute for expensive embroidery (*Reader's Digest*, 1979).

Needlework includes such a vast number of activities that this text can only partially cover the topic. Categories of needlework most commonly used in therapy will be discussed in this chapter. Occupational therapists need not limit themselves to these, but should ultimately choose those forms with which they are most familiar. In the exceptional case, the therapist may be able to teach a client a new skill or embark on a long-term project, but most treatment programs call for crafts that can be completed relatively quickly.

Tubbs, C., & Drake, M. *Crafts and Creative Media in Therapy, Fourth Edition (pp. 131-142).*

Types of Needlework

Simple Sewing

Simple sewing includes making, mending, or modifying clothing and home furnishings, usually with use of a needle and thread. Stitches range from the simple running or basting stitch, to the more difficult smocking, ruffling, and buttonhole stitches (Carroll, 1947). Today, much sewing is done on a machine, but some crafters prefer to do all hand-sewn work. Quilting, one popular form of needlecraft, can be done on a machine or by hand. It is a nostalgic American craft used in both home decoration and in making functional items such as blankets. Quilted objects or their designs are sometimes symbolic of marriage, friendship, and resourcefulness, or are representative of a region or culture. Historically, quilting provided a collaborative, social enterprise in a world where geographic isolation was the rule (Fidler & Velde, 1999). Today, it is also popular as an art form, and there are publications, museum displays, and quilt shows dedicated solely to its appreciation and perpetuation. Many stitches in quilting qualify as simple sewing, though the designs and color combinations of the fabric may be complex (*Reader's Digest*, 1979). Regardless of the product to be made, all occupational therapists should be familiar with simple hand sewing and basic use of a sewing machine. While useful in crafting, these skills are also sometimes needed for tasks such as making universal cuffs or adapting clothing for clients for unique needs.

Embroidery

Embroidery is a way of making a picture or design on cloth using a needle and thread. It can be either simple or complex, with dozens of different embroidery stitches from which to choose. One of the simplest and earliest stitches, often used in kits, is the cross stitch. Eighteenth century girlhood samplers were usually of the cross stitch variety (Banks, 1979; Creekmore, 1968). Other types of embroidery include crewel and counted cross stitch. Each embroidery style calls for a particular type of yarn or floss as well as a particular weight or weave of fabric. For example, in crewel embroidery, loosely twisted yarn (usually wool) is stitched on heavier fabric (Carroll, 1947), while thinner cotton floss is used in (counted) cross stitch. Counted cross stitch is popular among needlework hobbyists today, but it may be too difficult or time consuming for most therapeutic applications. A small stamped cross stitch kit or plastic canvas with a preprinted color-coded design may be a workable alternative. As with any craft, the popularity of a particular form or style of embroidery waxes and wanes over time. In most cases, therapists should try to choose projects with a contemporary look.

Needlepoint

Modern day counted cross stitch is an updated version of traditional needlepoint, a craft in which a single stitch type is used, but the number and arrangement of the stitches creates the design. While needlepoint is similar to cross stitch embroidery, it is done with a blunt needle (Figure 11-1) on a grid-like plastic or canvas backing that ensures uniform stitch size. Many of the world's fine tapestries were made using this method. Needlepoint has several advantages relative to its use in therapy. It requires less precise motor control than many forms of needlework, and since the needle is dull, it presents fewer hazards. Simple kits and patterns are available and the size of the yarn, needle, and canvas are easily graded. Needlepoint may serve as a reasonable substitute for someone who is unable to resume a more difficult form of needlecraft.

Knitting and Crocheting

Knitting and crocheting are both methods of using interlocking loops of yarn to make garments or articles for home use. Knitting is usually done in rows using two long, blunt-end needles (see Figure 11-1). Crocheting requires only one hook-like needle (see Figure 11-1) and stitching is also done in rows. Knitting and crocheting projects can include scarves, mittens, shawls, potholders, and afghans. Smaller thread can be crocheted into coasters, doilies, or tablecloths. Although both of these crafts, especially knitting, have experienced a recent resurgence in popularity, they require time and patience to master, and are therefore not used extensively in therapy. Some knitting hobbyists, however, highlight the stress-reducing quality of this craft (Pigza,

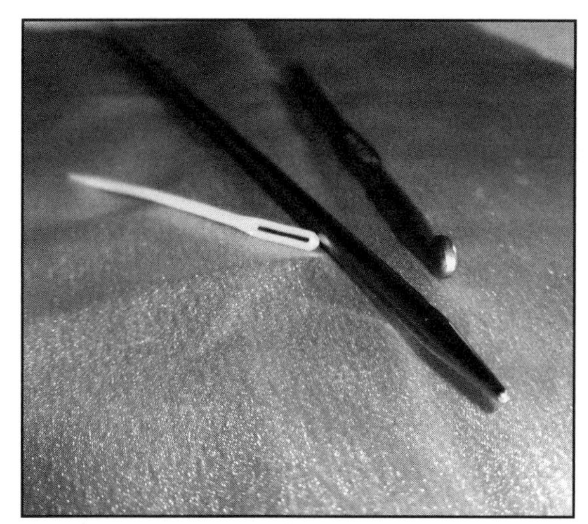

Figure 11-1. Various needlework tools: plastic needlepoint needle, knitting needle, crochet hook.

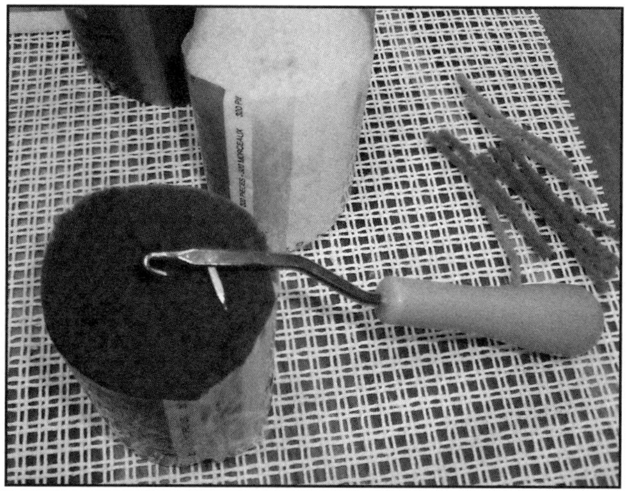

Figure 11-2. A latchhook.

2008) once the technique is mastered. Occasionally, the occupational therapist may encounter a client in rehabilitation who wants to continue or resume this pastime. Since the process may have to be adapted based on client limitations, it is advisable to at least know how the needles are handled in making basic stitches. The reader is referred to other sources for how-to instruction for knitting and crocheting.

Latchhook

Latchhook is a modern adaptation of a traditional style of rug making called knotting or Turkish knotting. Using a flat loom that holds the backing, yarn is pulled through two warp threads at a time using a rug hook. The knots are made in rows, and a thick pile is created (*Better Homes and Gardens*, 1966; Department of the Army, 1971; Moseley, Johnson, & Koenig, 1962). Today's carpets are made in essentially the same way, though done by machine. Some have cut pile, which is like Turkish knotting, and some have looped piles like hooked rugs (Department of the Army, 1971; Scharff, 1952). A latchhook (Figure 11-2) is a special kind of needlework hook with a small, hinged appendage on it that helps automatically knot the yarn as it is pulled through the rug canvas. The backing for most latchhook crafts is a heavy mesh cloth that can be bought in rolls, or comes in kits pre-cut and stamped with a design. The yarn pieces are 2 to 4 inches in length and are most often purchased ready-cut and bundled by color. Latchhook projects often take more time than is available for therapy sessions, but since the process is repetitive and easily learned, clients may be able to finish projects at home. Latchhook is most commonly used for making pillows, chair pads, and rugs and many kits on the market today are most suitable for children.

To make a latchhook stitch, insert the hook vertically into one hole and back out through the one immediately above it. Make sure the hinged latch goes all the way through both spaces. Slide a piece of yarn under the metal part of the hook handle, then grasp and hold both loose ends of the yarn and pull them up into the hook (Figure 11-3). Continue holding the ends of the yarn as you pull the hook back through the canvas. The latch will close around the yarn and it will be pulled back through the loop. Pull gently to tighten as needed. Start working the piece about an inch from the edge of the canvas and use the yarn color indicated by the stamped design. Continue this process, changing yarn color as needed, until the design is completed. To finish, fold each edge of the canvas over and stitch it in place. Using a latchhook requires more grip strength and force than most other needlework tools. Finishing the edge is also somewhat more difficult because the canvas is stiff and scratchy.

Locker Hooking

Locker hooking is somewhat of a hybrid of latchhook and needlepoint. It is done with fabric strips instead of yarn and uses a special tool called a locker hook. Loops of fabric are pulled up through the canvas grid, then locked into place by a locking medium, usually cotton twine. This needlecraft is useful for making items such as rugs, placemats, and trivets (Pulido, 2009).

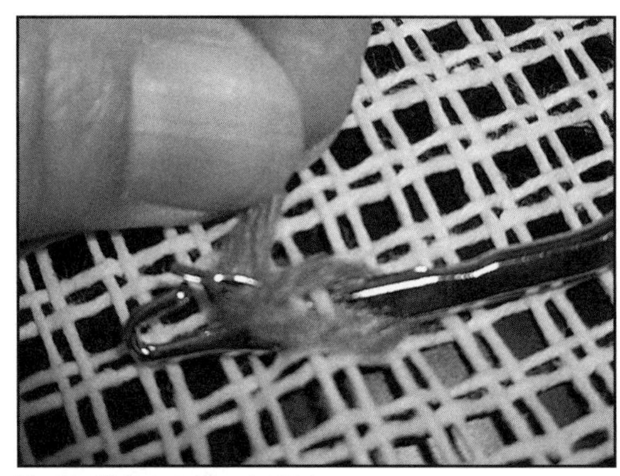

Figure 11-3. Latchhook stitch.

Needlefelting

Needlefelting is a method of embellishing or making stand-alone articles from a material called wool roving, a type of combed wool fiber. The wool is stabbed repeatedly with a sharp needle specially designed for this process; it causes the fibers to become enmeshed in a backing material (creating a surface decoration), or with the other fibers (creating a solid object). The needle is very sharp so should be used cautiously with clients, but the process itself is simple and repetitive. The reader is referred to the Resources at the end of the chapter for more information on method and projects.

Special Considerations and Precautions

Most needlework requires some degree of fine motor function, and visual acuity and perception are also necessary for some techniques. Due to the way the tools are used, it is not always possible to adapt them to accommodate poor grasp, but the demand varies with the style of needlework and the projects themselves can be graded. Clients with impaired visual skills may become frustrated when trying to follow a pattern or assess the accuracy of the stitches. Some clients may associate sewing more with work than with leisure, and therefore may prefer a different activity. Some sewing projects take time and may require multiple treatment sessions to complete, which is not feasible in some therapy settings.

Safety is another consideration in choosing needlework as a treatment media. Needles and scissors must be sharp to do the work efficiently, so clients using these tools should be closely monitored, especially those with blood-borne pathogens such as HIV or hepatitis. In a mental health setting, therapists must do a tool count before and after each session. Sewing machines present a similar danger; in addition, they are costly and easily damaged with misuse, so the therapist should always supervise clients in their use.

Tools and materials for needlecraft are inexpensive—with the exception of the sewing machine—and kits are readily available, so this makes it appealing as a therapeutic craft choice. Kits are more costly than raw materials, although those geared toward children tend to be slightly cheaper. The primary advantage of kits is that they simplify the preparation process and the selection is large. Because needlework is most often identified with women, men will be less likely to try it (Department of the Army, 1971).

Projects

To utilize needlecrafts as therapeutic activities, a clinic should be stocked with basic tools and supplies, such as left- and right-handed scissors, thimbles, a needle threader, different sizes of embroidery hoops, an assortment of needles (sewing, embroidery, needlepoint, knitting, and crochet), and a few types of fabric and thread. A three-way hoop that can stand on a table, be held between legs, or be clamped to a table for use by one-handed clients may also be useful. Some adapted embroidery stands also include a large magnifying glass that can be positioned over the work.

The project below is made using the tools of basic sewing but the concept can be adapted in myriad ways to make other items. Cotton is a suggested fabric; if fraying becomes a problem, the fabric can first be ironed to fusible webbing or cut with pinking shears.

Project—Table Runner

Plan It

As written, this project requires a sewing machine. The therapist should be sure to know how to thread it, how to change/fill the bobbin, and how to operate the machine. The runner could be made by hand, but it would be much more time consuming. Shop around for bargain fabric remnants; they are often available in one to two yard pieces.

Get Ready

Supplies

- Washable fabric, approximately 1 yard
- Thread of corresponding color
- Beads, optional (or pre-sewn bead strips, rickrack, or other decorative edging; if using beads, make sure that your sewing needle will fit through their holes)

Tools

- Sewing machine
- Scissors
- Sewing needle
- Fabric marking pen
- Measuring tape
- Straight pins
- Thimble

Do It

Process

1. Cut two pieces fabric to desired runner size (about 12 x 42 inches), allowing an extra 1/2 inch on each side. Iron each piece.
2. Lay the fabric pieces together with wrong sides facing, pin with straight pins to hold it secure, then stitch together both long sides and one short side with the sewing machine.
3. Turn fabric right side out. Fold in the ends of the remaining short side evenly to hide raw edges, iron, and sew together by hand using a whipstitch.
4. Using a sewing needle and thread, sew beads, evenly spaced, along the short ends. Start sewing at one corner and leave tag end of thread several inches long. Slide the needle through the bead, then run the needle down through the fabric, then back up where the next bead will be attached. After adding two to three beads, go back and knot the loose end of the thread around the first bead, tie, and cut as close to the knot as possible. Continue adding beads to the end. Repeat on the other short end of the runner (Figure 11-4).

If you are using a beaded strip, you will need to first pin it to the desired edges (beads facing in), on the right side of one of the pieces of fabric, then pin the other piece of fabric on top with the beads on the inside. Be sure right sides of fabric are facing and the seam is the same width as the strip of material holding the beads. This will ensure that only the beads will show when it is turned right side out. An easier option is to stitch the bead strip on the back after the pieces are completely sewn together, but the finished appearance will not be as neat.

If another decorative edging such as ribbon or rickrack is preferred, simply pin it to the top edge of the runner and stitch it all the way around using the sewing machine.

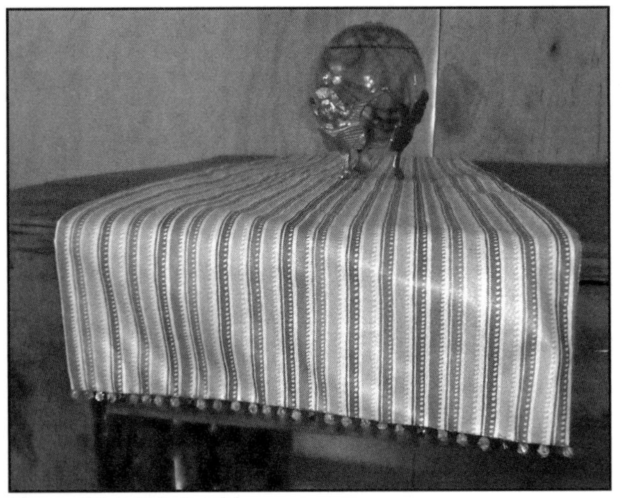

Figure 11-4. Fabric table runner.

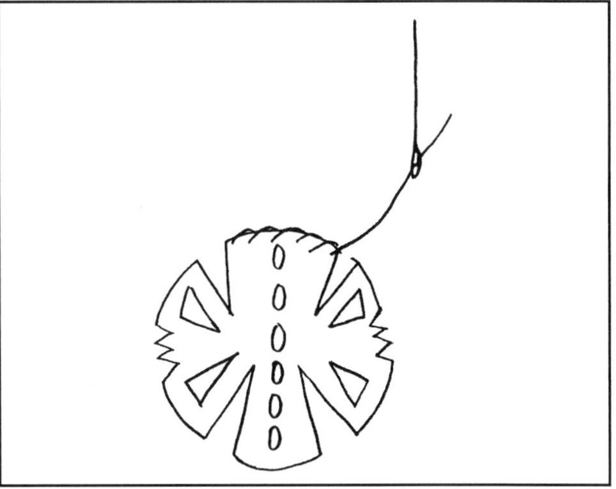

Figure 11-5. Appliqué using a whip stitch.

Change It

One way to modify the runner is to appliqué pieces of fabric of a contrasting color to the top piece of the runner (before sewing it to the back), either by hand or with the sewing machine. A variety of stitches and methods (Figure 11-5) can be used to stitch them down (Creekmore, 1968). Remember that any raw edges will probably fray when the material is washed; folding the edges under before sewing (or using a nonfraying fabric) will prevent this. There are a number of ways to grade this activity up, primarily by adding decoration to the top piece before sewing. Appliqué, mentioned above, is one method. Others are embroidery or cross stitch, or sewing on beads or sequins. A quilted runner can be made by first basting batting to the wrong side of one of the fabric pieces, sewing as described above, then quilting over the completed runner.

To grade the activity down, create a simple alternative that requires minimal "sewing" and can be completed in less than 30 minutes. Use only one piece of a nonfraying fabric such as fleece, felt, or burlap. One row at a time, fold the fabric lengthwise and cut small slits—evenly or randomly—along the fold. Do as many lengthwise rows as desired, or just go around each edge. Once the slits are completed, thread a length of ribbon—at least as long as the runner—in a plastic needlepoint needle (see Figure 11-1), then weave the ribbon in and out of the slits in each row (Figure 11-6). The ends can be left hanging, or can be secured under the edge with a stitch or two or with fabric glue. This adaptation would be useful for children or the elderly, especially if the therapist completes the step of preparing the fabric. Fabrics such as felt that don't fray and look the same on both sides are useful when simplicity is needed.

Document It

Below are examples of ways to document the use of needlework in order to demonstrate skilled intervention and application to areas of occupation.

- "During a sewing activity, the client was able to use tactile cues only to locate where to insert the needle, increasing efficiency in compensation for vision loss."
- "The client was able to create a supply list for her desired sewing project with only occasional cueing from the therapist. She utilized a cognitive strategy of "backward chaining" to recall all items needed."
- "The client consistently observed work simplification principles, using written reminders posted by the therapist, while working on a home sewing project."

Other Ideas and Grading

Many needlework projects are simple enough to be regularly included in the therapeutic activity arsenal. Items that can be easily sewn by hand or by machine include banners, windsocks, throw pillows, and tote bags, and some project ideas require no sewing at all. Articles such as baby bibs, table runners, napkins, and

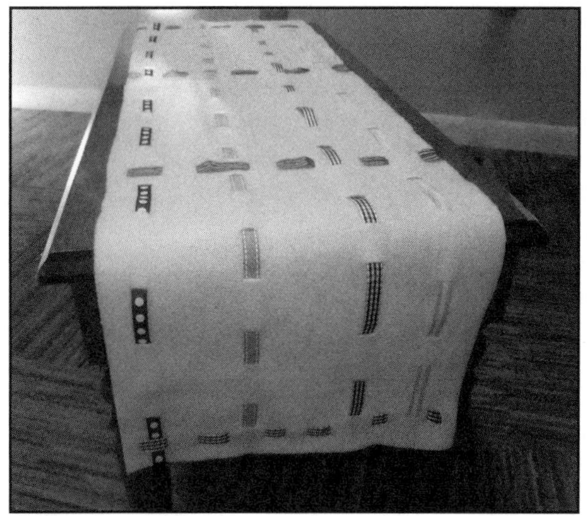

Figure 11-6. Ribbon-woven fleece runner.

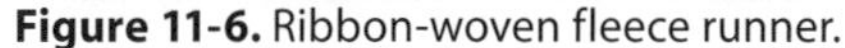

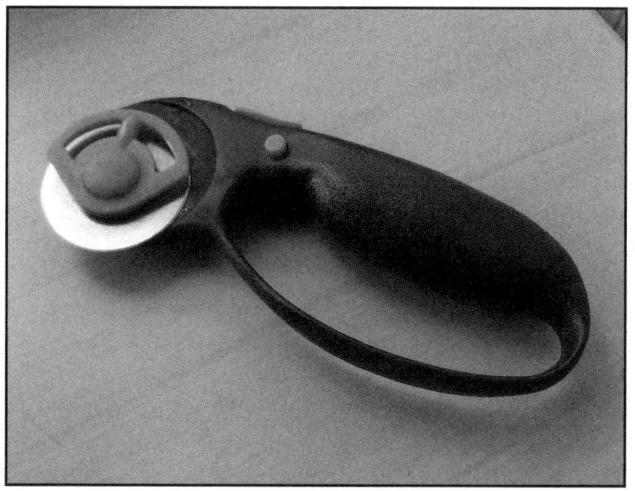

Figure 11-7. A rolling cutter for fabric.

pillowcases are good items for cross stitching and the designs can be copied or created by the client. Small needlepoint projects are plentiful: eyeglass cases, tissue box covers, coasters, bookmarks, and Christmas tree ornaments are just a few. Locker hooking, similar to both latchhook and needlepoint, uses strips of fabric in place of yarn and can be used to make attractive potholders, book covers, coasters, pillows covers, or small rugs. Rake knitting, another yarn craft, requires use of a loom-like device and may be easier for some clients than traditional knitting. Needlefelting is a recently popularized needlecraft that requires few tools and materials. The needle is extremely sharp, but the process requires little more than a repetitive stabbing motion, so an individual with less-than-normal dexterity could be successful with some projects. Weaving, technically more a fiber craft than a needle craft, is another way of using yarn or fabric that may be a good alternative for clients who have difficulty handling a needle. Simple weaving projects include making looper potholders and ribbon weaving (see Project Variation in this chapter). Other fabric crafts that eliminate the need for a needle are velvet embossing, fabric fusing, and felt making. Velvet embossing is done by placing the material over a raised design, such as a stamp, and ironing (Hall, 2001). Fusible fabric art is done with fabric scraps, fusible webbing, and an iron; no sewing is required (Walter, 1996). Felting is a process using wool batting and hot water to create a strong, no-fray fabric that can then be used in assorted ways. While the materials may be somewhat expensive for regular clinic use, scraps from old sweaters may be an affordable substitute.

Given the variety of needlework crafts, ways of grading are plentiful as well. The size of the needle, the weight of the yarn, and the work surface can all be changed to meet client needs. For example, doing needlepoint on plastic canvas with a plastic needle is usually simpler (and safer) than using a metal needle on a fine mesh canvas. For any method, designs can be plain or complex, stitch size can be large or small, and the project can encompass one or multiple steps. For instance, colorful napkins can be made by simply cutting and hemming fabric; or they can be embroidered or appliquéd and become much more complex. Clients can create their own designs and patterns, or can follow a preprinted one. Creations can be made with yarn or fabric and glue, without needle and thread, as in coiled yarn pictures. There are different styles of adapted scissors, embroidery hoops, lights and magnifiers, and other devices to compensate for physical limitations. For clients who cannot or should not use conventional scissors, rolling cutters (Figure 11-7) are a useful substitute for many functions. Be aware, however, that the blade is very sharp!

Main Therapeutic Applications

Physical Dysfunction

Needlework is the kind of craft that can be done easily by bed-bound patients. Small projects require little energy expenditure and can be done by frail or deconditioned clients. It can be stopped when the client becomes fatigued and resumed when the client is refreshed. Because the materials are inexpensive, they can be left in client rooms, for example if the client wants to work on the project outside of therapy, or in the case of isolation. Scissors are easily sterilized with disinfectants, but the therapist should dry them completely to prevent rusting. Larger needles and hooks can also be sterilized between clients, and smaller needles can be thrown away.

Needlecraft uses primarily distal joint and muscle actions but most projects involve some amount of elbow and forearm movement as well as proximal stability. Since it provides little resistance, clients with arthritic pain or deformities can still enjoy needlework, as long as it is structured to minimize long periods of static holding. Maintaining a static grasp for an extended period of time can damage an inflamed joint; resistive pinch and grasp should be avoided as well. Those with arthritis who desire to participate in needlework should be instructed to take frequent rest breaks and to respect pain (Melvin, 1998). A qualitative study done with a group of women with chronic physical conditions revealed many positive effects of engaging in needlework, including reduced anxiety and depression, relief from pain, development of social contacts, and creation of tangible proof of "good days" in the course of the illness or disability (Reynolds, 1997). Another study showed that women who sewed had decreased heart rate, blood pressure, and perspiration compared to women involved in other types of leisure activity (Reiner, 1995). Some forms of needlecraft are difficult if not impossible for the visually impaired, but some adaptations may allow the tactile sense to substitute for vision. Sewing projects are possible with the use of only one extremity, but adapted techniques and/ or equipment will likely be necessary. In the case of hemiplegia, the client may be able to use the affected extremity as a stabilizer and will thus receive important sensory input. Overall, the motor skills required for sewing can translate into many functional daily tasks such as dressing, grooming, and feeding (Bergman, 2010).

Mental Health

Embroidery can be very structured, as in cross stitch, or it can be a challenging, creative endeavor. Needlework can be used in the acute stages of depressive illness, as it requires little exertion and can be accomplished despite the fatigue reported by many depressed clients. In fact, people have traditionally used needlecraft, for example quilting, for relaxation. Due to the tangible and visual qualities of needlework, clients with difficulty focusing their thoughts may benefit from the repetition required in this craft (Brown, 2011). The therapist should carefully analyze the proposed activity to ensure as much as possible that the client will be successful, which may include assistance for certain steps (Early, 2009). This is important for maintaining a sense of control on the part of the client, as well as avoiding frustration or anger. Once the particular motor skills are learned, most people find needlework a relaxing occupation. Clients with mental retardation can be successful with projects that have simple, repetitive visual and motor patterns. All standard precautions for sharps should be observed for clients with any level of cognitive impairment.

Pediatrics

Needlework is a useful craft for both boys and girls, incorporating many perceptual and fine motor skills that children need to develop, such as hand-eye coordination, and for children under age 6 it usually has no gender connotations. Sewing cards—cardboard with holes punched along the outline of a picture—are often used for beginners. Sewing can be presented to children as just another way of making a picture. They can be shown how to draw an outline on cloth and then stitch over it. The activity can be structured to avoid too much repetition that may lose a child's interest. Burlap or other coarse cloth and large plastic needles are appropriate for children's needlework; cloth with a finer weave requires sharp metal needles that are not appropriate for young children. If a therapist plans to do such a needlework project with a group of children, it may be best to cut the yarn and thread all the needles before the children arrive, as they have trouble waiting their turn for help in threading their needle (Gaitskell & Hurwitz, 1975) and may become distracted playing with the yarn. Projects appropriate for children of different ages include wall hangings, puppets, placemats, and simple dolls or doll clothes. Children enjoy embellishing their creations with beads, buttons, sequins, and iron-on patches.

Adolescents

Unlike children, most adolescents do perceive needlework as a female occupation, and the therapist should respect their preferences and interests in activity selection. Many teens may view some forms of needlework as old-fashioned, yet may enjoy embellishing their clothing with beads, sequins, fur, or feathers. Adolescents could also work collaboratively on a group quilt or flag that displays a common theme or a sense of unity or belonging, incorporating needlework techniques in its construction. Or they may benefit from working together to make costumes for a group production. Apart from sewing as a craft, all school children of any age can benefit from knowing how to sew on a button or do other simple clothing repair using a needle and thread. Some adolescents may also be interested in learning how to use a sewing machine to make clothing or items for their room or home.

Older Adults

Many elderly women have sewn and mended for themselves and their families throughout their lives. While females will often willingly try a traditionally male craft, fewer men will participate in female-identified crafts such as needlework. Because many older women are familiar with sewing—either from necessity or as a hobby—it is usually easier to pique their interest in a needlework project. If there is a type of needlecraft with which they are already familiar, that may be the best place to start (Gould & Gould, 1971). If low vision interferes, as is common in elderly clients, using bright colors on a white background to create a contrast will make it easier for them to see. A clamp-on magnifying glass may be attached to the edge of the table if necessary. Full spectrum lamps are also available, some with magnifying lenses included. Individuals with peripheral neuropathy, common in diabetes, need to use extra care not to stick themselves with the needles. Since their sensation is an unreliable guide, using a thimble is recommended. In this population, any injury will take longer to heal, and an undetected injury could develop an infection. Other clients who warrant close supervision in the use of sharp tools are those taking blood thinners and those with dementia or other cognitive impairments that affect judgment or behavior regulation. If an elderly person wants to do a project that is too difficult, the therapist should make sure that a simplified substitute is not demeaning to that client.

Groups

Quilting has been a popular group activity for centuries, so there is a strong precedent for group sewing. Larger needlework projects, such as quilts or flags, are excellent choices for groups who may be together for a period of weeks or months, as in extended addiction treatment programs or residential facilities. For example, a group of adolescents may enjoy making a quilt out of their old T-shirts. These projects allow individual expression, yet result in a final product that signifies group unity and teamwork. The occupational therapist might provide a theme as a starting point, then group members can apply individual creative interpretations. Children could make squares by gluing, rather than sewing, fabrics and then work together to create a story from their designs. The storytelling may then serve as an outlet for negative feelings (Parham & Fazio, 1997).

Case Study

Virginia is a 79-year-old woman who suffered a stroke while on vacation with her family in Florida, and the left cerebrovascular accident (CVA) resulted in a right hemiparesis. Virginia completed the acute phase of hospitalization in Florida, but wanted to be closer to home for her long-term rehabilitation. She was transferred to a large rehab center approximately 50 miles from her hometown and her family. The planned length of stay was 2 to 3 weeks. Virginia's only son planned for her to move in with him and his family following her rehabilitation, but she fully hoped and expected to return to her own home.

The occupational therapist at the rehabilitation center used the Canadian Occupational Performance Measure (Law et al., 1994) to interview Virginia at her first therapy session. She discovered that Virginia's family had moved to the United States from Ireland while she was still a teenager. She stated that her family was hard working but never accumulated much financially. Virginia had worked for many years at a garment factory; she was widowed at age 62 and retired at age 72. She had remained active in many leisure pursuits, including social and volunteer activities, cooking, and knitting, and she identified all of these as valued roles during the interview. She had always lived frugally and described herself as independent and self-reliant. Her goals for therapy were to regain this independent and active way of life to the fullest extent possible.

During the objective portion of the evaluation, the occupational therapist found that Virginia's vision, cognition, and sensation were intact. Her dominant right upper extremity and lower extremity were hypotonic; she was unable to ambulate or use her right arm functionally, but she was able to transfer to and from her wheelchair with supervision. She followed instructions well and seemed like an excellent candidate for regaining function through compensatory methods. Initially, Virginia and the therapist made the following goals: to increase manipulation skills in the nondominant hand, to consistently use the right upper extremity as an active stabilizer, and to independently manage self-care tasks.

Virginia was quick to learn self-range of motion exercises and was faithful in correctly positioning her right arm. She persevered in trying to do things with her left hand and encouraged the therapist to challenge her. During one treatment session, Virginia saw another therapist using the clinic sewing machine to make a universal cuff. She asked her therapist if she could try sewing since it was already familiar to her. With Virginia's guidance, the occupational therapist gathered the needed items—a pattern, fabric, thread, straight pins, a rolling cutter, and a pair of left-handed scissors—and she began to work. During the process, the therapist suggested various compensatory techniques and was pleasantly surprised at Virginia's ability to cut out the pattern, pin it to the fabric, and cut the fabric, all with one hand. As she began to sew, her proficiency with her left hand was impressive, and with occasional instruction and cueing, she also began to use her right arm to help stabilize. She also exhibited good safety awareness throughout the project. With almost no assistance, Virginia was able to make herself a skirt with the use of only one hand. As the practice of positioning her right upper extremity for use as a stabilizer became habitual, Virginia also gained independence in self-care. By discharge, she was able to manage all her personal needs, and her son was willing to let her return to her own home on a trial basis.

Discussion Questions

1. What skills would a client need to possess to participate in this type activity, given the average therapist's limitations in providing one-on-one treatment? In what setting(s) would this craft be most useful and why?
2. Which needlecraft(s) would be the least likely to cause a needle puncture wound?
3. Which needlecraft(s) might be easiest for a client with low vision?
4. Do you perceive sewing to be a modern craft or a useful skill? Explain.

Resources

Kanzashi in Bloom: 20 Simple Fold and Sew Project to Wear and Give
By Diane Gilliland
Watson-Guptill Publications, 2009

Simply Felt: 20 Easy and Elegant Designs in Wool
By Margaret Docherty and Jayne Emerson
Interweave Press, 2004

Simply Needlefelt: 20 Easy and Elegant Designs
By Jayne Emerson
Interweave Press, 2009
Simple projects for a newly popular needlecraft.

Reader's Digest Complete Book of Embroidery
By Melinda Cross
The Reader's Digest Association, Inc., 1996
Contains an index, glossary, colored drawings, and photographs with patterns interspersed throughout the book. Excellent clarity of explanations.

The Good Housekeeping Illustrated Book of Needlecrafts
By Cecelia K. Toth (Ed.)
Hearst Books, 2001 paperback edition
A compendium of knitting, crotchet, embroidery, needlepoint, quilting, and rug making. Excellent color photo illustrations.

Sewing for Children
By Emma Hardy
Cico, 2010
Basic projects to teach kids beginning sewing skills.

Arts and Crafts Needlepoint
By Beth Russell
Anova Books, 2006
Updated version of an older book with classic needlepoint designs along with some art history.

Start Quilting With Alex Anderson, 3rd Edition: Everything First-time Quilters Need to Succeed
By Alex Anderson
C & T Publishing, 2009
Good book for beginners; includes projects.

The Complete Photo Guide to Crochet
By Margaret Hubert
Creative Publishing International, 2010
Full-color guide with instructions for many stitches and patterns for projects

The Chicks With Sticks Guide to Knitting: Learn to Knit with More Than 30 Cool, Easy Patterns
By Nancy Queen and Mary Ellen O'Connell
Watson-Guptill/Crown Publishing, 2008
Learn basic stitches, includes updated project ideas.

Hook, Loop 'n' Lock: Create Fun and Easy Locker Hooked Projects
By Theresa Pulido
Krause Publications, 2009
Instructions for basic techniques and lots of projects. Helpful pictures and clear instructions.

References

ABC Needlework & Crafts Magazines. (1984). *McCall's needlework and crafts: Scrap crafts*. New York, NY: Sedgewood Press.
Banks, M. (1979). *Anonymous was a woman*. New York, NY: St. Martinis Press.
Bergman, S. The use of needle crafts in occupational therapy. *TQS Articles*. Retrieved from www.thequiltshow.com/os/articles.php/articles_id/26.
Better Homes and Gardens. (1966). *Stitchery and crafts*. New York, NY: Meredith Press.
Brown, C., & Stoffel, V. C. (Eds.). (2011). *Occupational therapy in mental health: A vision for participation*. Philadelphia, PA: F. A. Davis Co.
Carroll, A. (1947). *The good house keeping needlecraft encyclopedia*. New York, NY: Rinehart & Company.
Creekmore, B. B. (1968). *Traditional American crafts*. New York, NY: Hearthside Press.
Department of the Army. (1971). *Craft techniques in occupational therapy*. Washington, DC: US Government Printing Office.
Earhart, C. A., Allen, C. K., & Blue, T. (1993). *Allen diagnostic module*. Colchester, CT: S & S Worldwide.
Early, M. B. (2009). *Mental health concepts and techniques for the occupational therapy assistant* (4th ed.). Philadelphia, PA: Lippincott Williams & Wilkins.
Fidler, G., & Velde, B. (1999). *Activities: Reality and symbol*. Thorofare, NJ: SLACK Incorporated
Gaitskell, C. D., & Hurwitz, A. (1975). *Children and their art* (3rd ed.). New York, NY: Harcourt, Brace, Jovanovitch.
Gould, E., & Gould, L. (1971). *Crafts for the elderly*. Springfield, IL: Charles C. Thomas Publisher.

Gregory, M. D. (1983). Occupational behavior and life satisfaction among retirees. *American Journal of Occupational Therapy, 37*(8), 548-553.
Hall, M. A., Wrobel, J., & Salamony, S. (2001). *Decorative crafts sourcebook.* San Diego, CA: Thunder Bay Press.
Hemphill, B. J., Peterson, C. Q., & Werner, P. C. (1991). *Rehabilitation in mental health: Goals and objectives for independent living.* Thorofare, NJ: SLACK Incorporated.
Law, M., Baptiste, S., Carswell, A., McColl, M. A., Polatajko, H., & Pollock, H. (1994). *Candian occupational therapy measure.* Toronto, Canada: Canadian Association of Occupational Therapists.
Melville, S. (1998). *Crafts for all abilities.* Tumbridge Wells, Kent, UK: Search Press Limited
Melvin, J., & Jensen, G. (1998). *Rheumatologic rehabilitation series: Assessment and management.* Bethesda, MD: American Occupational Therapy Association.
Moseley, S., Johnson, P., & Koenig, H. (1962). *Crafts design.* Belmont, CA: Wadsworth.
Parham, L. D., & Fazio, L. (Eds.). (1997). *Play in occupational therapy for children.* St. Louis, MO: Mosby.
Pedretti, L. S., & Early, M. B. (Eds.). (2001). *Occupational therapy: Practice skills for physical dysfunction* (5th ed.). St. Louis, MO: Mosby.
Pigza, J. (2008). *Craft therapy: Then and now.* Retrieved from www.drupal02.nypl.org/blogs/2008/05/07/craft-therapy-then-and-now.
Pulido, T. (2009). *Hook, loop, 'n' lock: Create fun and easy locker hooked projects.* Cincinnati, OH: Krause Publications.
Reader's Digest. (1979). *Crafts and hobbies.* Pleasantville, NY: The Reader's Digest Association Inc.
Reiner, R. H. (1995). Quick update: Stress reduction's common thread. *Journal of the American Medical Association, 274*(4), 291.
Reynolds, F. (1997). Coping with chronic illness and disability through creative needlecraft. *British Journal of Occupational Therapy, 60*(8), 352-356.
Scharff, R. (1952). *Handbook of crafts.* Greenville, CT: Fawcett Publications.
Walter, C. (1996). *Snippet sensations: Fast, fusible fabric art for quilted or framed projects.* Iola, WI: Krause Publications.

□ □ □ □ □ □ □ 12

Gardening and Nature Crafts

Objectives

The student should be able to:

- Discuss historical/cultural examples of the therapeutic uses of gardening
- List basic supplies and materials needed to do simple gardening/nature crafts
- Know how to complete and grade basic projects involving gardening and natural materials
- Explain advantages and limitations of gardening activities in therapy
- List precautions of gardening/nature craft activities
- Describe how gardening/nature crafts might be used with various therapy client populations

In looking for design and color ideas for creative projects—from home decorating to fine art—one need look no further than a neighborhood garden or wildflower-studded roadside. The beauty of nature is not only a source of rich artistic inspiration, but can also be a source of the actual materials used in crafting. Manipulation of flowers or other natural materials can produce decorative or functional objects every bit as attractive as those made from purchased materials. Cultivation of plants and flowers, while not a craft in the more traditional sense of the word, is nonetheless a creative, regenerative pursuit that has been shown to have highly therapeutic qualities (Wichrowski, Whiteson, Haas, Mola, & Rey, 2005).

Agriculture as a way of life has been around for thousands of years, but the use of leisure gardening and horticulture also has a long history, both as a hobby and as a part of therapeutic regimens. State hospitals for the mentally ill have used farming and gardening as work and rehabilitative activities since their inception; as early as 1768, Benjamin Rush proposed that digging in the soil had a curative effect (Relf, 1973). In fact, gardens were intentionally incorporated into the design of early asylum grounds because of their health-restoring properties (Spurgeon, 2005). The propagation and maintenance of houseplants probably developed as a hobby around the time of the exploration of the Americas. Ships traveling to distant, often tropical, lands were able to bring back exotic plant species, and Europeans built greenhouses and conservatories to replicate the environmental conditions necessary to maintain these plants year round. Many of today's common houseplants and outdoor flowering plants were imported from locales such as Africa, Japan, and China. Europeans were able to hybridize many of these varieties and featured them in elaborate gardens (*Reader's Digest*, 1979).

Tubbs, C., & Drake, M. *Crafts and Creative Media in Therapy, Fourth Edition (pp. 143-154).*

Incorporation of plants and other natural materials for ornamentation as an aspect of rituals and cultural festivities is also evident throughout history. American Indians used leaves, berries, and flowers to make natural dyes to decorate their homes, clothing, and even their skin. They used bones, seeds, feathers, and fur to create jewelry and headdresses, many with special ceremonial purposes or meaning. The popularity of the use of natural materials in crafts has fluctuated over the years but has always maintained a presence. A visitor to any craft fair will see many examples of this, from fine woven pine needle baskets to driftwood sculptures to dried flower wreaths and arrangements. This diverse group of media offers a wide array of affordable projects, with many of the materials as close as one's backyard. The therapist may even choose to start with the cultivation of plants—literally, from the ground up—and thereby create opportunities for both short- and long-term projects.

Currently, therapy clinics utilize horticulture/plant products in various ways, and numerous research articles and personal narratives substantiate their benefits. For example, a study published in 2005 demonstrated that, compared to a control group, cardiac patients who engaged in a horticulture program had lowered heart rates and improvement in their mood disturbance score. Other team members noticed positive results as well, such as increased and more animated interpersonal interaction (American Occupational Therapy Foundation [AOTF], 2005; Wichrowski et al., 2005). One outpatient physical dysfunction clinic has implemented a hay bale gardening program in which some clients plant and tend the crops, others build necessary components, such as trellises, and some pick and then prepare the vegetables in the rehab kitchen. Planting in hay bales instead of in the ground raises the plants to a more accessible height (Morris, 2005; see Agrability Project in Resources section). Other rehabilitation facilities keep houseplants for clients to tend; still others maintain outdoor gardening stations with raised planting tables or small flower gardens. State hospitals continue to use gardening in various levels of complexity for both leisure and pre-vocational goals. Some Alzheimer's programs utilize therapeutic gardens not only to afford opportunities for structured and routine activities, but also to provide an environment with abundant sensory stimulation for more impaired clients (Fisher's Center for Alzheimer's Research Foundation). Many nursing homes have courtyards with flower gardens, bird feeders, and birdbaths, and residents may be involved in their maintenance. Nature projects are also popular with children and can range from planting flower seeds to creating cards or pictures with found natural objects.

Special Considerations and Precautions

Horticulture Activities

While nature crafts require the same activity analysis as the crafts from any other category, gardening/horticulture has some unique aspects that require extra deliberation. If occupational therapists wish to implement long-term gardening projects, they must consider space, cost, the time required for planning and preparation, and administrative and peer support. A medium- or large-scale endeavor might require the work of several team members and significant start-up expense. Once the program is underway though, maintenance costs should be minimal. The out-of-doors, while beneficial for most, may pose hazards for some clients, for example those with plants or insect allergies or for whom exposure to sunlight is contraindicated. Use of fertilizers or pesticides is discouraged; if application of these products seems necessary, use the organic variety when possible. Indoor gardening projects are also an option; in addition to the above factors, the therapist must also consider available lighting and feasible plant selection. Both indoor and outdoor gardening are dirty activities, so both client and therapist should be prepared by wearing adequate protection for skin and clothing (e.g., gloves and aprons) and any indoor work areas should be covered as well.

Keep in mind that any project that involves plant cultivation is necessarily a long-term undertaking. This does not absolutely preclude it from use in shorter-term settings, but it must be structured such that the clients can easily discern, and benefit from, their individual roles in the process. In addition, not all gardening ventures have guaranteed success, so the clients should be able to tolerate (or even benefit from) some level of disappointment. Once established, therapeutic gardening projects take on a life and rhythm of their own; maintenance is often easier than the preliminary work.

Crafting With Natural Materials

In crafting with natural materials, precautions are the same as for other activities, for example, exercising care in the use of sharp tools, glues, and nonedible materials. Allergies and outdoor hazards should be considered if the project includes the gathering of items from a garden or forested area. Any plants with thorns should be avoided, and plant parts with other sharp protrusions, such as pinecones or holly leaves, should be handled with care. Leaves, sticks, rocks, and other items gathered from outside will be dirty, so hands should be thoroughly washed afterwards. Some natural objects, for example dried flowers, are relatively fragile, so the therapist should choose materials compatible with a client's handling skills. Naturally growing materials are free of cost; depending on how they are to be used, they can certainly be an economical craft choice.

Container Gardening Project—"Desert" Garden

Plan It

Some houseplants, for example Swedish Ivy, Pothos, and Wandering Jew, are easily rooted from cuttings, so are good choices for simple potting projects. Coleus, an outdoor annual, comes in many colors and also roots well from cuttings. The reader should refer to more comprehensive sources for other economical plant selections, as well as those that should be avoided. In general, avoid plants that require fastidious care, those that are thorny or poisonous, and those that might spread too rapidly and become a nuisance. The plants suggested in the project below require little water or other care and will grow from cuttings with no rooting necessary.

Get Ready

Supplies

- Flower pot or other planting container, about 8 inches in diameter, with drain hole; a shallow planter will also work well
- Saucer large enough to accommodate container (optional)
- Gravel or rocks
- Potting soil
- Succulent plants such as aloe vera, sedum, kalanchoe—can be snipped from larger parent plants
- Decorative rocks as desired

Tools

- Scissors or shears
- Small trowel or a large spoon
- Gloves

Time required: 20 minutes

Cost: Variable; small succulent plants are $2 to $3 dollars each, but cuttings from larger plants will work just as well

Do It

Process

1. In the container, spread a layer of gravel or rocks about 1 inch thick.
2. Add soil to within about 2 inches from the top.
3. Carefully insert plants, spaced 1 to 2 inches apart. Put shorter plants toward the front/outside, taller plants toward the back/middle (Figure 12-1).

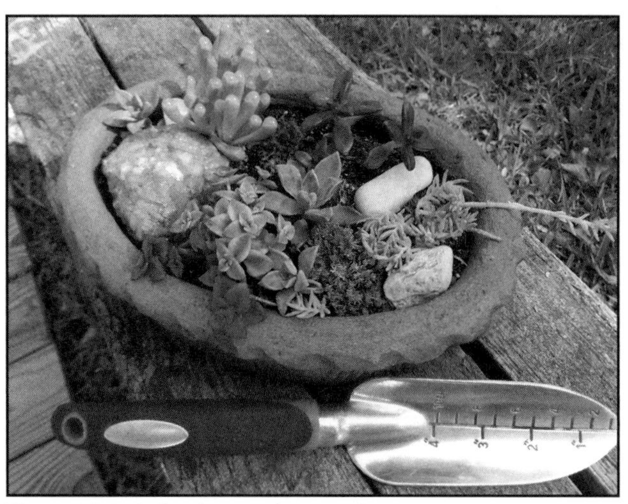

Figure 12-1. A simple succulent garden.

4. If desired, add stones, moss, large glass beads, or other decorative matter to fill the rest of the pot.
5. Water but allow it to drain completely before placing the pot in the saucer.
6. Instruct the client to water sparingly.

Change It

Ways to modify this project include using different plants or different types of pots, or decorating the pot in some way before planting. To grade up, have the client embellish the container before planting using terra cotta markers, paints, or mosaic or découpaging techniques. For example, spread an acrylic paint over a fern or other leaf, then gently place the leaf, paint-side down, on the exterior of the pot. Place a piece of newspaper over the leaf and, taking care not to let it move, press down over the surface of the leaf to transfer the paint.

To grade down, reduce the number of plants choices and the size of the pot. Or simply transfer a purchased plant from its plastic container into a new pot. The client could also arrange artificial plants or flowers if motor/dexterity deficits interfere with handling live plants.

Document It

The following are suggested ways to document a gardening or planting activity to represent work toward improving performance skills or areas of occupation.

- "The client was able to independently select and arrange plants in the pot without cueing for decision making."
- "The client worked on a planting activity in standing. He required minimal assistance for dynamic balance but tolerated 10 minutes of standing without rest."

Nature Craft Project—Wood Circle Ornaments

Plan It

This craft requires discs cut from a tree limb. Cutting them is simple with a chop or miter saw but this would almost certainly have to be done at another location ahead of time. This could also be done with a chain saw. The therapist without these tools will need to solicit help from a friend, lumberyard, or hardware store.

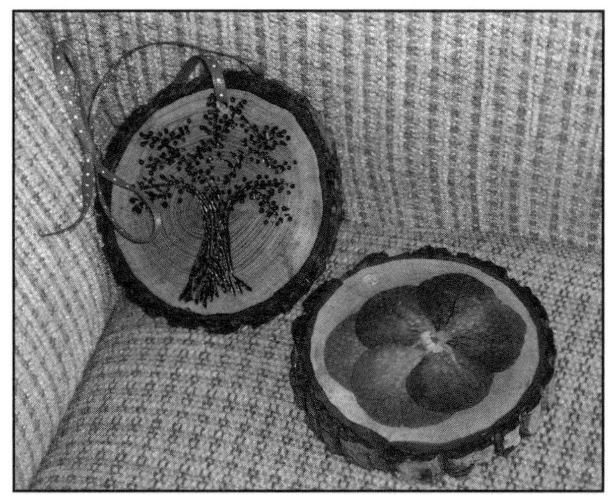

Figure 12-2. Wooden disc ornaments: wood-burned and with pressed flower.

Get Ready

Supplies

- Discs of wood cut from large tree branches (4 to 6 inches in diameter and about 1 inch thick), with or without intact bark
- Pencil or chalk
- Clear acrylic sealer
- Acrylic paint (optional)
- Ribbon or string for hanging, if desired

Tools

- Wood burner
- Hand drill
- Paint brush(es)

Time required: 20 minutes

Cost: None

Do It

Process

1. Have wooden discs pre-cut. If the therapist has no access to a suitable saw—such as a chop saw—smaller size discs can be cut with sharp pruning shears.
2. Sketch the desired design on the surface of the wood.
3. Drill a hole near the edge, at the top of the design, for the hanger, if desired.
4. Using the wood burner, go over the design. Follow directions with the wood burning tool for use of specific tips and safety precautions.
5. Spray or brush with clear acrylic sealer.
6. When thoroughly dry, tie a string or ribbon through the hole for hanging (Figure 12-2).

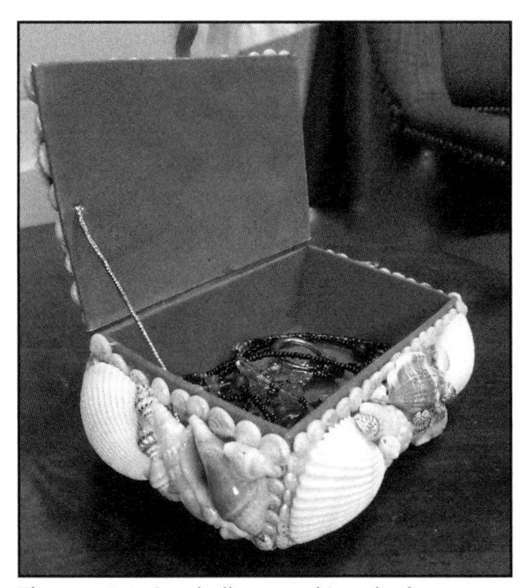

Figure 12-3. Seashell covered jewelry box.

Change It

For an easy variation, paint the design instead of burning it into the wood. To grade this activity up, increase the size of the discs and the complexity of the design. The therapist may want to have prepared designs from which the client can choose. Or do multiple smaller discs and then use them to decorate another object, such covering the edge of a picture frame or the outside of a flower pot (Wasinger, 2009).

To grade this activity down, have the client paint a design or glue items, such as seeds or pressed flowers, on the wooden disc (see Figure 12-2).

Other Ideas and Grading

Ideas for simple gardening/therapeutic horticulture and nature crafts are abundant and easy to find; see Appendices I and II and Resources at the end of the chapter. The Internet, homemaking magazines, and craft books with recycling or holiday themes are good places to look. The following options represent only a small sampling of the possibilities.

Pressed flowers can be used in making paper crafts such as greeting cards, bookmarks, or gift wrap, or can be used as decoration on other projects such as picture frames, flower pots, or in scrapbooking. Flat flowers like pansies work best for pressing; place flowers between paper towels and place them under several books for a few days. Flowers sealed under different types of semi-clear craft paper, such as vellum, create interesting effects (Hall, 2001). Whole flowers can also be dried by hanging or using dessicants, but remember that the drying process takes several weeks. Dried flowers can be used in arrangements, shadow box collages, or as ingredients in potpourri mixes. Colorful flowers or green leaves can be hammered between layers of light fabric to transfer their natural dyes.

Green leaves can also be used as the impression for rubbings or prints. For rubbings, hold paper securely on top of the leaf to keep it from sliding, then rub firmly across the paper with the side of a crayon, pastel, or pencil lead. Vary the design by using differently-shaped leaves or overlapping images. For prints, cover the surface of a fresh leaf evenly with ink or paint using a brayer. Carefully place the leaf, paint side down, onto paper. Place a scrap piece of paper on top and gently press all the way across the leaf. Green or colorful fall leaves can be pressed and dried in the same way as flowers, then used in similar applications. Leaves and flowers can also be used with sun-sensitive paper to create quick, simple nature prints.

Simple painted pinecones can be used in groupings or baskets to make easy table centerpieces. Or brush petal tips with glue and sprinkle with glitter. Natural materials such as berries, nuts, and pinecones, along with a glue gun, can turn a plain grapevine wreath into a seasonal wall hanging. Mosaic techniques can be used with shells, beans, seeds, pebbles, or eggshells instead of ceramic tiles (see Chapter 6), or these same items can be used to cover trinket boxes or picture frames (Figure 12-3). Natural objects, such as gourds, pieces of driftwood, or large rocks, can be painted with designs of choice then used as either indoor or outdoor decoration. Flowers and leaves can be cast in plaster to make garden plaques. Other ideas for outdoor ornamentation include stepping stones, birdhouses, or birdbaths.

There are a number of ways gardening and/or nature crafts can be used with a group. The following ideas provide general guidelines that can be adapted to individual circumstances. Start a therapy garden by having a group of clients plan and execute a gardening project of their choice. They can prepare a garden plot directly in the ground, or utilize planters, pots, hay bales, or other container system. They can choose to grow vegetables, annual or perennial flowers, or a combination. Planters can be painted or otherwise decorated; an ambitious group might even choose to enhance the entire garden area with bird feeders, banners, or art objects. Work on the project can be divided among members according to ability, need, and personal preference, and this may be structured as a long-term project involving multiple groups or individuals over time. Thorough planning prior to implementation will have the greatest assurance of success in both process and outcome. The therapist should have a basic knowledge of gardening, including planting techniques, watering and sunlight needs, and general time tables for growing common plants. Most plants, whether in the ground or in containers, require adequate drainage, so soil type or container design must accommodate this need. In deciding what to grow, consider later uses, such as for cooking (vegetable, herbs) or craft projects (dried or pressed flowers and leaves). A group garden project is ideal for a long-term setting but is also useful in the shorter term, especially if clients can return later to see the results of their work and its benefit to other clients.

A group of clients could also decorate a space or a bulletin board for a holiday, party, or other special occasion. Fall or Halloween celebrations are especially appropriate because of connections to harvest time. Clients could make wreaths from natural materials such as corn shucks—simply tie the shucks in half around a circular frame—berries, or dried fruit. Make a border for a bulletin board using a mosaic of beans or seeds or using leaf rubbings. Make table decorations with twig vases—glue small twigs around an empty vegetable or potato chip can—then fill with dried flowers and grasses; or iron leaves between waxed paper to make placemats. Again, planning is probably the most important component. Whatever project is chosen should provide a meaningful role for each participant.

Container gardening, an alternative for full-scale outdoor gardening, can take on various forms. Clients could choose cacti or succulents and add rocks or wood to create an artistic, southwestern, or Oriental look (see Figure 12-1). Mixed annuals can be artfully arranged in pots, window boxes, or hanging baskets and placed in courtyards, entryways, or hospital room windows. Depending on flower type, clients may be able to make small fresh flower bouquets or corsages from the plants they grow. Bonsai is another container gardening option, but it requires a special knowledge to do correctly. A therapist planning to utilize horticulture as a treatment option needs to be ready and willing to commit extra time to maintenance of plants and cleaning of the growing area, since there will be times that none of the clients have an interest in participating in this craft.

Horticulture activities can be graded or adapted in a number of ways. One popular gardening adaptation is the use of raised beds. Planters or terraced beds can be built to the necessary height to accommodate individuals in wheelchairs or those with limited standing tolerance. Some facilities have even more elaborate gardens that incorporate ramps and railings for full wheelchair accessibility (Bupa Health Information, 2005). Hay bale gardening is another relatively new and economical idea for raised bed gardening (Wise, 2005). For indoor gardening, the therapist can consider client ability and/or therapeutic goals and place pots accordingly. Plant containers can be large or small, light or heavy, purchased or made from recycled items. The primary requirements are that they can hold water—but also have a means of drainage—and that the material of which they are made can tolerate moisture over an extended period of time. For example, a metal or plastic coffee can serve as a flower pot if it has a few holes drilled through the bottom, but a cardboard box will deteriorate in a relatively short time.

Many adapted gardening tools are available from either online or traditional retailers. These tools help compensate for weak or inefficient grasp, inability to use an extremity, or poor overall endurance/generalized weakness. Choices include tools with ergonomically designed handles, ratcheting pruners, oscillating hoes, and one-handed flower snips (Bupa Health Information, 2005; Culver, 2005). See Appendices I and II and Resources at the end of this chapter for a listing of sources for both tools and gardening ideas.

Plant size and longevity, along with care needs (i.e., including light, water, and fertilization) should be considered when planning horticulture projects (Bupa Health Information, 2005). Some plants grow well despite some neglect and in less-than-ideal conditions; these are recommended for beginners or those with

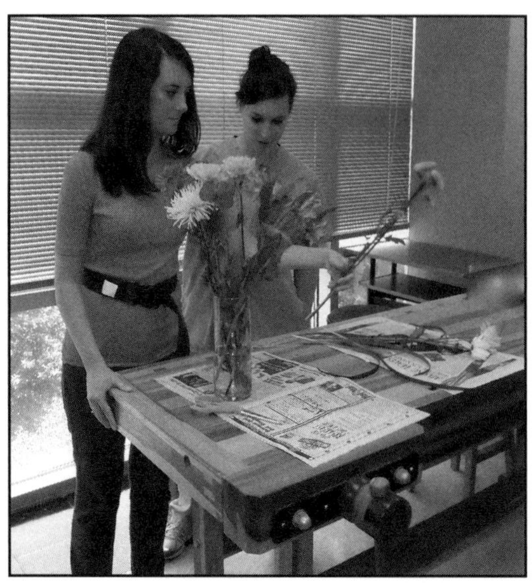

Figure 12-4. Working on reach and dynamic standing balance while arranging cut flowers.

limited time. Plants should be a manageable height—no more than 2 feet tall for raised beds. Many plants grow well from cuttings or seeds; these are good choices for the economy minded.

Crafts done with natural materials may fall into a number of different categories; therefore, it is a topic too broad for a generalized discussion of grading methods. The reader is referred to other chapters in this book for grading of various related craft types. As always, the complexity of projects can be graded based on number of steps, tools and materials required, qualities of the material to be handled, and the skill demands for each part of the process.

Therapeutic Applications

Physical Dysfunction

In using gardening activities or nature crafts, the therapist must choose the media based on the client's abilities and needs. These crafts, like many others in this book, incorporate fine motor skills such as grasp, pinch, and bilateral coordination, and both indoor and outdoor gardening hold opportunities for gross motor development, balance, and mobility work. Indeed, gardening activities can be structured to work on the whole body. The tasks of digging and planting are somewhat forgiving of deficits in dexterity or coordination and adaptations can be made for a client with mobility limitations if necessary. Outdoor gardening can be incorporated into a general exercise program and can improve physical stamina (Ecumenical Ministries of Oregon, 2005); bending and reaching components can be useful in remediation for static and dynamic balance, in either sitting or standing (Figure 12-4). Both working in and simply gazing at gardens seems to lower blood pressure and reduces stress (Wichrowski et al., 2005). Gardening activities can be graded such that they include other physical benefits such as opportunities for weight bearing, increasing muscle strength, increasing range of motion and flexibility, and general movement to promote circulation (Tose, 2005). Nature crafts can be suitable for most physical dysfunction settings and, if space allows, gardening programs can be a part of any rehabilitation program. This media category may be especially suited to the home health setting, where supplies are readily available and the activities are done in their natural context.

Mental Health

Horticulture has long been a part of mental health treatment; it is still commonly used in long-term facilities and appropriately so. Gardening activities offer opportunities for pre-vocational skill building (Palmer & Gatti, 1985), future-oriented thinking, leadership, and peer interaction. Though a structured process, it also allows for creativity and self-expression (Relf, 1973). Because clients with psychiatric problems often suffer from perceptual distortions and impaired reality testing, their thoughts may turn inward, and they may even physically isolate themselves from others. Gardening encourages a more external focus and provides reality-based, multi-sensory stimulation. It also helps restore a sense of control—often compromised during illness—and reduces stress and anxiety (Bruce & Borg, 2002). Successfully helping another living thing thrive will increase feelings of self-worth and teach concepts of interdependence. For clients with obsessive-compulsive disorder, the "dirty" aspect of gardening may be useful in desensitization treatment (Epstein, 1998). Clients experiencing an acute manic or depressive episode will need to be given short-term tasks, but as mood stabilizes, the long-term goal gardening will be especially therapeutic.

Pediatrics

Children are born explorers. Using materials and objects from nature, especially when the children can help gather them, is an excellent way to capitalize on this natural inclination while achieving a therapeutic objective. Most children relish time outdoors, particularly those children whose environments are often restricted due to disease or disability. Even children who may not be able to go outside due to their medical status can still enjoy participating in garden-related tasks, such as painting flowerpots, constructing birdhouses or scarecrows, or making stepping-stones. Planting and watching things grow is not only a practical learning experience, but also allows the child to be the nurturer and exert control over the environment. Like many other crafts, this treatment approach can foster creativity, self-expression, and self-esteem (Relf, 1973).

Adolescents

Like children, adolescents are still discovering themselves and the world around them, yet longing for independence and responsibility. Adolescents especially benefit from the care-giving aspect of horticulture activities; self-efficacy is enhanced successfully assuming responsibility for the welfare of another living thing (Early, 2009). Gardening activities can be structured for individual or group work, depending on the need; an intergenerational project can help adolescents work on interpersonal flexibility and building bridges of communication (James City County/Williamsburg Master Gardeners, 2005; Predny & Relf, 2004). Gardening is also an excellent way to evaluate and sharpen pre-vocational skills (Early, 2009). Use of nature crafts, in addition to benefits mentioned in previous sections, may also promote in adolescents the ideas of self-sufficiency and economy. In a consumer-oriented world, it may be helpful to highlight the beauty and usefulness of natural objects and instill a sense of respect for the environment (Carlson, 1993).

Older Adults

Therapeutic gardening is being used more and more frequently with individuals with Alzheimer's disease or other dementias. This activity is familiar and can be graded down to accommodate significant cognitive and physical limitations. Plant care provides the structure and routine important for maintenance of function in those with dementia. In addition, it helps maintain a tangible connection to the external world (Fisher's Center for Alzheimer's Research Foundation, 2005). Gardening can provide whole body exercise and stimulate multiple senses, facilitating both cognitive and physical well-being. For most people, spending time in a garden fosters feelings of peace and security, relieving anxiety. Some facilities also provide courtyard or "wandering" gardens where the residents can roam freely without fear of becoming lost. This is useful in managing the agitation and restlessness endured by some clients with Alzheimer's or other dementia. In this instance, the garden is a more sensory, less participatory experience. The temporal quality of growth may improve overall orientation and restore a sense of order to the often chaotic experience of dementia (Epstein, 1998). Older people may also enjoy nature crafts. The materials are familiar and may stimulate reminiscing discussions. The activities can be chosen and structured to work on a variety of motor, process, and communication skills.

Groups

Group work can be done in a number of ways using nature crafts or gardening. Clients can work together to plan projects and gather or shop for materials. They can work in parallel to create similar items, such as holiday decorations or gifts. As noted in the Projects section, growing vegetables or flowers is an excellent group venture. It allows for interaction and participation at diverse skill levels while creating a sense of interdependence and a collective goal mindset. Group gardening requires planning, division of labor, ongoing communication, and sharing of the results. Group members can be given assigned tasks and assume roles (Early, 2009) similar to those necessary in paid employment. Outdoor projects are especially useful, simply because of the scope and scale, but indoor group projects are also possible (e.g., beautifying the clinic or other areas in the health care facility). Gardening is also a good way to utilize heterogeneous groups, both in terms of age and ability. For example, master gardeners and schoolchildren may mix with elder adults in a community senior care program (James City County/Williamsburg Master Gardeners, 2005).

Case Study

Randy, a 21-year-old college student, was admitted to a private, long-term facility for brain-injured clients following a motor vehicle accident 1 month previously. He was a junior-year business major, living on campus at a nearby university. Before his accident, Randy enjoyed sports, outdoor activities, and socializing with peers. He had also showed an interest in art during high school, but had not formally pursued this in college. After the accident, Randy's parents held out hope he would be able to return to school, but they realized this was unlikely given the severity of his injury. If he remained unable to live independently, they planned to take care of him at home and take advantage of all possible rehab and/or pre-vocational services available.

At the time of admission, Randy was at level V on the Rancho Brain Injury Scale. He was awake most of the day, but had difficulty attending to a task and following verbal directions, and seemed to have a limited awareness of his surroundings (Trombly, 2002). Diminished verbalization made it impossible to accurately assess cognition, but Randy seemed to have global impairments. He had voluntary motion in both upper extremities, but a slight increase in flexor tone on the right affected gross motor coordination and fine motor manipulation skills. Randy could ambulate short distances with assistance, but his primary means of mobility was a wheelchair. Visual skills were also difficult to accurately evaluate, but he responded consistently to strong auditory and visual stimuli.

Randy's occupational therapist knew that if Randy were to actively participate, she needed to provide activities with enough stimulation and interest to hold his attention. She tried computer-based sports games, but he was unable to manage even a large switch and the visual tracking was too challenging as well. Because of his deficits in communication, he was unable to meaningfully interact with others in group activities. The therapist decided to see how Randy would respond to the facility garden; she reasoned that the multi-sensory input might arouse his attention without being over-stimulating. She found he did indeed visually attend to the colorful flowers and even tracked the occasional bird or butterfly that flew by. During each session, she increased the challenge by offering him cut flowers to hold and smell, and structuring opportunities to pull weeds, scoop dirt, or take short walks. Randy's attention and participation gradually improved, and after several weeks, he was able to complete structured planting activities with minimal cueing and assistance. Through intensive team rehabilitation services, his communication and motor skills were also gradually improving, enabling him to participate in more diverse activities. Eventually, the therapist gave him a chance to make decisions in a creative way by planting his own containers. He seemed quite pleased with the end result and requested more related activities. The occupational therapist showed him how to cut and arrange flowers, and he began to initiate making weekly arrangements for the dining room tables. Randy expressed hope of one day owning or managing a florist shop. While the therapist had some unspoken reservations about his potential to achieve this goal, she was pleased with his ability to think toward the future and identify definite interests. She began to use daily gardening chores as a means of establishing Randy's pre-vocational skills.

Discussion Questions

1. No theory or model was mentioned in this case; which one(s) do you think the therapist may have been using and why?

2. How might the therapist have used this type of intervention if the health care facility was without a garden?
3. What pre-vocational skills is Randy developing by working with plants?
4. What are some ways of minimizing the cost of starting a gardening program?

Resources

The Art and Craft of Pounding Flowers, Illustrated Edition
By Laura C. Martin
Rodale Books, 2003

Handmade Wreaths: Decorating Throughout the Year (Country Living Series)
By The Editors of Country Living
Hearst Books, 2001

Naturecrafts
By Gillian Souter
Three Rivers Press, 1996
Fifty gifts and projects, step-by-step. Some projects may be dated, but includes ideas for a lot of different materials.

The Complete Book of Gourd Craft
By Ginger Summit and Jim Widess
Sterling, 1998
Color photographs of completed projects and different types of gourds. Innovative ideas for both projects and many different decorative techniques.

Nature Printing with Herbs, Fruits & Flowers
By Laura Donnelly Bethmann
Storey Publishing, 1996
Includes many easy, yet innovative printing projects including how to print a spider web. Lovely color photos of materials and completed projects. Drawings show the process used.

Succulent Container Gardens: Design Eye-Catching Displays With 350 Easy-Care Plants
By Debra Lee Baldwin
Timber Press, 2010

References

American Occupational Therapy Foundation. (2005). *The gift of gardens and gardening.* Retrieved from www.aotf.org/portals/0/documents/Resources-WLWLibrary/Resource%20Notes/AOTF%20WLW%20Library%20Resource%20Notes%20-%20the%20gift%20of%20gardens%20and%20gardening.pdf.

Bruce, M. A. G., & Borg, B. (2002). *Psychosocial frames of reference: Core for occupation-based practice.* Thorofare, NJ: SLACK Incorporated.

Bupa Health Information. (2005). *Gardening for people with mobility difficulties.* Retrieved from www.bupa.co.uk/health_information/html/healthy_living/senior/gardening/adapted.html.

Carlson, L. (1993). *EcoArt.* Charlotte, VT: Williamson Publishing.

Culver, M. P. (2005). *Special garden tools help the physically challenged.* Retrieved from www.colostate.edu/Depts/CoopExt/4DMG/Garden/special.htm.

Early, M. B. (2009). *Mental health concepts and techniques for the occupational therapy assistant.* Baltimore, MD: Lippincott Williams & Wilkins.

Ecumenical Ministries of Oregon. (2005). *Patton home gardens project.* Retrieved from www.emoregon.org/Patton_home_gardens.php.

Epstein, M. (1998). The garden as healer. *The Seattle Daily Journal of Commerce.* Retrieved from www.djc.com.

Fisher's Center for Alzheimer's Research Foundation. (2005). *Therapeutic activities.* Retrieved from www.alzinfo.org/08/treatment-care/therapeutic-activities.
Hall, M. A., Wrobel, J., & Salamony, S. (2001). *Decorative crafts sourcebook.* San Diego, CA: Thunder Bay Press.
James City County/Williamsburg Master Gardeners. (2005). *Therapeutic gardening projects.* Retrieved from www.jccwmg.org/therapeutic.htm.
Morris, M. G. (2005, July 6). Health through hay: Patients rehabilitate with garden work. *Tupelo Daily Journal.*
Palmer, F., & Gatti, D. (1985). Vocational treatment model. *Occupational Therapy in Mental Health, 5*(1), 41-58.
Predny, M. L., & Relf, D. Horticulture therapy activities for preschool children, elderly adults, and intergenerational groups. *Activities, Adaptation and Aging, 28*(3), 1-18.
Reader's Digest. (1979). *Crafts and hobbies.* Pleasantville, NY: The Reader's Digest Association Inc.
Relf, D. (1973). Horticulture: A therapeutic tool. *Journal of Rehabilitation, 39*(1), 27-29.
Spurgeon, T. (2005). *Therapeutic horticulture: Growing for positive health.* Retrieved from www.positivehealth.com.
Tose, E. (2005). Therapeutic gardening. Retrieved from www.cmha-tb.on.ca.
Trombly, C. A., & Radomski, M. A. (2002). *Occupational therapy for physical dysfunction* (5th ed.). Baltimore, MD: Lippincott Williams & Wilkins.
Wichrowski, M., Whiteson, J., Haas, F., Mola, A., & Rey, M. (2005). Effects of horticulture therapy on mood and heart rate in patients participating in an inpatient cardiopulmonary rehabilitation program. *Journal of Cardiopulmonary Rehabilitation, 25*(5), 270-274.
Wasinger, S. (2009). *Eco-craft: Recycle, recraft, restyle.* New York, NY: Sterling Publishing Co./Lark Books.
Wise, S. (2005). No-stoop gardening. *Agrability Newsletter, Winter 2005.* Mississippi State University.

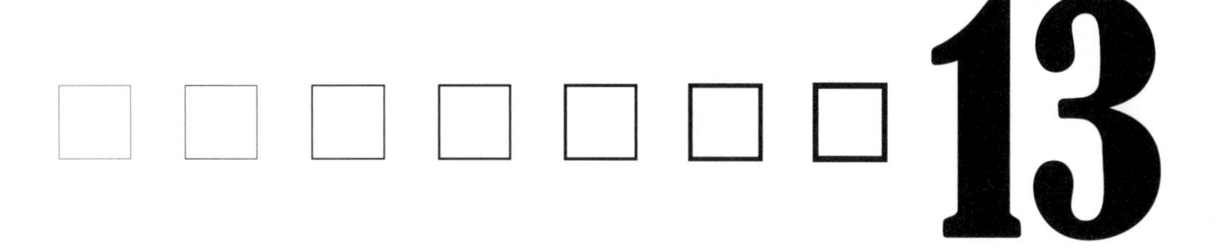

Cooking as a Craft

Objectives

The student should be able to:

- Discuss historical/cultural examples of cooking
- Know basic supplies and materials needed to do cooking and know how to complete and grade a basic project
- Understand advantages and limitations of cooking activities in therapy
- List precautions of cooking activities
- List ways to use cooking as a creative activity
- Discuss how cooking may contribute to occupational therapy assessment
- Articulate the application of cooking activities to various client populations

The definition of a craft—"an occupation or trade requiring manual dexterity or artistic skill" and, as a verb, "to make or produce with care, skill, or ingenuity" (Merriam Webster's Collegiate Dictionary, 10th ed., 1994)—justifies the inclusion of creative cooking as a craft category. Not only is food one of our greatest needs but in affluent societies, food preparation and presentation is also an art form. Food preparation, presentation, and consumption have a strong cultural component as well, lending them significance beyond survival. Cookbooks are a popular and frequently published category of text, and cooking is the most commonly practiced "craft" in occupational therapy clinics.

Everyone has to eat; human beings have consumed food for survival since the beginning of time. Early and primitive cultures likely lived primarily on wild, raw foods that were readily available. American Indians consumed berries and fruits from about 300 plants, and ate at least 59 varieties of greens (McBride, 1957). More than likely, a trial and error method was used to determine if something was edible or not, and the human digestive system evolved to process both animal and vegetable matter. Tales of the origins of cooked food abound: Charles Lamb's story says that a house fire burned a man's pig, which he then tasted and liked; another story states that natives consumed the flesh of deer and bear burned in a forest fire (Capron & Zucker, 2003). It is more probable, though, that the primates Homo Erectus already had the practice of intentionally cooking meat on top of coals. Neanderthals are thought to have made stews by hanging hides containing meat and water over fires (Beeuwkes, Todhunter, & Weigley, 1967; Ritchie, 1981). American Indians

Tubbs, C., & Drake, M. *Crafts and Creative Media in Therapy, Fourth Edition (pp. 155-166).*

made soups by drying, powdering, and boiling certain vines (McBride, 1957). Neolithic humans may have cooked grains by dropping hot stones into water with them. Refinement of cooking methods progressed along with the development of tools, such as metal utensils, ceramic pots, fireplaces, and eventually ovens. Advancements in techniques for food procurement and preservation also expanded the scope of cooking possibilities (Beeuwkes et al., 1967; Ritchie, 1981). For example, Native Americans developed irrigation techniques to increase crop yield (McBride, 1957). In today's world, agricultural and scientific innovations, improvements in transportation, specialization of tools and appliances, and the global exchange of information make methods of food production and its preparation almost limitless.

Our own cultural background greatly affects what foods we choose and how we view the occupation of cooking. Cultural food habits have developed over time and are influenced by climate, growing season, and regional soil and water, as well as economics, religious practices, superstition, means of processing and storage, exchange of ideas through travel, and even historical events (Capron & Zucker, 2003; Crowe, 2009; Hames & Joseph, 1986). How food is prepared and eaten is just as important—and also as culturally bound—as what is eaten. For example, an occupational therapist in the Navajo school system had her children prepare traditional fry bread. The activity not only facilitated motor skills of finger strength and dexterity, but also cognitive skills of sequencing and time awareness, all the while educating them about an important time in the history of their tribe (Crowe, 2009). Sharing and consumption of food has always been a group activity and continues to have social implications for participants. Today, food preparation is often a social activity as well. Many modern homes have a centrally located kitchen, often adjacent to or continuous with the family room, and it is a common gathering place. Factors such as who serves and in what order, who eats with whom, utensils and furniture, special preparation techniques, and use of religious blessings have social meaning and profoundly affect the eating experience (Capron & Zucker, 2003). Cooking or baking of special foods may be associated with certain holidays and evoke feelings of serenity or security. A food craving may also relate back to early food experiences. For example, peanut butter and graham crackers may recall images and emotions from childhood snack time and the individual unconsciously desires the former good feeling associated with eating that food. By repeating the food experience, the person seeks to get the same emotional experience (Hamilton & Whitney, 1979; Mosey, 1986). Not all associations with cooking or eating ex, however, are positive. Eating problems or disorders may relate to earlier negative psychological experiences, and for a person with an acquired physical disability, what once was a pleasure could now be a chore.

One way to think about food and cooking is to use Maslow's Hierarchy of Human Needs (see Figure 2-1). Food can be used in an attempt to fulfill needs expressed at all the hierarchical levels. At the lowest level, food and cooking are simply a means of nutrition needed for health/survival. At the next level, food availability or eating favorite foods affords a sense of safety and security. At the level of love and belonging, cooking may be associated with family dinners and a mother's care. At the next level, being able to eat in an upscale restaurant or to afford a professionally equipped kitchen may represent success and self-esteem. At the highest level, some people realize self-actualization by engaging in creative cooking activities. While a therapy activity involving food can appeal to a client's functioning at almost any level and can be used to accomplish a variety occupational therapy goals, the therapist should also consider and respect a client's negative reaction to this suggestion.

Cooking assessment has been a part of occupational therapy homemaking evaluations (see Table 2-1) for some time (Hopkins & Smith, 1978, 1983, 1988; MacDonald, 1960; Neistadt & Crepeau, 1998; Pedretti & Early, 2001; Trombly, 1983; Williard & Spackman, 1947) and examines a patient's ability to perform the physical and mental processes involved in food preparation. Historically, a cooking assessment was completed as part of the rehabilitation evaluation for the career (female) homemaker. As the roles of men and women have blended, however, the evaluation of cooking skills has become an important consideration for any adult not living in an institution with communal dining. Allen (1992) states that cooking should include planning and obtaining needed ingredients and equipment, as well as actually preparing the food. Since many component skills are the same as those used in self-care, craft completion (Klinger, 1997), and other daily activities, the occupational therapist can informally evaluate competence in multiple areas during a cooking activity. Depending on its complexity, food preparation can require cognitive skills such as memory, judgment, sequencing, and organization; physical skills such as endurance, balance, gross and fine motor movement, and coordination; or psychosocial skills such as patience, cooperation, and self-control. Several recent texts provide suggestions on how to adapt cooking tasks, as a part of home care, for various impairments (Brown & Stoffel 2011; Crepeau, Crohn, & Schell, 2009; Meriano & Latella, 2008; Pendleton & Schultz-Krohn, 2006), but it is seldom mentioned as a craft or creative pursuit.

Special Considerations

Although the projects presented in this chapter are of necessity limited in scope, certain precautions are common to most cooking activities. Some hazards are more obvious than others, for example, sharp knives and hot stove burners. Others are less so, such as dietary or swallowing restrictions. In planning food activities for children, be aware of foods that may present a choking danger, for example things that are small, round, long, or sticky (Capron & Zucker, 2003). Children may also have peri-oral sensory defensiveness or oral motor limitations, which can hinder chewing and swallowing. Adults, especially those with neurological impairments, may have similar problems and the occupational therapist is well advised to be familiar with all swallowing precaution guidelines. Elderly clients may have dentures, or partial tooth loss, so the therapist should be aware of what they can easily chew. For those with a reduced or distorted sense of taste, food—and therefore cooking activities—may be less enjoyable (Bonder, 2009). Special diets are common across the rehabilitation spectrum, so again, the therapist is responsible for assuring that these are observed in therapy. In using cooking activities with clients with psychiatric illnesses or acquired brain injuries, the therapist should be prepared for mood swings and even aggressive behavior. These clients may also have difficulty with organization, recognition of errors, anticipation of consequences, and recognition of safety risks (Klinger, 1997). Expectations of clients should be based on their cognitive level, for instance, a client functioning at a level 4 or below should not be expected to plan a dish or a meal (Allen, 1992). Other problems to anticipate with cognitively impaired clients include ability to differentiate edible from inedible; knowledge of utensil use, manners, and appropriate bite size; awareness of spillage and other safety or social hazards; and knowledge of safe storage and usability of food. For patients whose impairments are primarily physical, the therapist should be aware of client factors that may pose a safety risk such as decreased standing tolerance and balance, upper extremity strength and range of motion limitations, and decreased coordination or tremors. Vision loss also calls for increased attention to safety in the kitchen. For all clients, it is also important to remember that ability to participate in a dining experience has an impact on their acceptance in the larger community (Hemphill, Peterson, & Werner, 1991).

Food Project—Rolled Sugar Cookies

Plan It

The project presented here requires several ingredients, some of which have a limited shelf life, and it requires several steps to complete. The end product is edible, so the therapist needs to be sure it is not contraindicated in the client's diet, and common sanitary procedures, such as washing hands, should be observed. This activity demonstrates the scope of therapeutic objectives that can be achieved with a single activity and is also illustrative of the creative aspect of cooking.

Get Ready

Ingredients/Supplies

- 2 cups flour (plus extra flour for rolling out)
- 1 cup sugar (may use sugar substitute for all or part)
- 1/2 cup butter, softened
- 1 1/2 teaspoons baking powder
- 1/2 teaspoon salt
- 1 egg
- 2 tablespoons milk
- Assorted sprinkles, colored sugar, frosting as desired
- Tools
- Mixing bowl
- Measuring cups and spoons

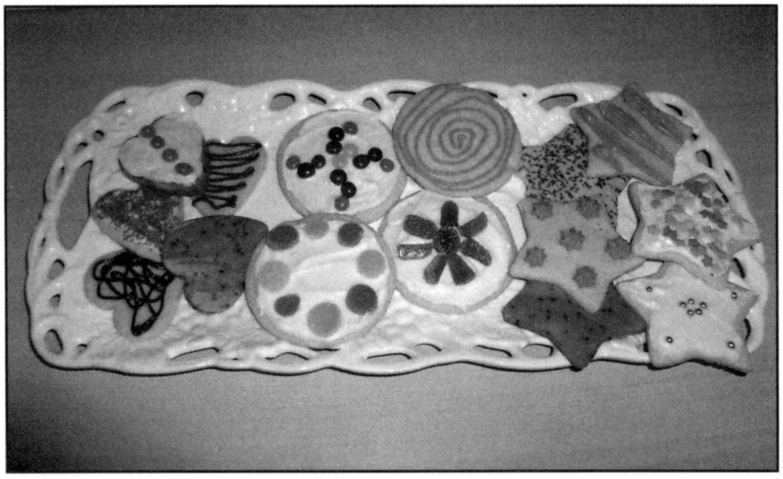

Figure 13-1. Cookie decorating ideas.

- Large spoon
- Rolling pin
- Spatula
- Cookie cutters
- Waxed paper or pastry rolling mat
- Cookie sheet
- Pot holder
- Electric mixer (optional)
- Oven or toaster oven
- Timer

Time required: 1 hour

Approximate cost: $2

Do It

Process

1. Preheat the oven to 300 degrees.
2. Thoroughly mix all ingredients using a spoon or electric mixer.
3. Turn dough out onto a sheet of waxed paper or pastry rolling mat that has been lightly dusted with flour. Gently roll the ball of dough back and forth a few times to coat the outside with flour. Roll the dough out with the rolling to about a 1/4-inch thickness.
4. Cut dough into shapes with desired cookie cutters. Carefully place the cut dough on an ungreased cookie sheet using a spatula. You may have to occasionally reposition the dough and/or dust the rolling pin or surface with more flour to keep it from sticking. You can also gather up the dough scraps and roll again to make more cookies.
5. Bake cookies in preheated oven for approximately 15 minutes or until lightly browned. If desired, apply sprinkles or colored sugar to dough before baking.
6. Baked and cooled cookies can also be frosted, or frosted and decorated with sprinkles, chopped nuts, small pieces of candy, or other small edible décor (Figure 13-1).

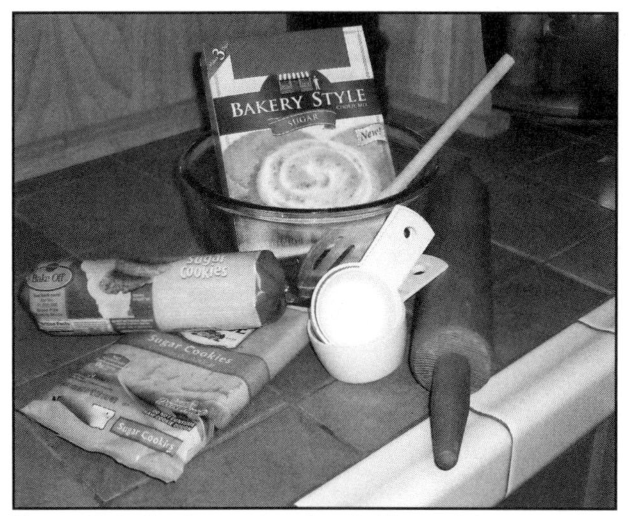

Figure 13-2. Grading options for a baking activity.

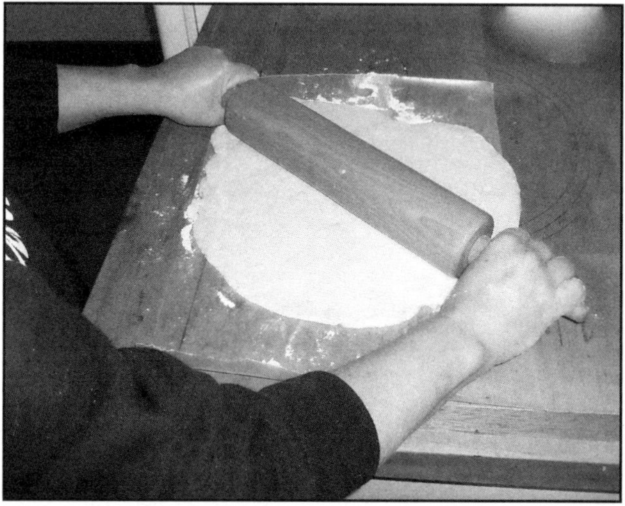

Figure 13-3. Rolling dough with a rolling pin facilitates bilateral gross grasp and coordination, weight bearing, and automatic actions.

Change It

To simplify this activity, start with a cookie mix, a roll of prepared dough, or even pre-cut prepared dough (Figure 13-2). Keep in mind, though, increased convenience usually equals increased cost as well. The therapist must also determine whether or not having the patient access the hot oven is a necessary to the therapeutic goals. For example, the therapist can choose to simplify the mixing component of the activity but still have the patient carry out the steps of the actual baking in order to work on safety issues. If there is no access to an oven of any kind, the therapist can provide already baked cookies for the patient to decorate. The therapist can also have the patient participate in the clean up portion of the activity; in fact, the cooking craft may only be a means to this end.

To grade the activity up, the therapist can have the patient cut the dough into more intricate shapes with or without a cookie cutter, and/or decorate them in various ways before or after baking. Application of frosting will require bilateral hand coordination or problem solving to execute with the use of only one hand. The addition of decorative elements can also be graded for level of fine motor demand. For example, colored sugar can be sprinkled on top without need for precision, but using a cake-decorating tool to create a special shape or image will require both strength and motor control. Initiating and terminating a task, copying a design or choosing colors, and sequencing the necessary steps are all cognitive elements that could be included in a more complex project. Plentiful resources are available for cookie decoration ideas, especially those with a holiday theme. See Figure 13-1 for some simple ideas or Resources at the end of the chapter for other creative cooking inspiration.

Document It

The following examples illustrate ways to report on using creative cooking in therapy.

- "The client was able to mix the ingredients independently, using the affected upper extremity to hold the bowl stable."
- "The client required only occasional cueing to remember to using learned joint protection techniques during the cooking and clean up process."
- "The client was able to successfully use the timer and posted signs (e.g., 'turn oven OFF' in the kitchen to compensate for memory deficits)."

Whether grading the activity up or down, the therapist should choose the method based not only on available time, tools, and supplies, but also on the objectives to be accomplished. For example, if the patient needs to work on upper extremity strength, weight bearing, or grasp (Figure 13-3) or following written directions, mixing the dough from scratch (or from a mix) and rolling it out will best achieve this. On the other hand, if the objective is facilitation of fine motor coordination, or an opportunity for self-expression, decorating pre-baked cookies will serve just as well. The therapist can use the appeal of a baking activity to engage the patient in working on a myriad of seemingly unrelated skills. A well-planned cooking activity can be a perfect choice for almost anyone, from an individual with bipolar disorder who needs skills in time management to one with rheumatoid arthritis who needs an opportunity to practice joint protection techniques.

Other Ideas and Grading

When it comes to food, the notion that presentation is as important as taste has led to the creation of a wide array of both tools and food products whose function is decoration. One need only visit a bakery or sushi bar to affirm that food can be as beautiful as it is tasty. Clients can not only create a work of art, they can eat it too! In addition, many decorative food projects can be done with little or no access to cooking equipment such as a stove or oven. Below are some ideas for "artistic" food.

- Decorate cupcakes or cakes with frosting and assorted candies. Cupcakes are particularly popular at the moment and may therefore hold more appeal. Use a basic cake decorating set to increase the complexity or to work on strength or grasp patterns in applying frostings. Use different colors of frosting and/or candy decorations to create holiday, cartoon, or other themed goodies. Or decorate a gingerbread house for Christmas; clients could make and assemble the gingerbread, or simply add the sweet embellishments. Larger craft stores usually sell an array of supplies for this type project and seasonal magazines and television programs provide great inspiration.
- Make a batch of crisp rice cereal treats, then mold the "dough" like clay into shapes and add decoration as desired. Food coloring can be added to the melted marshmallow/butter mixture before adding the cereal as well. Hands will need to be thoroughly washed, then greased, in order to handle the sticky mixture.
- Bread or roll dough can serve as a lower fat, lower sugar alternative to cookies and cakes. It can also be used in a variety of creative ways by twisting, shaping, or filling, and the baked item can be similarly decorated with glazes and fruits, nuts, or candy sprinkles.
- Make decorative garnishes using fruits or vegetables, such as radish roses, carrot curls, or carved melon bowls. Make a jack-o-lantern for Halloween. Resources for tools and ideas include home stores or departments, specialty cooking stores, bookstores, libraries, and of course, the Internet.
- Make fancy hors d'oeuvres with bases such as crackers, breads, or vegetable sticks, and add various spreads and toppings (e.g., cheeses or jams, olives, capers, pimentos, raisins, or nuts). Again, there are multiple sources of ideas, including cookbooks, magazines, and Web sites.

As illustrated by the single project in this chapter, cooking activities lend themselves to a broad range of grading possibilities: from one-step tasks to multi-course meals; from cold foods to hot or precisely timed dishes; from few ingredients and tools to a whole kitchen full of pots, pans, and utensils. The project and variations presented here focus on creativity/presentation and require a minimum of special tools or environments. Common dishes can be modified in many ways to increase or decrease the difficulty of their preparation. As previously mentioned, the ultimate choice of activity will depend on a blending of client interest and therapeutic objective.

Main Therapeutic Applications

Physical Dysfunction

For a person involved in rehabilitation to overcome a physical disability, cooking is often an appropriate treatment option. It is a familiar occupation to most, it requires multiple performance skills, and it can be graded in a variety of ways to hone in on specific problem areas. If the disability causes a disturbance in the eating process, helping the client learn to choose appropriate foods also becomes an important part of the activity. Planning meals and engaging in cooking can be milestone activities that clients need to gain confidence in their ability to surmount their problem and continue to enjoy life (Hopkins & Smith, 1983). Success in food preparation may also be one indicator for clients' families that they are capable of returning to independent living. For clients with neurological problems such as strokes, cooking can be useful in training on safety issues, mobility, balance, and use of the affected extremity or in remediation or compensation for cognitive deficits such as memory, judgment, and sequencing. Bread making, for example, is an excellent activity for a multitude of therapeutic goals. Kneading requires upper extremity weight bearing and strength, yet it can be successfully accomplished even with poor coordination and less than perfect movement patterns. The process requires the cognitive ability to follow written or oral directions, keep the tasks in sequence, read numbers, and remember time limits for rising and baking. It can also serve as an outlet for frustration or other negative feelings often experienced with a newly acquired disability. For clients with primarily orthopedic problems, the therapist can assess factors such as standing tolerance, range of motion, or adherence to joint protection and work simplification principles. For those with visual impairments, not only meal preparation, but successful management of the hazards in a kitchen, is of primary concern. Some clients with physical limitations will need compensatory strategies to enable food preparation; there are many aids and adaptive devices available, for example adapted cutting boards, pot stabilizers, and ergonomic handle utensils. Companies who sell adaptive equipment of this kind are listed in Appendix I. When using cooking as a therapeutic modality, the therapist must always consider weight control, diabetic, or other special diets in making food choices. While waiting for an item to finish baking, for example, patients may benefit from a discussion on food choices in keeping with a low fat, low sugar, or hypoallergenic diet plan.

Mental Health

Because food is so often tied to our early experiences of feeling loved and nurtured, cooking provides a rich opportunity for clients to learn to nurture themselves. While the therapist must be aware of those with both mental and physical deficits for whom food has become the focus of too much attention, cooking is often an excellent activity choice to address psychosocial concerns. Almost all cooking requires some level of planning and patience, yet is usually nonthreatening due to its familiarity. Depressed clients may have little appetite and may resist participation, but the involvement of a whole group in cooking may draw them in. Clients who are manic often want to cook elaborate dishes or meals but may become distracted long before it is completed. Clients with schizophrenia who have significant cognitive or perceptual difficulties may benefit from the concrete nature of cooking tasks but could need close supervision, verbal cueing, or physical assistance. For those who have eating disorders such as anorexia, bulimia nervosa, or obesity, a cooking activity is an opportunity to explore underlying reasons such as family dysfunction or early abuse. Special care must be taken with suicidal or aggressive clients if any sharp tools are being used (Allen, Earhart, & Blue, 1992; Early, 2009); a tool count should be completed after clean up but before clients leave the area.

For this population in particular, cooking provides an opportunity for teaching about nutrition. Individuals with long-standing mental illness may be on fixed incomes and tend to consume inexpensive but unhealthy foods. Those with dementia are particularly prone to mistake one ingredient for another or to add nonedible ingredients to the mixture. Such clients should be supervised closely during cooking activities. Clients diagnosed with substance use disorders may be fully independent in this daily occupation, but group meal preparation and consumption activities are opportune times to discuss how life will be different without drugs or alcohol, such as a change in eating habits or social challenges such as eating in restaurants that serve alcohol. Aside from cooking as part of life skills, they may benefit from the creative aspect alone. Clients with mild mental retardation may often live in situations where independence in basic cooking is expected; sometimes they marry and have families. Therefore, meal planning, cooking, and clean up are important skills to be developed with this population. Those with moderate mental retardation may enjoy cooking but need constant supervision. They usually live at home or in a group setting where others prepare meals and cooking independence is not necessary (APA, 1994; Robinson & Robinson, 1976).

Pediatrics

Bonding between infants and adults is most often associated with receiving and giving food. Early play experiences for children often involve playing house, making mud or sand pies, and having tea parties. Early work experiences may involve feeding pets, cleaning up after meals, or getting their own snack. Simple food preparation like stuffing celery or stirring chocolate drink mix into milk may be good for young children. Children from about 5 to 12 years of age may enjoy making cookies, sandwiches, or preparing frozen pizza.

For children with eating problems resulting from a physical or psychiatric illness, using puppets can be a means of exploring their feelings about food (Saunders, 1978). Many might also enjoy creative food constructions as discussed earlier in the chapter. Making holiday treats could instill feelings of security and continuity in addition to the other psychological and motor benefits of the activity. When cooking with children or adolescents, beware of food ending up on the ceiling or walls! Close supervision is recommended (Pratt & Allen, 1989).

Adolescents

Teenagers often benefit from completing the full sequence of tasks required for meal preparation—making a list, shopping, cooking, eating, and cleaning up. Those with mental health problems may be more acutely in need of life skills education. Mealtime can be a important social time for adolescents who are in the midst of deciding who they are and what they value, but it can also be a stressful occasion for those with body image concerns or low self-confidence (Brown & Stoffel, 2011). Young clients who are struggling with management of type I diabetes require special consideration. Pleasurable ways of preparing and increasing the visual appeal of healthy foods may facilitate better management of all of these conditions. Since consuming food is often a social activity, it may be an especially appropriate therapeutic activity for adolescents who have difficulty getting along with peers or authority figures. Completion of cooked or baked items teaches a lesson about patience and delay of gratification, but it also provides a tangible reward when instructions are correctly followed. Group cooking efforts, such as making pizza or decorating cookies for a party, are particularly useful with this population for both social benefits and role acquisition (Early, 2009).

Older Adults

The craft of cooking has great value for older clients. Since women represent a majority of the elderly population, and many have filled traditional roles of homemaking and meal preparation, elderly clients will often have a rich history of cooking from which to draw. Reminiscence groups may elicit accounts of favorite foods prepared in the past. Actual cooking experiences sometimes generate involvement from clients whose memory problems keep them from participation in many other activities. Sometimes the stimulation of the smell and taste receptors, via sensory memory, can trigger experiential memories that appear otherwise irretrievable (Zoltan, 2007). Cooking provides the diverse sensory stimulation and opportunity for familiar and meaningful activity that may be otherwise lacking in some health care settings.

Some deficits occur more commonly in the elderly population and many of these can impact their ability to cook efficiently or enjoyably, or may rob them of this role altogether. Visual problems can interfere with reading recipes, reading package ingredients, and setting oven dials. Hearing difficulties may make bell-type kitchen timers almost useless. Memory problems may cause an elderly person to forget to turn off an oven or burner. Pain, or decreased balance, strength or range of motion can make carrying dishes and ingredients hazardous (Bonder & Bello-Haas, 2009). In summary, the kitchen can be transformed from a place of cherished memories to a place of fear and frustration where accidents await. Some elderly clients will want to overcome these obstacles in order to return to independent living. Due to a move to a nursing home or other group living situation, other older individuals may not need to cook, but may nonetheless relish an opportunity to engage in this traditional way to give of and to oneself (Desnick, 1971; Mace & Robins, 1981; Wolff, 1970). For example, they may enjoy helping host parties and serving colorful, fun foods.

Groups

Cooking and eating foods in groups can be highly therapeutic. Improvement in inter- and intrapersonal functioning can be achieved along with all skills mentioned earlier—motor, cognitive, perceptual—through attention to such areas as communication, turn taking, reminiscence, and cultural identification. Since meals are historically social in nature, these activities are contextually appropriate. The diversity of component tasks in preparing a dish or a full meal allows for all group members to participate simultaneously at their own skill level.

Case Study

Iris is a divorced 56-year-old woman who is employed for childcare and homecare chores by a 35-year-old single mother and businesswoman. Although Iris has been on medication to manage her hypertension for several years, she ultimately suffered a left cerebrovascular accident (CVA) one day while at work. Her employer discovered her that evening and called an ambulance, which took her to a nearby university teaching hospital. The employer called Iris' children, who convinced her to undergo immediate carotid artery surgery to help prevent further damage. After this procedure, she was placed on the neurological intensive care unit (ICU).

The inpatient occupational therapist first evaluated Iris in the ICU. He assessed her passive and active range of motion, muscle tone, strength, oral motor function, visual perception, sensation, cognition, and general emotional state. She was found to have right hemiparesis in both upper and lower extremities with decreased proprioception as well as diminished tactile perception of sharp/dull, hot/cold, and two-point discrimination. She had a weak, nonfunctional grasp on the right and increased muscle tone interfered with smooth movement of the entire arm. The physical therapist planned to work on lower extremity facilitation/strengthening and gait. The speech therapist found that although Iris had some weakness in oral musculature, she could achieve lip closure and had no trouble swallowing. The theories underlying treatment in this inpatient clinic were the neurodevelopmental and rehabilitation models; consequently, treatment tended to be a combination of deficit remediation and teaching of compensatory techniques and equipment use.

During the interview, the occupational therapist could understand Iris' speech, even though she labored over each sentence. He found Iris to be somewhat depressed and, in particular, worried about losing her job. She feared that her employer would have to replace her before she recovered. She had enjoyed her work, thought her pay and benefits were above average, and also genuinely liked her employer. Iris' daughter thought she could partially take over her mother's job temporarily by rearranging her own work schedule and the occupational therapist called on the case manager to help with this issue as well.

Eventually, Iris was moved out of ICU and onto the rehab unit. The occupational therapist and Iris decided she should participate in a functional (cooking) evaluation to see how much she could use her affected upper extremity and how well she could compensate for her motor deficits. In the adapted kitchen, Iris was able to manage her wheelchair and access the sink, stove, and counters. Iris expressed concern that her employer's kitchen had high countertops and a microwave over the stove, but the therapist reassured her that she would probably have more motor return and she could also learn adapted techniques to compensate for lost abilities. Iris had already begun to gain control in her right upper extremity, but she still required moderate assistance for ambulation with a hemi-walker. During the cooking assessment, Iris was able to wash a celery stalk but had trouble trimming and chopping it. She also had difficulty using the electric can opener. The therapist showed her several helpful techniques, such as using her affected extremity to stabilize the bowl in her lap for mixing, and using an adapted cutting board for chopping.

As Iris worked, she began to talk about her job and family life. She told of preparing elaborate meals for her employer's dinner parties, and sometimes staying overnight at her employer's home on these late evenings. Since two of her own grown children still lived with her in her small house, she enjoyed an occasional night away. She had worked in her present job for 5 years, and described it as interesting and fulfilling. She had never felt as much a part of a family for whom she worked as she did on her current job. She reiterated that her primary goal was to get back to work.

The occupational therapist had Iris participate in a number of therapy sessions in the kitchen. She not only worked on functional meal preparation skills, but the therapist also structured opportunities for Iris to work on weight bearing on her affected arm and utilizing normal movement patterns in grasping and reaching. She also showed her a variety of adapted tools such as a pot stabilizer, one-handed jar opener, and large-handled utensils. Iris did many activities from the wheelchair, but could now come to standing independently when necessary. By the end of her second week, she could prepare her own lunch with only minimal assistance.

Prior to her discharge, Iris independently made decorated cupcakes for the therapy staff.

Functional use of her right hand had gradually improved and she tried to use it as much as possible in placing jellybeans and sprinkles on top of the cupcakes. In spite of the fact that she had to do a great deal of cooking as part of her job, she still enjoyed baking for friends and family during her free time.

Iris eventually started back to work on a part-time basis. She moved into the guestroom at her employer's house until she was able to resume driving. Her employer allowed her to assume duties as she was able and by the end of 7 months, Iris was working full-time again. She and the child spent some afternoons baking cookies or playing games together that afforded Iris enjoyable ways to practice using her right hand more skillfully.

Discussion Questions

1. Describe how the activity of cooking is a component of more than one area of occupation for Iris.
2. What other assistive devices might you recommend? In what other ways could you have facilitated functional use/positioning/normal movement of her right upper extremity during cooking activities?
3. You would like to have Iris participate in a cooking group to plan, prepare, and eat a pizza. How could you adapt this activity for a group member who is on a salt-restricted diet? A diabetic diet? A low-fat diet?
4. Clients taking the antidepressant drug called MAOIs are prohibited from eating many foods because they could cause a hypertensive crisis. Using another source to identify these foods, make a list of commonly eaten foods/dishes that these clients should NOT eat.

Resources

The Decorative Art of Japanese Food Carving: Elegant Garnishes for All Occasions
By Hiroshi Nagashima and Kenji Miura
Kodansha International, 2009

Nibbled: 200 Fabulous Finger Food Ideas
By Katy Holder, Tim Robinson, and Sara DeNardi (contributor)
Thunder Bay Press, 2005

Food Art: Garnishing Made Easy
By John Gargone
Schiffer Publishing, 2003

Crazy About Cookies
by Krystina Castella
Sterling Publishing, 2010

Hey There Cupcake
By Clare Cresp
Mulcher Media, 2004

Finger Food
Edited by Katherine Gasparini
Laurel Glen, 2002

Betty Crocker's New Cake Decorating
John Wiley and Sons, Inc., 1999

Betty Crocker's Christmas Cookbook, 2nd Edition
Wiley Publishing, 2006
Festive holiday foods, including items to make as gifts.

Better Homes and Gardens New Junior Cookbook, 7th Edition
By Better Homes and Gardens Books
Better Homes and Gardens, 2004

Cartoon figures introduce sections on the basics of measuring, safety, menu planning, table-setting. Also includes a glossary and drawings of tools, pots, and pans. There are sections on the various meals and special foods such as desserts. The recipes take from two to eight steps, thus allowing for different levels of complexity.

References

Allen, C. K., Earhart, C. A., & Blue, T. (1992). *Occupational therapy treatment goals for the physically and cognitively disabled.* Bethesda, MD: AOTA, Incorporated.

American Psychiatric Association. (1994). *Diagnostic and statistical manual of mental disorders* (4th ed.). Washington, DC: American Psychiatric Association.

Beeuwkes, A. M., Todhunter, E. H., & Weigley, E. S. (Eds.). (1967). *Essays on history of nutrition and dietetics.* Chicago, IL: The American Dietetics Association.

Bonder, B. R., & Bello-Haas, V. D. (2009). *Functional performance in older adults* (3rd ed.). Philadelphia, PA: F. A. Davis Co.

Brown, C., & Stoffel, V. C. (Eds.). (2011). *Occupational therapy in mental health: A vision for participation.* Philadelphia, PA: F. A. Davis Co.

Capron, M. E., & Zucker, E. (2003). The ultimate cooking companion for at-home caregivers. Upper Saddle River, NJ: Prentice Hall.

Crepeau, E. B., Cohn, E. S., & Schell, B. A. B. (2009). Willard and Spackman's occupational therapy (11th ed.). Philadelphia, PA: Lippincott Williams & Wilkins.

Crowe, T. K., & Hong, N. (2009). Culturally rich, meaningful occupations. *Advance for Occupational Therapy Practitioners, 25*(10), 8.

Desnick, S. G. (1971). *Geriatric contentment.* Springfield, IL: Charles C. Thomas.

Early, M. B. (2009). *Mental health concepts and techniques for the occupational therapy assistant* (4th ed.). Philadelphia, PA: Lippincott Williams & Wilkins.

Hames, C. C., & Joseph, D. H. (1986). *Basic concepts of helping: A holistic approach* (2nd ed.). Norwalk, CT: Appleton-Century-Crofts.

Hamilton, E. M., & Whitney, E. (1979). *Nutrition concepts and controversies.* St. Paul, MN: West Publishing Company.

Hemphill, B. J. (1988). *Mental health assessment in occupational therapy.* Thorofare, NJ: SLACK Incorporated.

Hemphill, B. J., Peterson, C. Q., & Werner, P. C. (1991). *Rehabilitation in mental health: Goals and objectives for independent living.* Thorofare, NJ: SLACK Incorporated.

Hopkins, H. L., & Smith, H. D. (1978). *Willard and Spackman's occupational therapy* (5th ed.). Philadelphia, PA: Lippincott Williams & Wilkins.

Hopkins, H. L., & Smith, H. D. (1983). *Willard and Spackman's occupational therapy* (6th ed.). Philadelphia, PA: Lippincott Williams & Wilkins.

Hopkins, H. L., & Smith H. D. (1988). *Willard and Spackman's occupational therapy* (7th ed.). Philadelphia, PA: Lippincott Williams & Wilkins.

Klinger, J. L. (1997). *Meal preparation and training: The health care professional's guide.* Thorofare, NJ: SLACK Incorporated.

MacDonald, E. M. (1960). *Occupational therapy in rehabilitation.* London, UK: Bailliere, Tindall, and Cox.

Mace, N. L., & Robins, P. V. (1981). *The 36-hour day.* Baltimore, MD: Johns Hopkins University Press.

McBride, M. M. (1957). *Harvest of American cooking.* New York, NY: Putnam's Sons

Meriano, C., & Latella, D. (2008). *Occupational therapy interventions: Functions and occupations.* Thorofare, NJ: SLACK Incorporated.

Merriam Webster (Ed.). (1994). *Merriam Webster's collegiate dictionary* (10th ed.). Springfield, MA: Merriam-Webster, Incorporated.

Mosey, A. C. (1986). *Psychosocial components of occupational therapy,* New York, NY: Raven Press.

Neistadt, M. E., & Crepeau, E. B. (1998). *Willard and Spackman's occupational therapy.* Philadelphia, PA: Lippincott Williams & Wilkins.

Pedretti, L., & Early, M.B. (Eds.). (2001). *Occupational therapy: Practice skills for physical dysfunction* (5th ed.). St. Louis, MO: Mosby.

Pendleton, H. M., & Schultz-Crohn, W. (Eds.). (2006). *Pedretti's occupational therapy: Practice skills for physical dysfunction* (6th ed.). St. Louis, MO: Mosby.

Pratt, P. N., & Allen, A. S. (1989). *Occupational therapy for children* (2nd ed.). St. Louis, MO: Mosby.

Ritchie, C. I. A. (1981). *Food in civilization.* Sydney, Australia: Methuen Australia Pty., Ltd.

Robinson, N. M., & Robinson, H. B. (1976). *The mentally retarded child: A psychological approach.* New York, NY: McGraw-Hill.

Saunders, F. M. (1978). *Your diabetic child.* New York, NY: Bantam books.

Trombly, C. A. (1983). *Occupational therapy for physical dysfunction* (2nd ed.). Baltimore, MD: Waverly Press.

Willard, H. S., & Spackman, C. E. (1947). *Principles of occupational therapy.* Philadelphia, PA: Lippincott Williams & Wilkins.

Wolff, K. (1970). *The emotional rehabilitation of the geriatric patient.* Springfield, IL: Charles C. Thomas.

Zoltan, B. (2007). *Vision, perception, and cognition: A manual for the evaluation and treatment of the adult with acquired brain injury.* Thorofare, NJ: SLACK Incorporated.

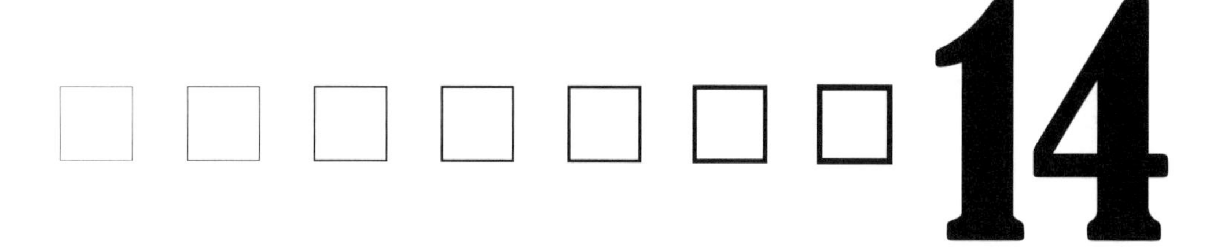

Crafts From Found and Recycled Materials

Objectives

The student should be able to:

- List basic supplies and found or recycled materials useful in making craft projects
- Complete and grade simple projects from found/recycled materials
- Describe advantages and limitations of using found/recycled materials for crafting
- List a variety of projects that can be made using found/recycle materials
- Articulate how crafts from found/recycled crafts can be used therapeutically with various client populations

Although this chapter was originally written with the home health therapist in mind, the idea of using recycled or commonly available materials to create functional or decorative crafts is no longer the exception, but rather an approach embraced by many. Repurposed items incorporated into creative works could be considered environmentally responsible and, in some instances, even chic. The craft ideas presented here are equally appropriate for either home-based therapy or in clinical or other community-based settings, and include projects made from common household items along with projects for the home. Home décor is a popular topic in various current crafting forums and for that reason may be appealing to clients.

While occupational therapy has been a part of home health care services for many years, this area of practice has proliferated in the last two decades as hospital stays have been abbreviated in order to contain costs. Clients are sent home in spite of remaining health care needs (Joe, 1996; Levine, Corcoran, & Gitlin, 1993; Meyers, 2010) and the treatment/outcome emphasis is on functional limitations and the efficiency with which they are addressed. While a home setting may be a hindrance to more medical approaches, a client's home is the ideal location for occupational therapy since occupational needs can be assessed and adapted for in their natural context. The home is also the best place to empower the client; therefore the therapist's role as teacher for both patient and family is paramount. Although treatment approaches may be modified in this setting (Atchison, 1997; Levine et al., 1993; McGuire, 1997; Meyers, 2010; Stahl, 1998), the same core values of occupational therapy still apply (Opacich, 1997). Crafts incorporate many skills and behaviors that can generalize to many areas of function or they may be ends in themselves as the therapist helps the client explore alternative leisure options at home. Leisure or other productive use of sometimes newly available time is often a neglected aspect of function both during and after hospitalization;

Tubbs, C., & Drake, M. *Crafts and Creative Media in Therapy, Fourth Edition (pp. 167-182).*

incorporation of crafts in therapy may facilitate the client's independent pursuit/follow-through of these activities after discharge. Crafts are sometimes easier to plan for in home health since the treatment is intermittent over a longer period of time and an activity can be spread over several sessions if needed. In addition, some clients may even have projects already begun and/or have supplies and materials available. If not, though, one way to contain costs is to use found art and craft materials rather than expensive commercial materials. Cost containment is an unavoidable aspect of practice today and must be considered in planning treatment.

Found Materials

The term *found materials* refers to articles, materials, or supplies not intentionally prepared for use in crafting. Creative therapists have always devised ways to use things that others might simply discard, and the current cultural emphasis on recycling has made this more acceptable, even desirable to the general public. Many Internet craft sites devote an entire category to "green" or recycled crafts and Appendix II and Resources listed at the end of this chapter offer plentiful ideas. One program in New York has made affordable adaptive equipment for pediatric clients using materials such as corrugated cardboard, wood, plastic, and foam (Hendrickson, 2005) and therapists practicing in impoverished countries regularly make use of what the average therapist would consider unconventional materials (Werner, 2009). Fazio describes a pre-vocational program implemented with homeless, mentally ill, HIV-positive clients. The participants "manufactured" handmade paper from scrap paper materials, then used the paper to make greeting cards and wrapping paper to sell. This project was chosen in part because of the low cost of implementation, a necessity in many community-based programs that rely heavily on grants for funding (Fazio, 2008). The current economic climate makes some recycling almost mandatory, regardless of setting, if the therapist wants to include crafts in treatment on a regular basis (Breines, 1998; Ehrlich & Piersol, 1997). Considering the price of a simple craft kit averages around $3.00, it is easy to see how using prepared materials could become cost-prohibitive over time. Found materials are especially convenient in home health practice since it is impossible for a therapist to carry a full spectrum of crafts from place to place. A few basic craft tools and supplies, however, can be kept in a box in the car—similar to a first aid kit—allowing the therapist to improvise on-the-spot from found materials that are usually present in every household (Adams, 1989, 1991a, 1991b). The therapist can also collect items ahead of time to facilitate activity planning.

Tools and Supplies for Basic Crafting

- Scissors
- Needle nose or other pliers
- Various glues (e.g., white glue, super glue, glue gun, spray adhesive)
- Needle and thread
- Masking and cellophane tape, string, rubber bands
- Sandpaper
- Pressing iron
- Hammer
- Sponge
- Brushes, cotton swabs
- Water-based paints, washable markers
- Toothpicks (Stribling, 1970)

Types of Found Materials

Household Items

The items listed below may become components of the completed project but some can also be used as tools in the process. For example, plastic lids make good paint palettes, or eggs cartons can keep materials, such as beads, separated.

- Plastic lids, paper plates, coffee filters
- Empty milk or juice containers, plastic or cardboard; yogurt containers
- Cardboard toilet paper or paper towel rolls
- Sewing thread spools
- Plastic soda bottles, container caps
- Styrofoam trays (e.g., from meat, cookies, etc.), egg cartons
- Empty glass jars with lids, glass bottles
- Aluminum pie tins, small metal candy tins, cupcake liners
- Tin cans, coffee cans
- Used candles or crayons
- Coat hangers; liquid starch, clothes pins
- Oatmeal boxes, shoe boxes, cereal boxes
- Strawberry baskets
- Flowerpots (plastic and clay)
- Popsicle sticks

Pantry Items

- Flour and salt
- Dried beans, pasta, rice, popcorn
- Whole cloves, cinnamon sticks
- Corn husks
- Cornstarch
- Potatoes
- Peanuts in the shell

Natural Materials

- Driftwood, twigs, small branches
- Seeds, seed pods
- Leaves, flowers, grasses
- Seashells, eggshells
- Feathers, bones
- Stones
- Gourds
- Pinecones

Scrap Paper Products

- Discarded wrapping paper or greeting cards
- Old magazines or catalogs
- Old puzzle pieces
- Wallpaper sample books
- Newspaper
- Brown paper bags
- Shredded newspaper or other packing material
- Cardboard (from boxes, shirt packing)
- Tissue paper
- Paper napkins, doilies

Fiber and Fabric

- String, yarn
- Sequins, buttons
- Gift or fabric ribbon
- Old socks, old pantyhose
- Fabric scraps, lace scraps
- Embroidery floss
- Discarded clothing
- Old curtains
- Ragged dishtowels

Project Ideas Using Found Materials

- Greeting cards
- Picture frames
- Collages, posters
- Christmas or other holiday ornaments
- Window decorations
- Sculptures, mobiles, wall hangings
- Bird feeders, planters
- Candles, candle holders
- Decorated containers
- Masks, puppets, dolls

To introduce or implement crafting in the client's home, a therapist might ask a client to choose from a list of possible projects, such as the list above, and then assist the client in finding the materials to make it. Even the lack of certain supplies or materials may offer a therapeutic opportunity for adaptation or problem solving. The client's culture may influence what crafts will be of interest, therefore the decision to use crafts may offer the therapist the additional insight needed for culturally competent service provision (Piersol, 1998; Weinstein, 1997). An understanding of the impact of a client's culture on occupational performance is essential for best practice in occupational therapy (Pendleton & Schultz-Krohn, 2006).

Crafts can also be utilized to teach knowledge of and appreciation for other cultures. For example, Native Americans were, by necessity, especially resourceful at utilizing natural materials. Children often enjoy making Native American objects and clothing and the process allows them to learn about Native American culture as well as gain respect for the beauty and function of natural materials (Carlson, 1994; Leftwich, 1970). The concept of using found materials also fits with environmentally responsible practices such as recycling, appropriate to all client populations.

Candles

Candle making is included in this chapter because it possible to use old or partially used candles and broken crayons as a wax source, and molds and most other necessary tools and supplies can be improvised with household items. Candle making also has some of the same activity demands as cooking and most homes will have the necessary equipment available. Although now considered a leisure craft, candle making was once vitally important in providing illumination and for fulfilling certain ceremonial functions. Early candles were made from tallow—rendered animal fat—or more expensive beeswax. The Romans are credited with inventing the first wick candles (Abadie, 2002). Until the molding technique was developed, candles were made by hand using the dipping method. Candles were first mass produced in the 1830s; the modern candle-making process is little changed since then (Abadie, 2002; Bardey, 1999). Although candles are no longer needed for illumination, they have retained their importance in religious and other ceremonies and rituals. Candles are popular as gifts and home décor items, are used to create moods and aromas, and can, of course, still provide light when the power goes out.

While candle making may not be a common craft in occupational therapy clinics, it has definite therapeutic possibilities because it is low cost and requires few specialized tools and materials. Wax is also malleable at low heat levels, and can be melted over and over, so a satisfactory end product can usually be achieved. Basic methods of candle making are pouring, dipping, and rolling. Essential supplies and equipment for poured and dipped candles are wax (usually paraffin or beeswax), a heat source and suitable container (usually a double boiler) for melting the wax, wicking, measuring tools, molds or containers, pot holders, and a wax thermometer. Other items that may be helpful include a funnel for pouring wax; a hammer for breaking large chunks into smaller pieces; a paring knife or scissors; some type of probe for stirring and inserting wicks; and clean up items such as newspaper, paper towels, and aluminum foil or waxed paper (Larkin, 1998). Finally, dyes, scents, and decorative materials can also be used to make more creative, customized candles. The basic pouring procedure is described in the project instructions below. After just a few trials, the therapist will have the equipment and methods fine tuned.

Project—Molded Ice Candle

Plan It

This activity is time-sensitive, both in the fact that the melted wax will begin to quickly harden once it is poured, and that the ice will melt in the mold if it is not added right before pouring in the hot wax. It is recommended that the therapist go through the process at least once before doing it with a client. If the client is unhappy with the result, though, the wax can be re-melted and used in a new mold. Stearin is not absolutely essential, but will improve the overall quality of the candle. Different types of molds can be used, but some form of waxed cardboard container is the simplest since it can simply be torn away once the wax has hardened.

Get Ready

Supplies

- Wax (candle remnants or paraffin wax), plus stearin or other hardener
- Square wicking, primed
- Mold seal or sturdy tape
- Color (e.g., broken crayons or old candle remnants), scent (optional)
- Small cubes of ice

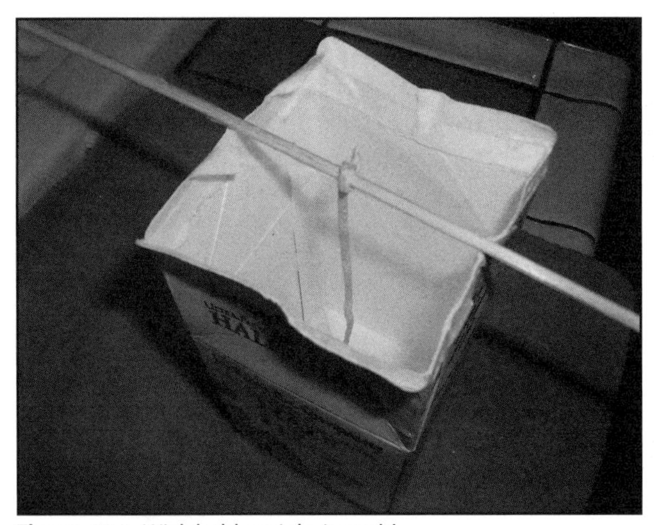
Figure 14-1. Wick held upright in mold.

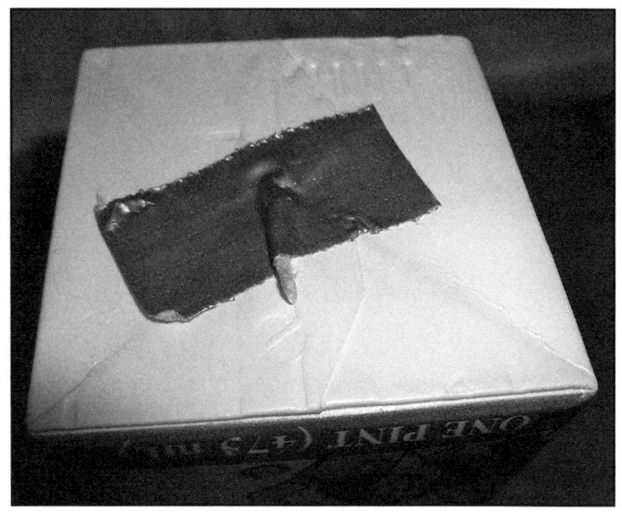

Figure 14-2. Wick secured at bottom of mold.

Tools

- 1-pint cardboard milk carton (the mold)
- Double boiler or pot with melting container
- Heating element
- Scissors
- Funnel
- Small dowel or bamboo skewer

Time required: 45 minutes

Approximate cost: $2 (or much less if old candles are used instead of purchased paraffin)

Do It

Process

1. Cover work area with newspaper.
2. Prepare the mold; cut the top section off, make a small hole in the center of the bottom.
3. Insert wick through the hole with an inch or so protruding and run the straight pin through it to hold secure.
4. Lay the dowel across the top of the mold and wrap the wick around it, secure with a piece of tape if needed (Figure 14-1). Be sure not to pull the wick out of the hole in the bottom.
5. From the bottom of the mold, make sure the wick taut, then seal the hole completely with the mold seal or securely tape over the hole and protruding wick (Figure 14-2).
6. Melt the wax to 160 degrees; add hardener per package instructions; add color and scent as desired.
7. Pour 1 to 2 inches of wax into the mold.
8. Add some ice cubes, then more wax, then more ice cubes, and so on until the mold is full. Take care to keep the wick centered during the process.
9. As the candle cools, poke a probe down the center of the candle near the wick, and refill the cavity with wax, using a funnel if necessary for more precise pouring. The wax used for refilling should also be at 160 degrees.
10. Let the candle cool completely.

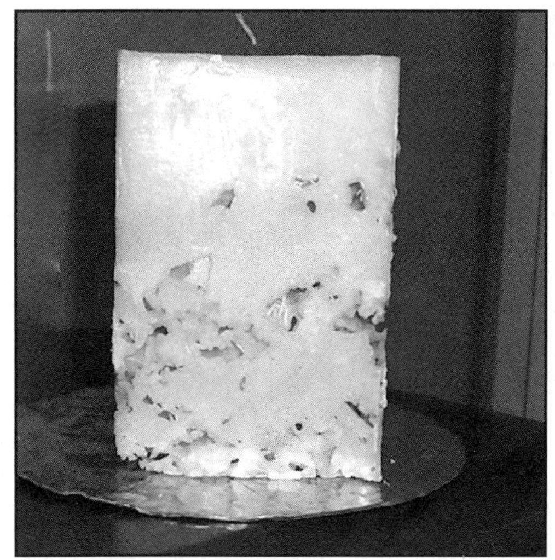

Figure 14-3. Completed ice candle.

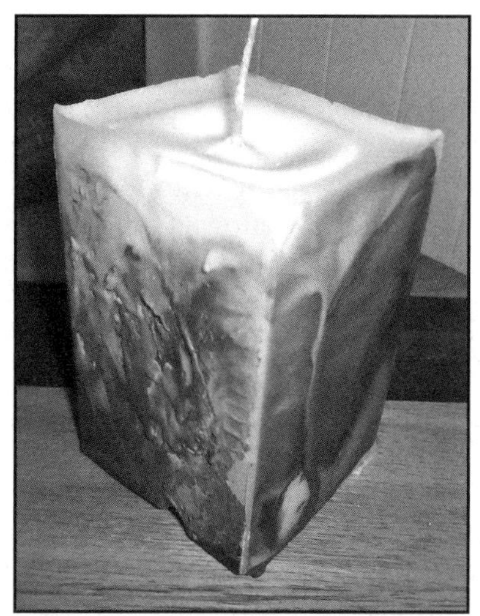

Figure 14-4. Candle decorated with melted crayons.

11. Remove the wick from the dowel. Tear away the mold, trim the wick flush with the candle bottom, and trim the top wick to about 1 inch in length. Rub the sides with a piece of old nylon stocking to give it a shinier finish (Figure 14-3).

Change It

This candle can be varied by using a differently shaped mold, by not using the ice, or by adding color during the melting process or after the candle has hardened. For example, lay a few crayon pieces on a waxed paper lined baking sheet and allow them to melt at a low temperature in an oven or toaster oven. Then simply dip each side of the candle in the melted crayon for a swirl effect (Figure 14-4). To grade the activity down, the therapist can have the client prepare the mold and choose colors or scents, but assist with the melting and pouring. Simpler still, the client could merely decorate the outside of the candle after it has been prepared by carving or painting designs with melted wax. To grade the activity up, omit the ice and have the client pour the wax in layers, using a different color for each one. Or cut colored wax in chunks and fill the mold with them before pouring in the melted (white) wax.

Document It

Since several aspects of this activity are similar to steps in cooking, there are multiple ways to relate it to occupational goals in documentation. Examples are as follows:

- "The client was able to safely manipulate the hot container, using hot pads as needed, and remembered to turn off the stove without cueing."
- "The therapist provided the client with a written, step-by-step checklist for the procedure which he was able to follow independently."
- "The client was inattentive and impulsive during the candle-making activity, indicating that she may be unsafe to return to independent cooking at this time."

Multiple techniques for creating unique and interesting candles can be accomplished—either during the pouring/molding process or after the basic candle is formed—with common household materials. For example, use unusual containers or molds such as egg shells, large sea shells, or shaped aluminum foil that has been stabilized in a bed of sand. Or fill the mold with chunks of colored wax or crayon pieces before pouring the melted wax; this will create a mottled appearance in the finished candle. Another idea is to place a pre-made pillar candle in the center of a mold, then surround it with trinkets or natural materials (non-flammable) before adding melted wax to fill the mold, producing a "treasure" candle (Larkin, 1998). Use cardboard juice containers, toilet paper rolls, or waxed milk cartons to make tear-away molds. Candles can be poured in layers; tilt to one side during hardening for an angled effect. Dyes and oils are available for coloring and scenting candles to the maker's preference.

After a candle has been poured and hardened, decoration can be added to the outside by using melted wax as "glue" to attach cinnamon sticks, shells, or pressed flowers. Warm wax can be whipped in a bowl using a whisk or hand mixer; the whipped wax is then spread on the top and/or sides of a candle to resemble icing, foam, or snow. Create cupcake candles by using muffin tins as molds, then "frosting" with whipped wax. Pillar or ball candles can be dipped in melted wax of different colors (e.g., crayon pieces) to create an outer shell, or different colors can be dripped around the edge. Or first cover some areas with masking tape, and then roll the outside of the candle in the melted wax. After cooling, peel off the tape (*Reader's Digest*, 1979). Thin sheets of wax warmed in an oven can be cut and appliquéd to the outside of pillars as well, but must be worked fairly quickly. You can even use paints or carving to embellish the outside. In summary, decorating the exterior of the candle is one way of enabling someone to participate in this craft at a simpler level (Webster, 1972). Rolled candles are another simple variation, requiring only beeswax sheets, wicking, a cutting tool, and a blow dryer, but the wax sheets must be purchased and are probably too expensive for regular use in a therapy setting. This method is simple but less conducive to adding creative elements.

Certain precautions should be taken when making candles. The principal danger is the risk of burns from the hot wax or from the heat source itself. The therapist should be sure that any client making poured candles has adequate muscle strength and control to manage the container during pouring and it is advisable to use pot holders or mitts. Dipping candles is somewhat less hazardous, but still involves exposure to hot wax. Rolling candles poses little or no risk to the client. Although some people use candles only as decoration, they are meant to be burned, and the occupational therapist should keep this in mind when suggesting this craft to a client. The therapist should feel reasonably confident that the client has adequate judgment or supervision to use the candle safely at home. Hospital settings prohibit the burning of candles of any kind, so the therapist should give the client possession of his or her creation only upon discharge. Another option is to have the client make candles as gifts for others. Tools used intermittently in making candles can also pose hazards. As with any activity, precautions should be taken when using pointed or sharp implements. If a client is unable to use such tools safely, the therapist will need to assist with these steps of the process.

Paraffin costs approximately $3.00 per pound; beeswax is considerably more expensive (Triarco Arts and Crafts, 2011). Depending on the form in which wax is purchased, certain ingredients such as stearin may need to be added, which will slightly increase the cost. Colors, scents, and wicks are an additional but not significant expense, especially if purchased in bulk. Although a variety of molds and containers are available on the market, many common household items can be used just as well.

Making candles can be messy so it is advisable to cover the work area with newspaper. Remove wax from clothing by pouring hot water over it; remove wax from carpet by rubbing it with an ice cube, then scraping with a dull knife. Hot water will also remove wax from objects such as tools and containers, but wax should never be poured down a drain. Wax is flammable, so it should never be melted in a container in direct contact with the heating surface, should never be left unattended, and the water level in the double boiler should be monitored. If melting wax does catch on fire, immediately cover the container. Never attempt to extinguish burning wax with water as this can scatter the flames. Keep a vessel of cool water handy, though, in case hot wax contacts the skin. Even this rarely causes anything more than temporary discomfort, and cooled wax will easily peel off of skin (Bardey, 1999). It may be helpful to use disposable containers such as metal coffee cans for melting wax to minimize clean up time (Larkin, 1998). One nice quality of wax is that it can be re-melted and remolded without affecting its integrity. If the client is unhappy with the end-product, it can simply be thrown back in the pot, melted, and poured anew. A professional-looking finish can be achieved by rubbing the cooled candle with a piece of old pantyhose material (Abadie, 2002).

Project—Clove Orange

Supplies

- Orange(s)
- Whole cloves
- Ribbon (optional)

Tools: Scissors (optional; for cutting ribbon)

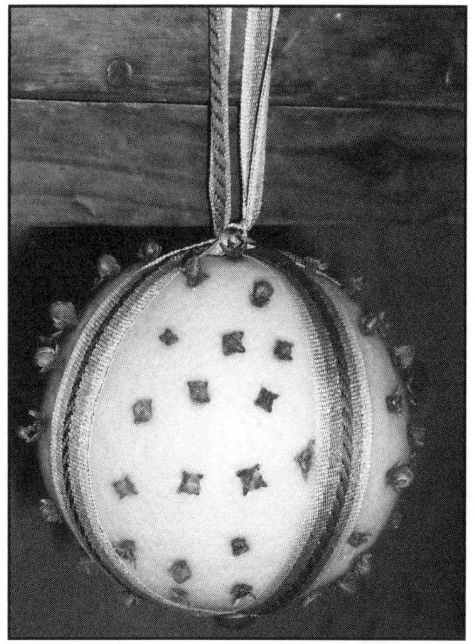

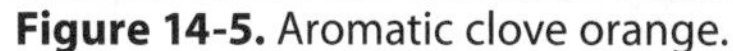

Figure 14-5. Aromatic clove orange.

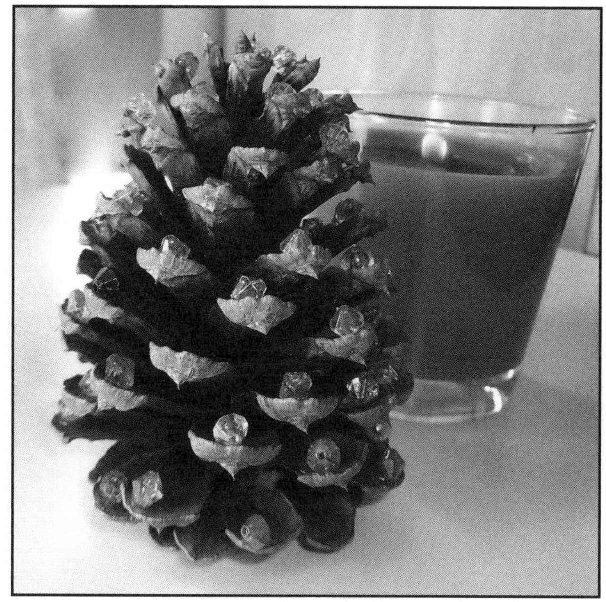

Figure 14-6. Pinecone Christmas tree.

Process

1. Push the sharp, pointed ends of the whole cloves into the orange rind. This can be done in a pattern or in a random arrangement with as few or as many cloves as desired.
2. To hang the completed clove orange, wrap a ribbon snugly around the center, tie in a knot at the top, and tie another knot a few inches up the ribbon to form a loop for hanging (Figure 14-5).

Clove oranges are extremely easy to make and their pleasing aromatic scent makes them popular during the fall and winter holiday season. This activity might be good for a client diagnosed with hemiparesis who is learning to incorporate the affected extremity as a stabilizer and/or to improve the dexterity in the nondominant hand. Whole cloves can be expensive, so shop the bargain racks, especially at the end of the holiday season.

Project—Pinecone Christmas Tree

Supplies

- Large pinecone
- Tacky glue or glue gun with glue sticks
- Beads, seeds, sequins, or other small items for decoration

Tools: No tools are required, although tweezers may be used

Process

1. Stabilize the pine cone, large end down, by setting it in a glass or other container slightly smaller than the base of the pine cone. Or remove enough bottom scales (if necessary) so it will sit flat.
2. Place a small drop of glue on individual scales and add a bead or other decoration. Continue in this fashion until you like the look of the "tree" (Figure 14-6).
3. Other options are to spray paint the pine cone first. Or dot the ends of the scales with glue and sprinkle with or roll in glitter.

You can make a "forest" full of trees, or vary the color and style of decorations to complement certain décors or holiday themes. This activity might benefit a client working on fine motor, visual scanning, or visual discrimination skills.

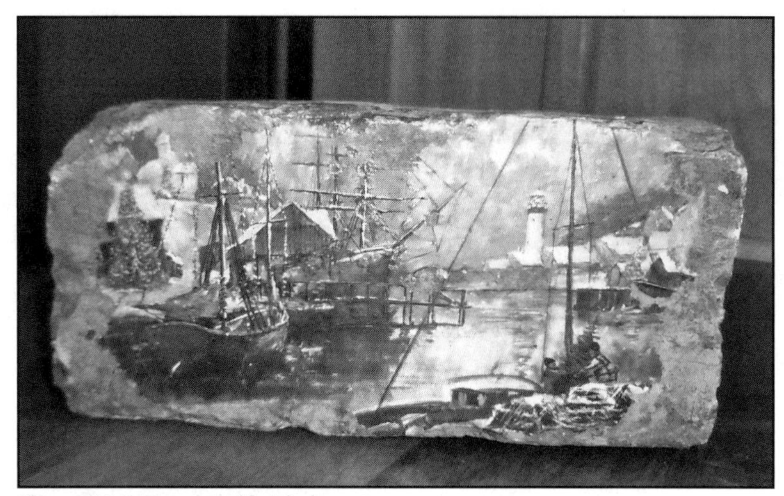

Figure 14-7. Decorated brick doorstop.

Project—Brick/Greeting Card Doorstop

Supplies

- A brick, old or new (can have cracked or chipped areas)
- Greeting card with image of a size and orientation suitable to the size of the brick
- White glue
- Felt, at least 2 x 8 inches (or large enough to cover bottom of brick)
- Acrylic sealer, optional

Tools

- Sponge
- Scissors
- Foam or bristle paint brush

Process

1. Cut the back flap off the greeting card and discard. Clean the brick thoroughly. If using water, be sure to let it dry completely.
2. Moisten the back side of the greeting card picture, allow it to sit for several minutes under a damp cloth or sponge. Then, using a damp sponge or finger, gently rub away the layers of paper until only a thin sheet with the image remains. Rub carefully so as not to tear the picture, but small tears can be patched.
3. Gently tear around the edges of the picture to the size and remaining image desired. The image should be no larger than the face of the brick. Let the card dry.
4. Spread a generous layer of glue on the face of the brick, then attach the card image, smoothing all the edges as flat as possible. The glue will be clear when it dries, so there is no concern about getting it on top of the picture.
5. Seal the image by applying additional coats of white glue (drying between each coat) or by spraying or brushing with acrylic sealer according to product directions. The brick/glue will need to dry before the sealer is applied.
6. Glue a strip of felt to the bottom of the brick to prevent it from scratching flooring.

The choice of images to use on the doorstop is virtually endless. The thinner the paper and the less defined the edges, the more it will blend and look like the image is printed on the brick surface (Figure 14-7).

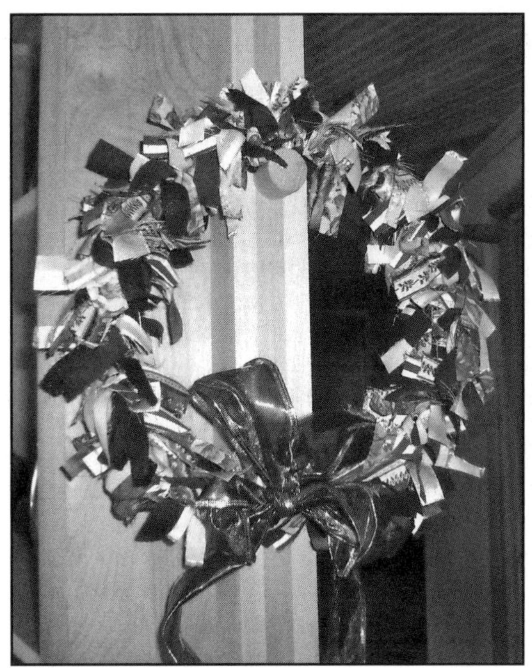

Figure 14-8. Fabric strip wreath.

Motor control is needed to keep from tearing through too much of the wet paper, but the client can work slowly and the paper can be remoistened as necessary. The activity may be good to work on grading the amount of force applied.

Project—Fabric Strip Wreath

Supplies

- Scrap fabric
- Metal ring or wooden embroidery hoop, 8 to 10 inches in diameter
- Yarn or string for hanging

Tools

- Scissors or rolling cutter
- Cutting mat (if a rolling cutter is used)

Process

1. Cut or tear fabric into strips, approximately 1 x 6 inches. The number needed will vary, but it will probably take 200 or more. Fabric style and color will depend on the creator's taste and where the wreath will be used. If a rolling cutter and mat are used, the fabric can be folded such that several layers can be cut at one time.
2. Tie the fabric strips snugly around the ring (but knotting is not necessary), occasionally sliding them together to create a full look.
3. When finished, tie on a looped length of yarn or string for hanging (Figure 14-8).

(Adapted from C & T Publishing's Design Collective, 2010)

The fabric wreath can be used as a holiday decoration or as an everyday wall decoration. The size or colors can be easily varied and beads, feathers, or other decoration can be added by tying or gluing on. This project can be especially useful when the client needs to work on repetitive reaching, endurance, or finger strengthening. The height of the work can be easily adjusted to achieve the therapeutic goal.

Other Ideas for Found Materials

The craft possibilities with found and household items are only as limited as the imagination of the occupational therapist and client. Because the materials were likely not intended for crafting in the first place, the creativity door is wide open. Boxes of all types can be painted, decoupaged, wrapped, or covered with papier-mâché to hold photos, jewelry, or other keepsakes. Glass jars or wine bottles can be painted, or covered with glass mosaic or colored tissue paper to form votive candle holders or vases. Pressed flowers, grasses, or ferns can be added to homemade cards or wrapping paper (Hall, 2001). Cut, paint, or stamp plain lunch sacks to make unique gift bags. Plastic lids or juice container lids can become coasters; cardboard milk cartons make excellent candle molds. Pasta can be used to make children's necklaces, Christmas tree garland, or mosaics; they can be spray painted or mixed with other media. Use carved potatoes to stamp tote bags, T-shirts, or journal covers. Construct Popsicle sticks or clothespin halves into miniature buildings or furniture or make them into picture frames and decorate with old puzzle pieces. Backs of greeting cards can be moistened and peeled away; the remaining thin picture can cover Styrofoam balls for ornaments, or become part of a collage. Or arrange and laminate several cards to make colorful placemats. Salt dough can be molded much like clay, then baked, painted, and varnished to make a multitude of decorative items such as refrigerator magnets or tree ornaments. Bring new life to old lampshades by covering them with thin patterned paper and découpaging (Dahlstrom, 2004). Make yarn pictures by coiling different colored yarns according to a pattern. Paint candy or breath mint tins a solid color, then decorate with beads, shells, or buttons.

It is also possible to make basic craft supplies from household ingredients. Natural dyes can be extracted from leaves, berries, and certain vegetables such as beets. Homemade paper can be made from paper scraps and water. Make glue or finger-paint from flour or cornstarch, "yarn" from strips of old clothes, or stencils from plastic carton pieces (Carlson, 1993). The list goes on and on. The therapist is encouraged to explore other craft books (see Resources section) and be observant when attending craft fairs and festivals. Books with children's crafts, nature crafts, or a "trash to treasure" focus all have excellent—and almost always affordable—ideas.

Home Decorating

Home design and decorating is currently a popular topic in magazines and television programs, and some clients may be interested in attempting a simple project, especially in their home setting. In this case, it will be especially important that the client choose the activity but the therapist may offer guidance and suggestions based on individual abilities, goals, and supplies and time available. Some clients may already have an interest in home decorating or may have projects already underway; this is an ideal opportunity for the therapist to help the patient problem solve to resume desired occupations and to do so in the natural context. The realm of home decorating is rich with opportunities for gross motor involvement, including activities that require standing, bending, and reaching. Clients can fabricate small home décor items such as some listed in preceding paragraphs—vases, pillows, candles/candleholders, and more—or they can try more ambitious endeavors such as stenciling a border in a room or sewing a set of curtains. Clients could also make small furniture accessories, recover dining chairs, etch a glass door or mirror, or paint a cabinet. As always, the therapist is responsible for ensuring that the activity demands are realistic in terms of therapeutic objectives and that there is a reasonable chance of success, but this type of thinking "outside the box" may be the difference that motivates a client to his or her full potential.

Case Study

Agnes, an 82-year-old retired school principal, is receiving home health occupational therapy for a Colles' fracture of her left wrist that she sustained from an assault during a burglary. Agnes still lives in the home she shared with her husband while they raised their three children. Although Agnes has been a widow for 15 years, she has chosen to stay in her neighborhood where she is close to friends, familiar stores, and her church. The neighborhood is gradually changing, though, as elderly neighbors die or move into assisted-living residences. Some older homes are being sold at reduced prices and some have been allowed to run down or are abandoned altogether. Agnes had felt safe until a someone broke into her house late one afternoon. When she confronted the burglar in her kitchen, he knocked her down, fracturing her radius as she attempted to break her fall. The burglar hit her several times, causing several large bruises and a black eye. He took her purse, which was lying by the telephone in the kitchen, and ran out the backdoor, leaving her for dead. Agnes eventually heard the mailman on her porch, called out to him, and he used his cell phone to summon the police.

Agnes spent 2 days in the hospital for evaluation and treatment; she was seen only twice in occupational therapy before discharge. Since the treating therapist divided her time between inpatient treatment and home health, all services components of the same Preferred Provider Organization (PPO), she planned to continue seeing Agnes at home. Agnes' wrist was immobilized in a cast, but her fingers were free. The initial evaluation included sensory testing of Agnes' fingers, assessment of proximal range of motion, and circumferential measurement of all fingers to check for edema. Since the Model of Human Occupation was the underlying theory in this occupational therapy department, the therapist planned to do a more thorough assessment of roles and habits at the client's home.

Through conversation, she had already learned that Agnes enjoyed a variety of crafts, talking on the telephone with her friends, attending church, and visiting with neighborhood children. Over the years, she had taken great pleasure in teaching the children about cooking, gardening, and making things with their hands. She expressed some anxiety about returning home, but was determined not to be frightened away. Along with home health occupational therapy, Agnes' physician recommended she also consult a psychologist to help her heal emotionally from the trauma.

Agnes' daughter, who lives 2 hours away, took a week of leave from her job to be with her mother during her first days at home. During that week, the occupational therapist made her first visit, with a level II fieldwork student accompanying her. They found Agnes' home to be neat, with a minimum amount of dust and clutter. The therapist had the student assist the client in completing the Occupational Self-Assessment (OSA; Christiansen & Baum, 2005). Agnes described her involvement in the recent garden club project in which they made dried flower wreaths for a community craft fair. She had cut and dried flowers from her own garden to use in the wreaths. She spoke of how much she still enjoyed her neighborhood, in spite of some of the changes. She knew her daughter and her friends would now want her to move into a retirement residence, but she resisted this idea. Agnes was unable to think of any specific goals she had for her therapy or her future, except being able to stay in her own home. She was able to do all of her self-care except bathing. Although the home health nurse had shown her how to put a plastic bag over her cast to protect it from moisture, she still felt insecure in getting in the shower. The occupational therapist and student also evaluated her home for safety hazards and made a few minor recommendations such as removing throw rugs (Collins, Beissner, & Krout, 1998; Piersol, 1998).

During the second occupational therapy visit, Agnes spoke of missing her grandchildren, who all lived in other cities, and continued to mention all the activities she had done with the neighborhood children. It occurred to the fieldwork student that Agnes might be able to utilize found or recycled craft materials to continue to do projects with the children without having to buy items she could ill afford. Agnes showed the student items that she had saved to reuse or recycle, including clean styrofoam trays, empty glass jars, and plastic strawberry baskets. Agnes explained she had always saved such things—probably due to growing up during the Depression—and made a habit of being frugal due to the limitations of her fixed income. During a craft activity, Agnes was able to hold items with her casted left hand while cutting and placing items with the right. The occupational therapist knew this movement, however limited, would be good for minimizing edema in the affected extremity. At the end of the session, the student again talked with Agnes about goals for therapy. The activity session had prompted her to think further about her current limitations and hopes for the future. Her first goal was to recover the full use of her left hand and arm once the fracture was healed and the cast removed. Complete self-care independence was her long-term goal. She then thought she ought to have a goal of being able to interact with the neighbor children each day so she would not be lonely; for the time being, she was confined to the house unless someone could drive her. To better ensure her safety and give her peace of mind, she hoped to have wrought iron safety doors installed for both the front and back exits. This will allow her to stay in her house with greater peace of mind.

The third occupational therapy home health visit was the last, since the PPO case manager determined that Agnes could get the most benefit from outpatient visits (when her cast was removed) for upper extremity strengthening as well as visits to the psychologist if needed. Prior to the final visit, the fieldwork student and occupational therapist spent a good deal of time planning. They needed to use the allotted time efficiently to teach Agnes whatever she needed to know to manage her daily activities in her home and community. They decided that making a written plan outlining ways to continue doing crafts and other projects with the neighborhood children would be most beneficial for maintaining her activity level, promoting use of her left hand, and preventing social isolation. They had Agnes make a list of places where she could assist children with crafts on a regular basis, including in her own home. With only a little cueing, Agnes was able to name the neighborhood school, a Sunday school class, and the local community center recreation program. They assisted her in finding the phone numbers needed to contact these places, as well as the transportation service of the area Agency on Aging so she could get to these locations.

Discussion Questions

1. How was the occupational therapy approach consistent with the stated theory, the Model of Human Occupation?
2. List some specific craft projects you think would be appropriate for Agnes and the children.
3. How can the therapist and student document what they did with Agnes to show the importance and benefit of her continued crafting with children?
4. In our multi-cultural communities, what differences might be expected in clients' receptivity to this therapeutic approach?

Resources

Candle Making
Basic Candle Making (Basic Book Series)
Edited by Eric Ebeling
Stackpole Books, 2002

Candle Making (Step-by-Step Crafts)
By Cheryl Owen
Creative Publishing International, 2001

The Encyclopedia of Candle Making Techniques
By Sandie Lea
Quarto Publishing, 1999

Candle Making Secrets: Insider Tips and Advice on How to Make Perfect Candles, Every Time
By Jennifer Furgeson
CreateSpace, 2010

Found and Recycled Materials
Eco-Craft: Recycle, Recraft, Restyle
By Susan Wasinger
Lark Books, 2009
Projects for modern decorative and functional items using materials that most people throw away.

Fantastic Recycled Plastic
By David Edgar and Robin Edgar
Lark Books, 2009
Clever and imaginative projects made from plastic containers.

The Big Green Book of Recycled Crafts
Leisure Arts Series
Leisure Arts, Inc., 2009

Fabulous Jewelry from Found Objects
By Martha LeVan
Lark Books, 2005

Best Friends Forever
By Laura Torres
Workman Publishing, 2004
Fun, inexpensive crafts for kids and teens to make for each other.

Easy Crafts to Make Together (Better Homes and Gardens Series)
By Susan M. Banker
Meredith Books, 2004
Crafts designed for parents and children to make together.

Jewelry From Nature
By Cathy Yow
Sterling Publishing, 1999

The Decorative Egg Book
By Deborah Schneebeli-Morrell
Lorenz Books, 1998

Trash to Treasure: The Recycler's Guide to Creative Crafts
By Anne Childs (Ed.)
Leisure Arts, Inc., 1996.
How to give a second life to boxes, buckets, felt-pens, styrofoam packing, empty food containers, furniture, paper bags, pinecones, and vines. Seven pages of patterns for drawing or painting.

Easy-to-do Holiday Crafts From Everyday Household Items
Edited by Sharon Dunn Umnik
Boyds Mills Press, 2005
Simple, inexpensive projects for children.

References

Abadie, M. J. (2002) *The everything candlemaking book*. Avon, MA: Adams Media Corporation.
Adams, G. (1989). *How to make craft recipes*. Green Oaks, IL: Oak Springs Publications.
Adams, G. (1991a). *How to make craft projects from nature*. Libertyville, IL: Oak Springs Publications.
Adams, G. (1991b). *How to make craft projects from recycled materials*. Libertyville, IL: Oak Springs Publications.
Atchison, B. (1997). Occupational therapy in home health: Rapid changes need proactive planning. *American Journal of Occupational Therapy, 51*(6), 406-409.
Bardey, C. (1999). *Making candles and potpourri*. New York, NY: Black Dog and Leventhal Publishers, Inc.
Breines, E. (1998). The case for recycling "stuff." *Advance for Occupational Therapy Practitioners, 14*(24), 5.
Carlson, L. (1993). *EcoArt*. Charlotte, VT: Williamson Publishing.
Carlson, L. (1994). *More than moccasins: A kid's activity guide to traditional North American Indian life*. Chicago, IL: Chicago Review Press.
Christiansen, C., & Baum, C. (1991). *Occupational therapy: Overcoming human performance deficits*. Thorofare, NJ: SLACK Incorporated.
Collins, J., Beissner, K. L., & Krout, J. A. (1998). Home health physical therapy; Practice patterns in western New York. *Physical Therapy, 78*(2), 170-179.
Dahlstrom, C. F. (Ed.). (2004). *Better homes and gardens easy crafts to make together*. Des Moines, IA: Meredith Books.

Design Collective. (2010). *Little birds*. Lafayette, CA: C & T Publishing. 91-93.
Ehrlich, P., & Piersol, C. (1997). How you can succeed as a home care therapist. *Advance for Occupational Therapists, 13*(43), 12.
Fazio, L. S. (2008). *Developing occupation-centered programs for the community* (2nd ed.). Upper Saddle River, NJ: Pearson Prentice Hall.
Hall, M. A., Wrobel, J., & Salamony, S. (2001). *Decorative crafts sourcebook.* San Diego, CA: Thunder Bay Press.
Hendrickson, C., & Lesser, S. (2005). Building on possibilities. *Advance for Occupational Therapy Practitioners*, 21(9), 23-25.
Joe, B. E. (1996). Homecare; growth and change. *OT Week, 10*(45), 14-15.
Larkin, C. (1999). *The book of candlemaking: Creating scent, beauty, and light.* New York, NY: Chapelle, Ltd., Sterling Publishing Company.
Leftwich, R. L. (1970). *Arts and crafts of the Cherokee.* Cherokee, NC: Cherokee Publications.
Levine, R. E., Corcoran, M. A., & Gitlin, L. N. (1993). Home care and private practice. In: H. L. Hopkins & H. D. Smith (Eds.). *Willard and Spackman's occupational therapy* (8th ed.). Philadelphia, PA: Lippincott Williams & Wilkins.
McGuire, M. J. (1997). Documenting progress in home care. *American Journal of Occupational Therapy, 51*(6), 436-445.
Meyers, S. K. (2010). *Community practice in occupational therapy: A guide to serving the community.* Sudbury, MA: Jones and Bartlett Publishers.
Opacich, K. J. (1997). Moral tensions and obligations of occupational therapy practitioners providing home care. *American Journal of Occupational Therapy, 51*(6), 430-435.
Pendleton, H. M., & Schultz-Krohn, W. (2006). *Pedretti's occupational therapy: Practice skills for physical dysfunction.* St. Louis, MO: Mosby Elsevier.
Piersol, C. V. (1998). How is OT in the home unique? *Advance for Occupational Therapists, 14*(8), 7.
Reader's Digest. (1979). *Crafts and hobbies.* Pleasantville, NY: The Reader's Digest Association Inc.
Stahl, C. (1998). Putting pediatric home care in better focus. *Advance for Occupational Therapists, 1*(14), 32-33.
Stribling, M. L. (1970). *Art from found materials.* New York, NY: Crown Publishers.
Triarco Arts and Crafts. (2010). *2010 Catalog.* Minneapolis, MN: Triarco Arts & Crafts, LLC.
Webster, W. E., & McMullen, C. (1972). *The complete book of candlemaking.* Garden City, NJ: Doubleday and Company, Inc.
Weinstein, M. (1997). Bringing family-centered practices into home health. *OT Practice, 2*(7), 35-38.
Werner, D. (2009). *Disabled village children: A guide for community health workers, rehabilitation workers, and families.* Berkely, CA: Hesperian.

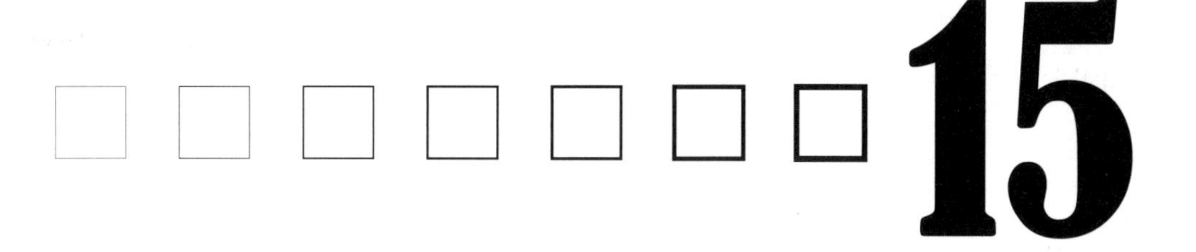

Paper Crafts

Objectives

The student should be able to:

- Discuss historical/cultural examples of paper crafts
- List basic supplies and materials needed to do paper crafts and know how to complete and grade a project
- Understand advantages and limitations of paper crafts activities in therapy
- List precautions of paper crafts
- Describe ways that paper craft activities can be used with various client populations

Paper was invented in China sometime between 200 and 100 B.C. Other materials had been used to write on for many centuries before that—wet clay, tree bark, cloth, and papyrus, from which the word *paper* comes—and early paper was used almost solely for this purpose. The Arabs learned about paper from their conquests in Asia and introduced it to Europe. Paper was still being made by hand at the time of the invention of the printing press in the 15th century. In the 18th century, a machine was invented that could make paper from wood pulp, though it did not become widely used for another 100 years (Lively, 2004). During this time, the Chinese developed glues they used in fashioning many paper crafts. The Japanese originated the craft of *origami*, or paper folding, which has evolved into a sophisticated art form. Today there is a tradition of groups joining together to fold 1,000 paper cranes as expressions of peace and love. Other cultural examples of paper crafts include intricate and colorful Mexican paper cut-outs, and the East Indian craft of papier mâché.

Paper, aside from its important function for writing, offers a world of craft delight for all ages (Department of the Army, 1971; Moseley, Johnson, & Koenig, 1962; *Reader's Digest*, 1979). Paper crafts may conjure memories of growing up, for example, our earliest party and holiday decorations may have been done with paper chains and crepe paper, or we may have aggravated our teachers by folding and flying paper airplanes. The commonplace nature of paper crafts may minimize their perceived value for some occupational therapists, but their versatility enables adaptation for almost any client population. One advantage of paper is its low cost and ready availability. Almost every office has a supply of paper, as well as pencils, glue, scissors, tape, staples, and paper clips—everything necessary for many projects. Several crafts whose principal material is paper will be discussed in this chapter. These include papier mâché, paper making, paper folding and

Tubbs, C., & Drake, M. *Crafts and Creative Media in Therapy, Fourth Edition (pp. 183-200).*

construction, paper cutting, collage and découpage, scrapbooking, and assorted ideas for decorating the paper itself. Due to the diversities in form, ideas for projects and grading suggestions are scattered throughout the text rather than grouped in one section.

Special Considerations

Most types of paper are inexpensive in comparison to other craft supplies, so an assortment can be stocked in most clinics. Even normally discarded items such as newspapers or old magazines are useful in many paper projects. Because of the low cost, the therapist can allow the client to make multiple attempts without worrying about waste. Specialty papers are more expensive and the occupational therapist may have to consult catalogs or art supply stores to find them, but basic office/school paper is available in most any general merchandise store. A glance at "paper" in the index of a craft catalog—more than 70 listings in some—will quickly reveal the broad scope of paper craft possibilities. This guarantees variety, but the therapist should be familiar with the products and their uses before making a selection. For example, some types are thin and delicate while others are thick enough to hold up to stamping, gluing, or other treatments; some are thicker still and best used for construction. Some papers have a translucent or metallic quality for use in more decorative applications such as greeting cards. Buying in bulk is usually more economical, but frequency of use and storage capacity should be considered as well as cost.

Paper crafts are generally very safe; paper cuts are always possible, though, so the therapist should caution or monitor clients with decreased sensation. Scissors may be used with some paper crafts, so standard sharps precautions should be observed. Some glues or solvents used in special processes may require extra ventilation or use of gloves, but this would be the exception rather than the rule. Depending on the form, paper crafts may or may not be messy; area preparation and clean-up time should be considered for projects requiring glue, paste, or paints.

Papier Mâché

The art of papier mâché (French for "chewed paper") was born centuries ago during a time when paper was a valuable commodity as a means of conserving/recycling this material (*Reader's Digest*, 1979). Although its earliest forms were probably developed in China, it was elevated into a fine art in the Far East (Lively, 2004). France was the first country in Europe to adopt this craft and is the source of its common name today. Papier mâché can be made by several different processes: by soaking pieces of torn up newspaper and mixing it with cooked starch; by using commercially prepared papier mâché mix; or by using the strip method. The last method will be described here, in the creation of a papier mâché bowl.

Project—Papier Mâché Bowl

Plan It

This project requires minimal dexterity and is a good choice for someone with a short attention span because each layer can be completed in a short period of time. One disadvantage is that it will require several sessions to complete due to drying time. The application of the wet strips may prove challenging for a client with sensory defensiveness but at the same time may be a good way of reducing tactile sensitivity. It is also a handy idea for a setting with few material resources.

Get Ready

Supplies

- Plastic bowl
- Newspapers
- Masking tape
- Liquid white glue

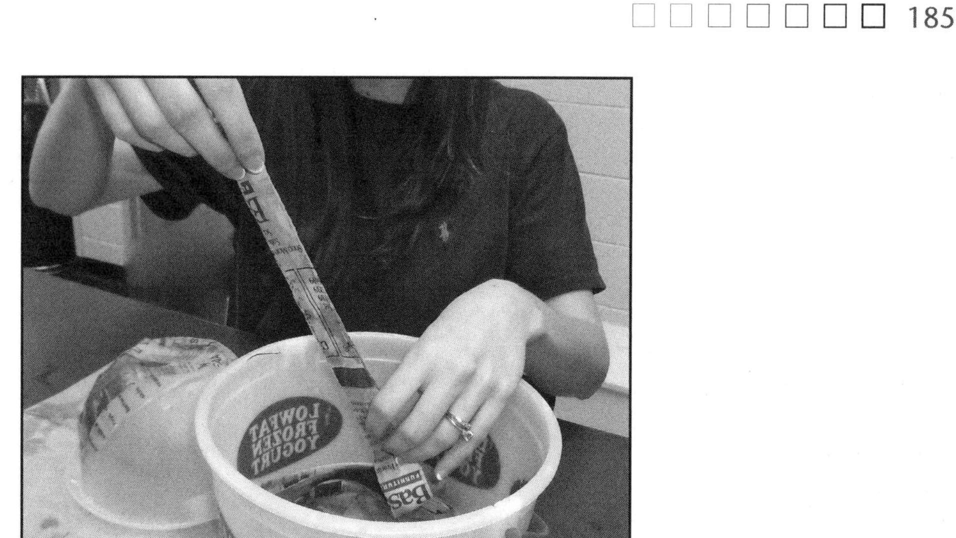

Figure 15-1. Client works to tolerate tactile input during papier mâché activity.

- Tissue paper, or paper cut-outs
- Petroleum jelly or plastic wrap
- Lacquer

Tools
- Bowl to mix glue
- Brushes for paint and lacquer
- Foam paint brush (for lacquer)

Time required: 3 to 4 sessions of about 30 minutes each for a medium-sized bowl

Approximate cost: Less than $1

Do It

Process
1. Cover the workspace with several layers of newspaper.
2. Invert the bowl on the work surface (this serves as the mold) and coat it with petroleum jelly or surround it with plastic wrap (as smoothly as possible) and secure the edges with tape.
3. Tear up one sheet of black and white newspaper into strips approximately 1 inch wide and 3 to 6 inches long.
4. In the bowl, mix one part white glue to one part water.
5. Put several strips in the glue/water mixture to coat them. Remove them, one at a time, pressing out excess liquid with the fingers (Figure 15-1), and apply to the bowl, smoothing as much as possible. Allow it to dry.
6. For the next layer, tear strips from the colored comic strip section of the newspaper and dip and apply in the same way. Using a different color paper will enable the maker to see that the whole surface has been covered with the second layer. Allow this layer to dry as well. Add at least one more layer of plain black and white newspaper strips. Additional layers can be added if desired, allowing time to dry after each.
7. After the last layer is dry, smooth the bowl by lightly sanding the surface or by adding additional strips to smooth any rough spots.

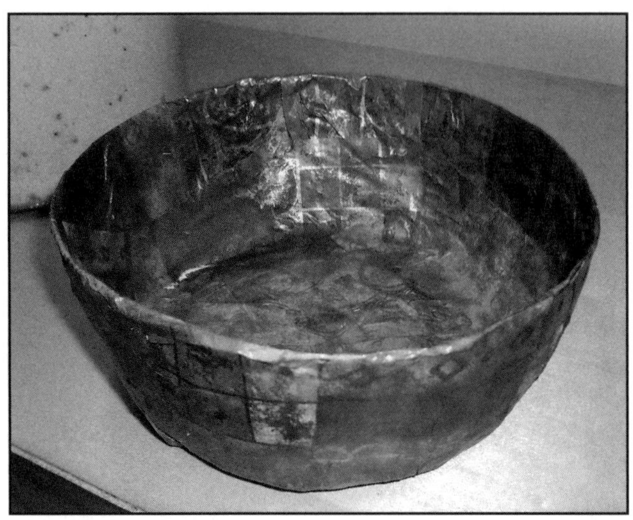

Figure 15-2. Papier mâché bowl, decorated with printed tissue paper.

8. Remove the paper bowl from the mold and paint as desired with any water-based paint, or decorate with other methods described below.
9. Lacquer the bowl for durability. This bowl is not suitable for direct contact with food.

Change It

Surface decoration variation is one means of grading the project up or down. To grade down, glue torn pieces of colored or printed tissue paper (Figure 15-2) to the surface instead of painting. This requires less precision than manipulating a paintbrush to paint a design. If tissue paper is too difficult to manage, strips of colored copy paper will work as well. To grade up, have the client cut pictures of choice from magazines and glue on the bowl in the fashion of a collage. For a faster project, soak shredded office paper in water for several hours, squeeze out excess moisture, process in a blender, then knead and press like clay over the mold (Wasinger, 2009). This process is similar to that of paper making described below, and can be done in one session but requires advance preparation and a greater amount of hand strength.

Document It

The following are a few examples of ways to communicate the therapeutic application of this craft:

- "The patient was able to tolerate touching the wet paper strips with her fingers for 2 to 3 minutes at a time before requesting to wash them." (see Figure 15-1)
- "The patient required cueing to visually scan the surface to see if all areas had been covered."
- "The client was able to use (affected) open hand to smooth strips into place with guiding by the therapist."

Paper Making and Paper Casting

A less common craft activity is paper casting; this involves making a pulp from soft tissue or using ready-prepared fibers. The pulp is then pressed into a terra cotta clay mold and allowed to dry. These castings can be painted and sealed to make hanging or other decorations (Barron, 1992). The pulp can also be formed around a mold, such as a bowl (Wasinger, 2009) or allowed to dry flat in sheets and used for other projects such as pictures, note cards, and gift tags.

Project—Handmade Paper

Supplies
- Scrap paper
- Water
- Torn leaves, flower petals, grass (optional)

Tools
- Blender
- Plastic dishpan
- Screen (sized to cover bottom of the dishpan)
- Towel
- Sponge
- Fabric sheets; scrap is okay
- Iron (optional)

Process
1. Tear paper into pieces and soak in water overnight.
2. Put soaked paper into blender, fill about halfway with water, and blend in short pulses. You may have to experiment with proportions of paper and water.
3. Put screen in the bottom of the dishpan; add several inches of water.
4. Pour paper pulp into dishpan. Swirl around, then lift straight up on screen.
5. Lay screen (with pulp) on an old towel to drain.
6. Cover paper pulp with fabric. Using a sponge, press down on fabric to remove water. Continue this process, squeezing out sponge as needed, until the fabric/pulp is as dry as possible.
7. Holding the fabric in place, flip the screen over and remove it. Allow pulp to dry; or place another piece of fabric on top and iron until dry.

(Adapted from Carlson, 1993)

Paper Folding

The traditional Japanese craft of origami, in its simpler forms, is a creative way to work on motor performance skills such as bilateral coordination, dexterity, and strengthening (Breines, 2006), and cognitive performance skills such as sequencing and following verbal or written directions. Combinations of hundreds of traditional folds transform paper into animals, flowers, puppets, boxes, or abstract forms (Lively, 2004). It is recommended that the therapist master a few constructions so they can be easily and skillfully demonstrated (Brienes, 2006). The cat shown in the following illustrations is one of the simplest figures. Special origami paper can be used, but any thin paper (cut to the proper dimensions) such as typing paper will usually serve just as well in a therapy application.

Project—Origami Cat

Plan It

This activity is particularly good for working on following written or demonstrated instructions in a specific sequence as well as fine motor skills. Advantages are the low cost and availability of the material. Young children will have to be instructed one step at a time and may need help for folding neatly. This activity is highly structured, therefore little creativity is allowed or needed.

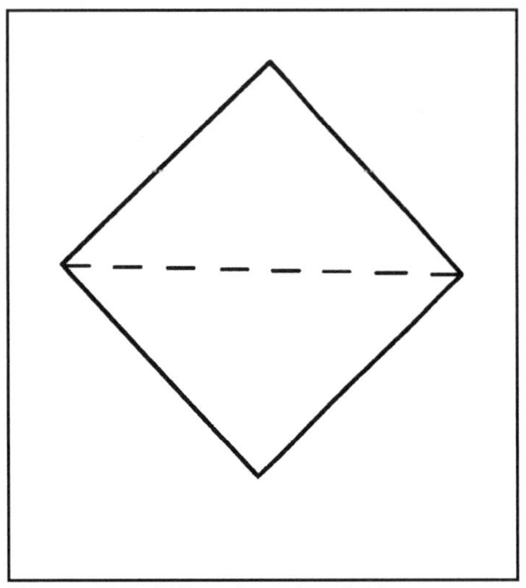
Figure 15-3. Origami cat, first fold.

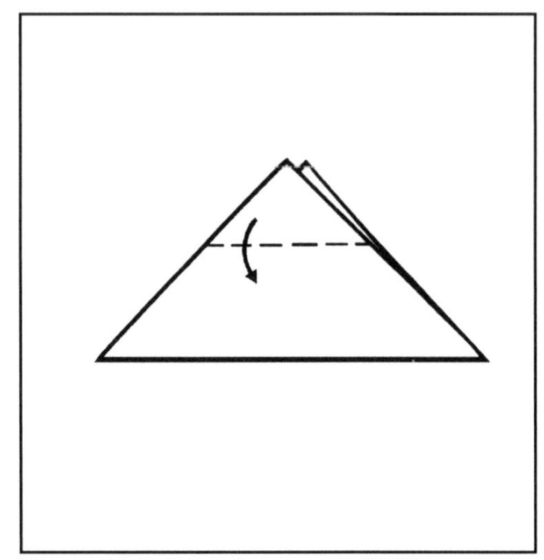
Figure 15-4. Origami cat, second fold.

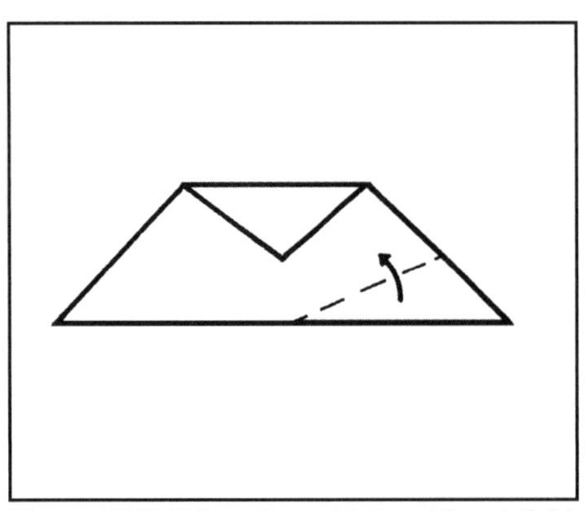
Figure 15-5. Origami cat, third and fourth fold.

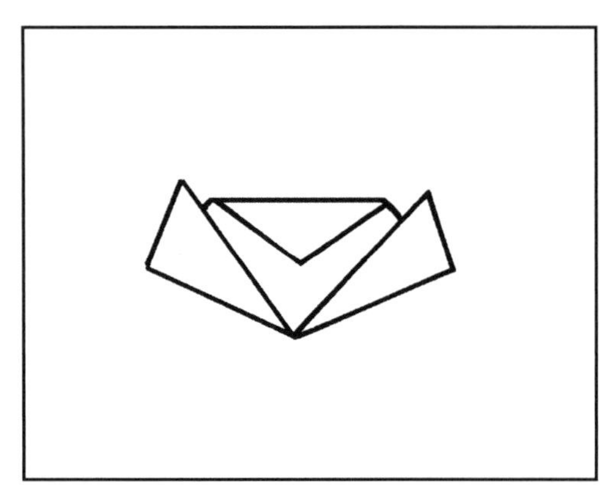
Figure 15-6. All folds completed.

Get Ready

Supplies
- Paper

Time required: Less than 15 minutes

Cost: Pennies

Do It

Process
1. Fold an 8-inch square of paper from corner to corner (Figure 15-3).
2. Fold down the top corner as shown (Figure 15-4).
3. Fold up the bottom corners as shown (Figures 15-5), to form ears. When all folds are completed (Figure 15-6), turn the cat's head over.
4. Draw eyes, nose, mouth, and whiskers (Figure 15-7; Sakade, 1958).

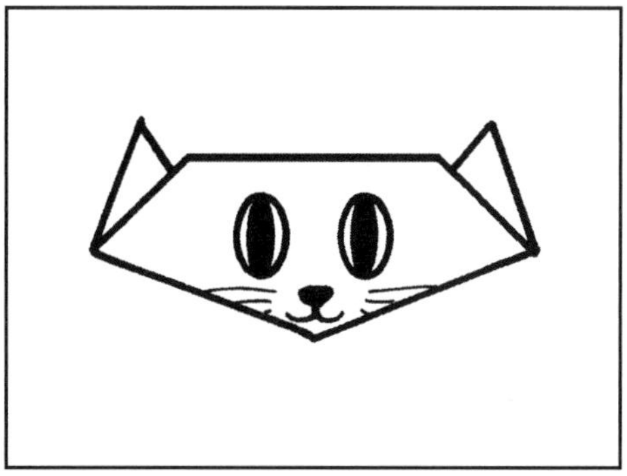

Figure 15-7. Front of origami cat face drawn with a felt pen.

Change It

To vary the activity and allow for some individuality, decorate the cat's face in different ways by using markers or gluing on facial features This activity can be graded by changing the size or thickness of the paper, by pre-folding the paper, by using glue to hold down corners or edges as needed, or by choosing a simpler or more complex pattern (Breines, 2006).

Document It

Below is an example of reporting a therapeutic application of this craft.

- "The client had difficulty aligning edges due to visual deficits. After cueing by therapist to use fingers to feel the edges (tactile compensation), client performance improved."

Paper Sculpture

Paper sculpture offers an array of possibilities for stimulating creativity. Sculpture implies that it is a three-dimensional object and the subject can be realistic or abstract, functional or decorative. Besides a paper product, glue is the most important material for this kind of sculpture (Bottomley, 1983; Fabri, 1966). Sculpture can be constructed entirely of paper, or it can be built by adding paper to an understructure.

Project—Corrugated Cardboard Frame

Plan It

Paper construction can be graded and adapted to fit most any therapeutic objective. The primary caution with this activity is safety using the sharp cutting tool. To achieve an attractive end product, some degree of precision is needed for measuring, and cutting requires both control and strength. Construction or sculpture of more abstract forms might be better suited for a client with impaired coordination or apraxia. On the other hand, the material is inexpensive and this may be a useful craft for a client working to improve fine motor function.

Get Ready

Supplies

- Corrugated cardboard, different colors if desired
- Glue
- Markers or paint

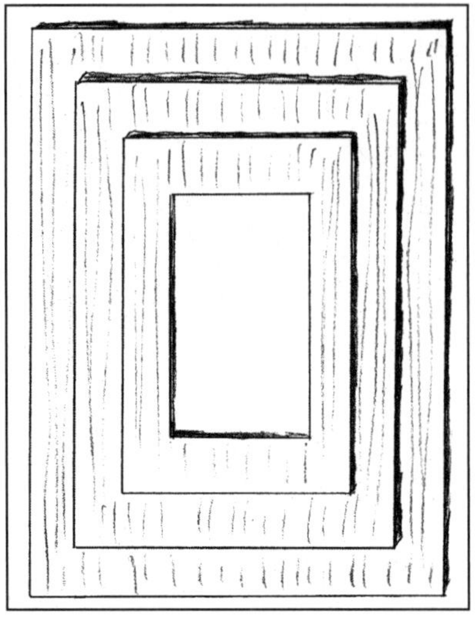

Figure 15-8. Corrugated cardboard frame.

Tools

- Scissors
- Utility knife or craft knife
- Paint brushes, optional

Time required: 30 to 45 minutes

Cost: Less than $1

Do It

Process

1. Cut three rectangles of cardboard, each successively smaller, for example, one 7 x 9 inches, one 6 x 8 inches, one 5 x 7 inches.
2. In the smallest rectangle, cut a centered 3½- x 5½-inch hole using the utility knife; this will accommodate a 4- x 6-inch photograph.
3. Glue the medium sized rectangle, centered, onto the largest rectangle. Glue the small rectangle onto the medium, but glue only the outer edges of the sides and the bottom (Figure 15-8). The top edge should be left open for the insertion of the picture.
4. Decorate the frame with markers or a light brushing of paint

Change It

The frame size can be altered to accommodate any size picture and once constructed, the creator can make a stand using a folded strip of cardboard glued to the back and/or decorate the front in some way. To grade this activity down, make the frame from card stock or some other thinner paper material that can be cut with scissors instead of a utility knife. Use different colors to eliminate the need to paint it after assembly. The cardboard can also be colored easily by rubbing over the corrugated surface with the side of a crayon, creating a lined effect. To grade the activity up, decorate the frame with small shapes cut from leftover cardboard, or with paper beads or quilling (methods described below).

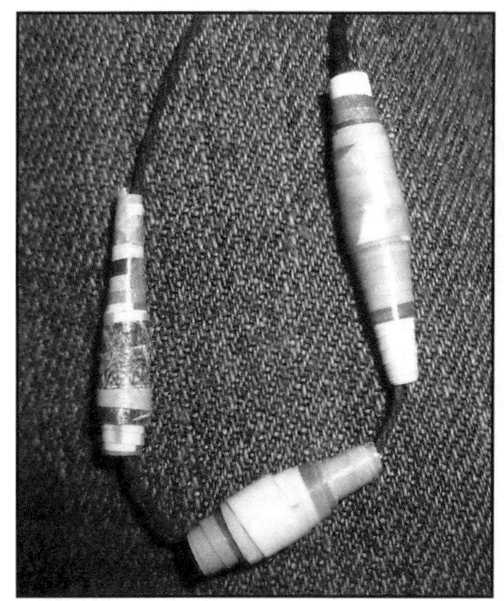
Figure 15-9. Paper beads.

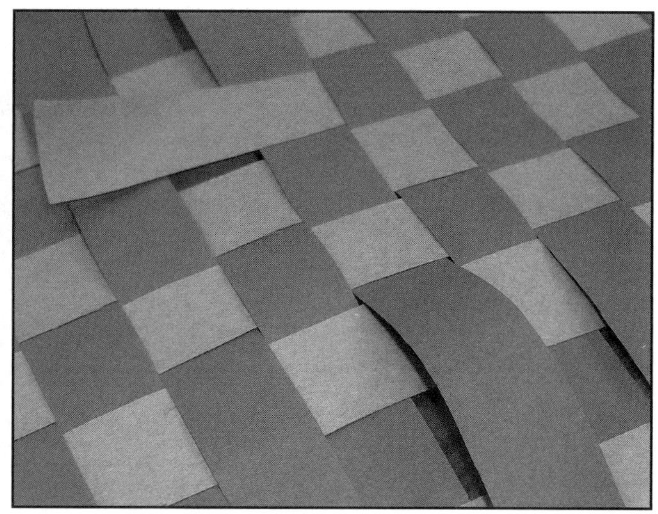
Figure 15-10. Paper weaving.

Document It

The following are a few examples of ways to document functional skills addressed by using this craft:

- "The patient was able to hold the exacto knife in the affected hand and control it as he cut along the outline."
- "With therapist assistance, the client was able to use his affected upper extremity to hold the ruler in place as he drew the lines for cutting."

There are numerous other forms of paper construction. Quilling is a process in which very narrow strips of paper are coiled into shapes and glued to a flat surface to create pictures of varying complexity. Paper beads (Figure 15-9) can be made by cutting narrow, elongated triangles from colorful, preferably glossy paper (such as a page from a magazine), then rolling it tightly around a small dowel such as a toothpick, starting with the wide edge. Glue the pointed end and let dry. The beads can then be used for stringing or as a surface decoration on other objects. Paper weaving is another paper craft that can be modified to make it appropriate for almost any age group. It can be used as assessment or intervention in areas such as spatial relations, fine motor dexterity, and ideomotor praxis. To do paper weaving, cut slits in a whole sheet of paper, making sure to keep all four edges intact. Cut a second piece of paper (of the same size) into strips and, one at a time, weave the strips through the slits in the other sheet, alternating the over/under pattern (Figure 15-10). The weaving can be done with bright or glossy papers and the completed sheets can be used in other projects, for example, they can be laminated and used as placemats or glued onto other surfaces such as trays or box tops. Another interesting variation is to make a photocopy of a colored picture, then complete the weaving process described above using the two pictures—one in color and the other in black and white (Figure 15-11). Still another example of paper construction is the creation of paper flowers. There are numerous methods and they may incorporate tissue paper; crépe paper; or stiff, semi-transparent papers. The only other supplies usually needed are glue, scissors, and stem material such as pipe cleaners or florist wire.

Construct "stained glass" window panels using black construction paper and colored tissue paper. Simply cut shapes from the construction paper using a craft knife, leaving borders of approximately 1/2 inch between each section. Then glue tissue paper into each section, preferably without extending into the adjacent section. For a more finished look, cut two sheets of the black paper exactly alike to make a front and a back. Hang in a window so the light can shine through the tissue paper. Refer to Resources section at the end of the chapter for places to find other paper construction ideas.

Paper Cutting

Paper cutting, another paper craft with origins in the Far East, eventually spread to Europe and became popular in German, Swiss, and Polish cultures. It was customarily used to make silhouettes and religious

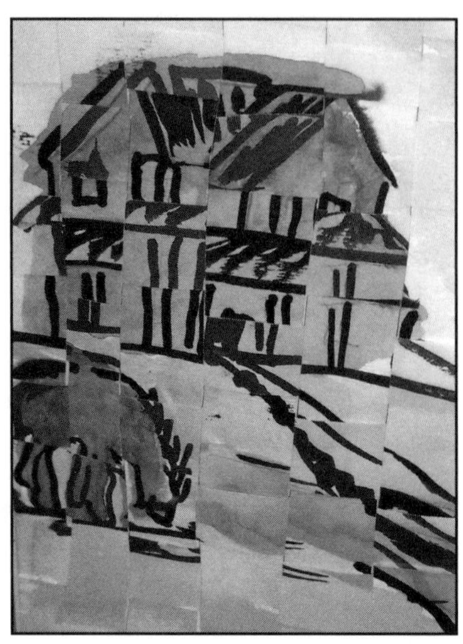

Figure 15-11. Paper weaving using a color/ and black and white image.

depictions, as well as scenes from everyday life (Lively, 2004). Paper cutting requires only paper and small, sharp scissors or a craft knife. Some designs are intended to be cut from folded paper, others from flat paper. Because this craft requires the use of both hands and some degree of precision, it is useful for fine motor work and the intricacy can be graded according to client ability.

Collage

Collage is derived from the French verb *coller*, which means *to glue*. This art form had an important influence on 20th century art (*Reader's Digest*, 1979). Collages can be made of most any material, but paper may be the most common. Essential supplies are paper, glue, and a mounting surface, and the basic process is simply cutting or tearing and gluing. Various colors and textures of paper can be mixed to create interesting effects, using designs that are abstract or pictorial. Collage can be used to decorate other objects such as boxes, lamp shades, or greeting cards, or used to simply create a picture (Lively, 2004).

Découpage

While this paper craft, like so many others, probably originated in China, the term *découpage* was first used in France and Italy and derived from the French word, *couper*, meaning to cut. It became highly popular there in the 18th century and was used as an inexpensive way of reproducing the look of lacquer ware. Pictures were cut out and glued to objects, then covered with clear lacquer to simulate the hand painted designs on oriental furniture. Its use as a decorative technique quickly spread to other countries (Bower, 2011). Though the original method took a great deal of time to complete, modern products have made it a simple and satisfying craft for clients. New one-coat finishes have been developed that simulate those that formerly required multiple coats of varnish or lacquer (Bodger & Brock, 1976; *Reader's Digest*, 1979; VanZandt, 1973); however, some authors still recommend several coats of varnish for the best surface protection (Lively, 2004). Decoupage can be applied to glass, porcelain, or wood.

One advantage of decoupage is that a nice product can be achieved with only a few steps and a low-functioning client can be successful. Most decoupage finish is neither flammable nor toxic, so it is nonhazardous. It can be used to preserve personally valuable mementos like graduation or birth announcements. The primary drawback is the series of waiting periods while the glue or finish dries; the client may be discharged before the finish is completely dried. The therapist should be sure that the project can be completely finished (and dry) before the client is discharged.

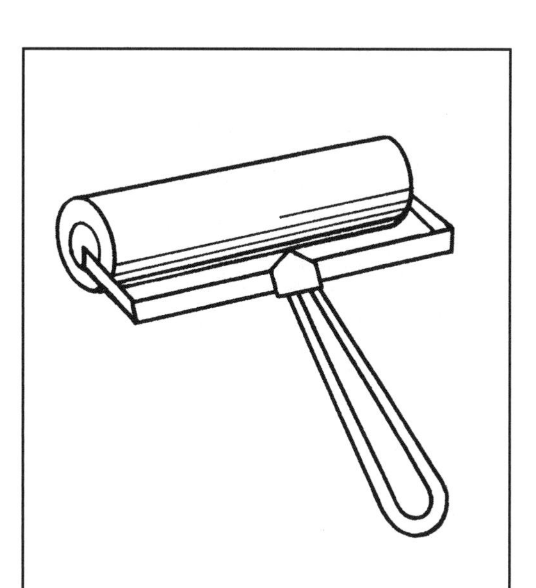

Figure 15-12. Brayer.

Scrapbooking

Scrapbooking is currently an extremely popular craft and some craft stores devote several aisles exclusively to scrapbooking supplies. Scrapbooking is essentially a paper craft in which an individual's photographs or other memorabilia are combined with decorative elements and compiled into book form. To create a scrapbook, the first requirement is some type of binder, large journal, or blank scrapbook. The maker may also want to use clear plastic sleeves to protect the finished pages. Other supplies commonly used are paper of various weights and colors, adhesive tabs, double-sided and regular tape, special scissors (for cornering, scalloping, and pinking edges), decorative hole punches, assorted stickers and stamps, marking pens, and photo corners (Dahlstrom, 2004). Avid scrapbook fans use numerous other tools and materials to embellish pages as well. Tools and supplies generally available in a therapy clinic/office, such as rulers, paper cutters, and stencils, will also come in handy.

To reiterate, the general idea of scrapbooking is to create attractive pages to display personal photos. Techniques often utilized include framing or borders around pictures or sections of text, and thematic enhancement of the rest of the page (Dahlstrom, 2004). Scrapbookers usually try to achieve visual balance and complementary color schemes, but this may or may not be a concern for most clients. It will be helpful to have sample layouts that the client can simply duplicate, possibly choosing different colors or embellishments. Purchased scrapbooking supplies can be costly, but found or natural materials, as described elsewhere in this text (Chapters 12 and 14) are certainly an option. Basic supplies are available in most clinic settings, particularly those that routinely use crafts. This paper craft can be easily graded and results in an end product that is personalized and meaningful to the client. Scrapbooks help to "cement oneself in history" and reinforce a sense of identity (Fidler & Velde, 1999); see Chapter 2 for a personal occupational therapy testimony on the therapeutic benefits of this activity (Johnson, 2005). As a variation, have a group or individual create a bulletin board like a giant scrapbook page, containing photos of facility events, parties, or field trips.

Paper Decoration

Paper can be decorated in multiple ways and some processes, such as block printing, were staples of early occupational therapy practice. Other common and simpler techniques include stamping and stenciling. Block printing is a process in which a design is carved into a flat wooden or linoleum block. The block is covered with ink using a brayer (Figure 15-12) or roller and then pressed onto the paper. A simplified version involves the use of stamps, which can be purchased or made with assorted everyday items from sponges to potatoes. This is currently a popular craft and a large variety of stamps are available for purchase in most hobby stores. The monochrome stamped design can be left plain or colored with colored pencils. Stenciling, like stamping, can be done with pre-made patterns, or they can be custom cut from heavy paper, lightweight cardboard, or plastic sheets specially designed for stencil templates. Other forms of paper decoration include layering and carving, cutting and curling, crumpling, salting, stitching, staining, or texturing with paste; the list is virtually endless (Hall, 2001). The references and Resources in the chapter are excellent sources for a plethora of inexpensive paper projects.

Main Therapeutic Applications

Physical Dysfunction

Paper crafts can be structured for almost any treatment or activity setting and any level of function. They are especially appropriate for home health clients, as the materials are usually available and affordable. Most of the paper crafts emphasize distal upper extremity movement; the amount of dexterity needed will depend on the method. While little strength is required in most cases, endurance (and patience) may be required for repetitive processes or for keeping pieces in a position until the adhesive dries enough to hold. Paper crafts are especially good for cardiac and respiratory clients, as little exertion is required. One practitioner even described using holiday paper crafts in an acute rehab setting. Clients were able to socialize and make the facility festive while simultaneously working on gross motor, fine motor, and perceptual skills (Schroeder, 2007). Paper crafts may be difficult for clients with hypertonia or lack of fine motor control, since paper is easily bent or crushed. Although many paper crafts normally require bilateral hand function, they are a good activity choice for practicing adapted techniques, since the materials are inexpensive enough to throw away and start over. Another advantage is that they present few dangers such as fumes, dust, or sharp edges.

Mental Health

Paper craft is potentially frustrating, since paper is easily torn or crushed, and the therapist should be alert to those clients who have a low tolerance for failure. On the other hand, paper is cheap, which would allow trial and error if the client is willing to persist in the task. Clients with cognitive impairment or a tendency to perseverate may have difficulty judging how much glue to use; applying the glue with a small brush may remedy this problem. Activities with only a few steps, such as stamping, stenciling, simple cutting, or collage can be accomplished with minimal attention or decision-making or problem-solving skills. In community settings, or those where clients have a longer length of stay, paper crafts are good for making holiday decorations. The holiday mood of a clinic, dayroom, or communal gathering place is greatly enhanced by the addition of colorful items such as hanging ornaments, flowers, garlands, streamers, and mobiles.

Simple paper folding can be used to assess cognitive function such as ability to follow directions, perceptual skills, and emotional regulation, including frustration tolerance. Paper sculpture can be used as a projective test in that clients can be asked to describe their sculpture and what meaning it has for them. One such example is the Magazine Picture Collage, a traditional occupational therapy psychiatric assessment used with adults. The client is asked to create a collage from self-selected magazine pictures and the therapist then makes inferences about mood and other mental health factors based on picture choices and overall task performance. There is some evidence of inter-rater reliability in interpretation of results (Hemphill, 1999).

Pediatrics

Paper crafts are especially good for children; the material is familiar and they can use their own creations as imaginative toys. An older occupational therapy assessment, the Lafayette Clinic Battery, uses paper craft to assess developmental skills (Llorens, 1969). They are useful in gaining fine motor skills needed for activities related to academic success such as scissors use and handwriting (Henderson & Pehoski, 2006; Kuhaneck, Spitzer, & Miller, 2010). Very young children can tear paper and as they begin to want to try cutting, rounded scissors minimize safety concerns. Encouraging children to embellish their paper craft with paint or crayon will foster creativity and exploration of materials and outcomes. They can build a world, destroy it, and rebuild it, as they do in their fantasies. They can make paper puppets or paper bag puppets that do their talking for them, which is especially appropriate for children having difficulty communicating. They can do paper sculpture, papier mâché, or simple decorated paper projects with little fear of failure. One of the most common problems for children doing paper crafts is using too much glue. Paste or glue sticks may be better for young children, though they do not adhere as well. Children are prone to form top-heavy sculptures, so the therapist may have to assist them in making an adequate a base. As children approach adolescence, they want to make more realistic sculptures. See Resources at the end of the chapter for sources of ideas for pediatric and adolescent projects.

Adolescents

Because paper constructions are often abstract, teens desiring realistic representations may prefer drawing or painting. On the other hand, they may excel at making masks and origami (Gaitskell & Hurwitz, 1975) and origami can be used with this age group to foster cooperative or creative behaviors (Breines, 2006). Adolescents, especially girls, are likely to enjoy making their own cards, wrapping papers, and gift tags. They can make handmade paper and incorporate it in collages on items to decorate their rooms. Because the materials are inexpensive and many of the processes are quick, the adolescent can feel free to experiment until he or she achieves the look he or she wants. Picture collages are an excellent means of expressing one's identity or feelings. Teens may also enjoy making paper bead jewelry, paper flowers, or creating a scrapbook of family and friends. Again, the low-cost feature of paper crafts makes them ideal for children or adolescents who may be hospitalized long term; other crafts may be too expensive to use on a daily basis.

Older Adults

Paper can sometimes be used for processes similar to those previously done with fabric. Quilt patterns and appliqué that may have been used by the clients in the past can easily be adapted to paper designs. As a rule, older clients are less likely to enjoy experimentation and those with cognitive deficits can struggle with new learning, so projects that have a familiar structure are most appropriate (Bonder & Bello-Haas, 2009). Even some of the most disabled clients in nursing homes can successfully complete a simple paper activity such as gluing precut holly leaves onto a cardboard wreath. Making paper toys for children may provide satisfaction for some elderly clients. When selecting the type of paper craft, the therapist should consider visual demands, such as having to copy a design, and cognitive demands, such as the number of steps or the need to following written or verbal directions. For example, after set-up, papier mâché is a simple repetitive process that requires little or no vision and few cognitive skills, yet provides upper extremity exercise and tactile stimulation. Origami may be difficult for some clients due to the precision and sequencing required and making the well-defined creases could be stressful to the small joints of the hand. Although they may seem minor, paper cuts can be painful and annoying and have the potential to create greater problems for elderly clients who heal more slowly.

Groups

Paper crafts are a good choice for group activity. Large projects like bulletin boards can be done as a collaborative effort, or individuals can work on separate items for a community purpose, such as holiday decorating or making paper flower bouquets for table centerpieces. Groups of elderly clients could make greeting cards for sick children, or vice versa. The concept of making something for others will often entice someone to participate who would otherwise decline the activity (Breines, 2009). Clients could make papier mâché or other paper masks to use in a group dramatic production, or could make abstract paper constructions such as collages as a means of sharing thoughts or feelings in a social interaction session.

Case Study

Rosa is a 9-year-old second grade student attending a public school. She has struggled to keep up with the work each year and has been kept back twice since starting first grade in spite of scoring in the normal range on general intelligence tests. She has few friends and doesn't seem to want to go out and play after school like most of her peers. Rosa's teacher referred her for evaluation by occupational therapy, reasoning that undetected learning, motor, or sensory integration problems may be the source of her difficulties. The occupational therapist tended to use the sensory integration frame of reference and initially evaluated Rosa by administering the Bruininks-Oseretsky Test of Motor Proficiency and the Sensory Profile, as well as by observing her in the classroom and talking with her, her parents, and her teachers. The therapist learned that Rosa is the only daughter of parents who are both East Indian and immigrated to the United States before Rosa was born. Both parents are medical professionals, perplexed at their daughter's apparent slowness, and anxious to use any means available to help her succeed. Rosa's teachers report some problems with attention in class, but mostly a seeming unwillingness to participate in written and other work. On the Bruininks-Oseretsky Test, she scored slightly below normal on the gross motor sections, but markedly below normal on the fine motor tests. She also complained of pain in her hands when discussing her performance with the therapist. Upon closer physical examination, the occupational therapist noticed slight redness and swelling in Rosa's wrists and some of her finger joints. She later discussed her findings with the parents and recommended a visit to the pediatrician.

Rosa returned to school with a diagnosis of juvenile rheumatoid arthritis. The parents expressed feeling guilty for not recognizing this clinical picture before; they were both busy professionals and had simply failed to notice the signs. Both they and the therapist understood that this would be a life-long battle, so reasoned that Rosa should learn management techniques as early as possible. Because the therapist was accustomed to using a sensory approach, she had to refresh her skills on arthritis management techniques. At the same time, she knew she needed to choose fun activities in order to gain Rosa's interest in learning new techniques and methods. The occupational therapist chose to engage Rosa in paper crafts as a fun way of learning and practicing joint protection principles. She varied the projects in order to incorporate many different motor demands. As the child worked, the therapist showed her how to use loop scissors for cutting; how to use the heel of her hand to accomplish stamping and folding; how to use her palms instead of fingers when squeezing the glue bottle; and showed her how to adapt pencils and other tools for providing a larger grasping surface. The therapist also instructed Rosa's parents in these techniques so they could be reinforced at home.

With medication, regular mobility exercises, pain management strategies, and the use of joint protection techniques, Rosa successfully completed the second grade and has become much more socially active. The therapist checks on her regularly to monitor for any new symptoms or functional problems.

Discussion Questions

1. Of the paper crafts discussed in this chapter, which type do you think would be best for Rosa as a play/leisure activity and why?
2. Should the occupational therapist have done other assessments? If so, which ones and why?
3. Why was paper craft an appropriate choice for school system practice?

Resources

Trash Origami: 25 Folding Projects Reusing Everyday Materials
By Michael LaFosse and Richard L. Alexander
Tuttle Publishing; DVD edition, 2010

Visual Quick Tips: Paper Crafts
By Rebecca Luden and Jennifer Schmidt
Visual, 2008
Basic information and lots of different techniques and ideas.

Start Scrapbooking: Your Essential Guide to Recording Memories
By Wendy Smedley
Memory Makers, 2010
Good for beginners.

The Michaels Book of Paper Crafts
Edited by Dawn Cusick and Megan Kirby
Lark Books, 2005

Beginner's Guide to Paper Making
By Mary Reimer and Heidi Reimer
Sterling Publishing, 2005

Origami Flowers: Popular Blossoms and Creative Bouquets
By Hiromi Hayashi
Kodansha America, Inc. through Oxford University Press, 2003

Arnold Grummer's Complete Guide to Paper Casting
By Arnold and Mabel Grummer
Krause Publications, 2002

The Usborne Book of Papercraft
By Alastair Smith
E. D. C. Publishing, 2002

It's All About Cards and Tags (from *Memories in the Making* scrapbooking series)
By Nancy M. Hill
Leisure Arts, 2004

Papercraft: 50 Extraordinary Gifts & Projects, Step by Step
By Gillian Souter
Crown Trade Paperbacks, 1997
Colored photographs show paper making, papier mâché, paper weaving, paper folding, cut paper, sculpture, decoupage, and surface coloring techniques such as marbling, stenciling, and printing. Nice variety of crafts for a beginning crafters. Good index.

Creative Paper Cutting: Basic Techniques and Fresh Designs for Stencils, Mobiles, Cards and More
By Shufunotomo (Ed.)
Trumpeter, 2010
Simple projects, appropriate for children, with clear instructions.

Origami in Action: Paper Toys that Fly, Flap, Gobble, and Inflate
By Robert J. Lang
St. Martins Griffin, 1997
Sequential drawings of how to make 39 different figures. Each project is designated as easy, intermediate, or hard. A black and white photo shows the completed figure of each origami toy.

A Year of Crafts for Kids
By Kathy Ross
Millbrook Press, 1996
Page after page of crafts organized by holidays, such as Earth Day, Hanukkah, Christmas, and Kwanzaa. Most crafts require about six common items like scissors, glue, tape, paint, a stapler, and paper or plastic containers. Each section has an introductory cultural explanation of the holiday. Bright color pictures show the process.

Classic Origami
By P. D. Tuyen
Sterling Publishing Co., Inc., 1995
Vietnamese author relates this art to his Vietnamese childhood. He discusses the origins of this craft and current trends. Thorough, clear sequential drawings of the process for the 26 animals which are listed in the index.

Papier Mâché Style: 100 Step-by-Step Designs
By Alex MacCormick
Chilton Book Company, 1995
Explains the history of this paper craft. Describes materials, processes for mold making, jewelry, paper making, and finishes. Wonderful full-page photographs and an index. Has a list of English artists.

Origami Animals
By Hector Rojas
Sterling Publishing Company, Inc., 1993
Wonderful photographs of real animals plus photographs of dioramas that include the origami animals. The book progresses from simpler to more complex projects. Some of the diagrams are small, which makes them more difficult to understand. This book is for the more accomplished paper folder.

Sculpture in Paper
By Nicholas Roukes
Sterling Publishing, 1993

The Art and Craft of Papier Mâché
By Juliet Bowden
Chronicle Books, 1995
Tells the history of papier mâché with photos of antique examples of the craft, folk art objects and modern papier mâché art. Illustrations are drawings of processes for making vessels, jewelry, whimsical sculptures, and decorator items. Has a list of English artists and a good index.

The Art and Craft of Collage
By Simon Larbalestier
Chronicle Books, 1990
Large color photographs of collages from dried flowers and greeting cards to plastic doll heads.

Crafts for the Classroom
By Earl W. and Marlene M. Linderman
MacMillan Publishing Co., Inc., 1984
Discusses developmental skills for art with children. Contains many paper projects for children.

Creative Origami
By Kunihiko Kasahara
Sir Issac Pitman and Son, Ltd., 1977
Clear diagrams and photos of traditional forms as well as new artistic creations. One hundred different designs.

References

Barron, D. (1992). *Paper casting: A beginner's guide*. Norcross, GA: Plaid Enterprises, Inc.
Bodger, L., & Brock, D. (1976). *The crafts engagement calendar 1976*. New York, NY: Universe Books.
Bonder, B. R., & Bello-Haas, V. D. (2009). *Functional performance in older adults* (3rd ed.). Philadelphia, PA: F. A. Davis Co.

Bottomley, J. (1983). *Paper projects for creative kids of all ages*. Boston, MA: Little, Brown and Company.
Bower, L. (2011). *History of decoupage from life 123*. Retrieved from www.life123.com/hobbies/scrapbooking/decoupage/history-of-decoupage.shtml.
Breines, E. B. (2006). *Origami: Folding magic*. Retrieved from www.occupational-therapy.advanceweb.com/Editorial/Content/PrintFriendly.aspx?CC=96509.
Breines, E. B. (2009). Giving as motivation. *Advance for Occupational Therapy Practitioners, 25*(20), 6.
Carlson, L. (1993). *EcoArt*. Charlotte, VT: Williamson Publishing.
Dahlstrom, C. F. (Ed.). (2004). *Better Homes and Gardens fast scrapbooking*. Des Moines, IA: Meredith Books.
Department of the Army. (1971). *Craft techniques in occupational therapy*. Washington DC: U.S. Government Printing Office.
Drake, M. (1999). The evaluative process in occupational therapy. In B. J. Hemphill (Ed.), *Assessments in occupational therapy mental health: An integrative approach*. Thorofare, NJ: SLACK Incorporated.
Fabri, R. (1966). *Sculpture in paper*. New York, NY: Watson-Guptill Publications.
Fidler, G., & Velde, B. (1999). *Activities: Reality and symbol* (p. 97). Thorofare, NJ: SLACK Incorporated.
Gaitskell, C. D., & Hurwitz, A. (1975). *Children and their art* (3rd ed.). New York, NY: Harcourt, Brace, Jovanovitch.
Hall, M. A., Wrobel, J., & Salamony, S. (2001). *Decorative crafts sourcebook*. San Diego, CA: Thunder Bay Press.
Hemphill, B. J. (1999). *The evaluative process in psychiatric occupational therapy*. Thorofare, NJ: SLACK Incorporated.
Henderson, A., & Pehoski, C. (2006). *Hand function in the child: Foundations for remediation* (2nd ed.). St. Louis, MO: Mosby Elsevier.
Johnson, K. (2005). *The therapeutic value of scrapbooking*. Retrieved from www.seniority.co.uk/contributions/homeandhobbies/artsandcrafts.
Kuhaneck, H. M., Spitzer, S. L., & Miller, E. (2010). Activity analysis, creativity, and playfulness. In H. M. Kuhaneck, S. L. Spitzer, & E. Miller (Eds.), *Pediatric occupational therapy: Making play just right*. Sudbury, MA: Jones and Barlett Publishers.
Lively, K. (2004). *Making great papercrafts: Origami, stationery, and gift wraps*. London, UK: Hermes House.
Llorens, L. A. (1969). An evaluation procedure for children 6-10 years of age. *American Journal of Occupational Therapy, 21*(2), 64-69.
Moseley, S., Johnson, P., & Koenig, H. (1962). *Craft designs*. Belmont, CA: Wadsworth.
Reader's Digest. (1979). *Crafts and hobbies*. Pleasantville, NY: Reader's Digest Association, Inc.
Sakade, F. (1958). *Origami book two: Japanese paper-folding*. Rutland, VT: Charles E. Tuttle Company.
Schroeder, S. (2007). *Deck the halls with OT crafts*. Retrieved from www.occupational-therapy.advanceweb.com/editorial/content/editorial.aspx?cc=103010.
VanZandt, E. (1973). *Crafts for fun and profit*. London, UK: Aldus Books.
Wasinger, S. (2009). *Eco-craft: Recycle, recraft, restyle*. New York, NY: Sterling Publishing Co./Lark Books.

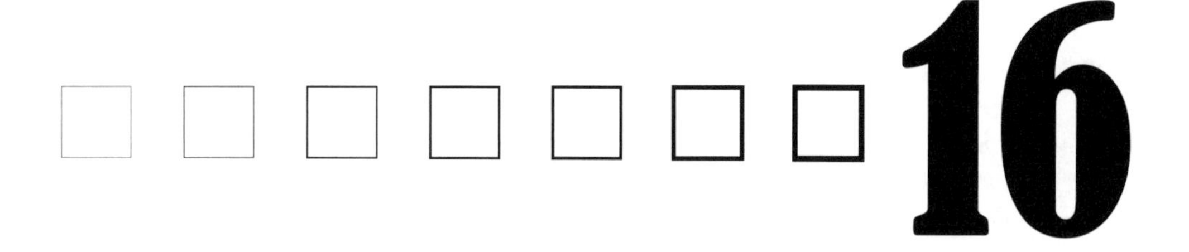

Bead and Wire Work

Objectives

The student should be able to:

- Discuss historical/cultural examples of beadwork
- Know basic supplies and materials needed to do beadwork/wirework and know how to complete and grade a project
- Understand advantages and limitations of beading activities in therapy
- List precautions of beading/wirework activities
- Describe ways to use beading/wirework activities with various client populations

Beadwork, like many other decorative crafts, has been around for thousands of years. Beadwork was found at the tombs of Ur, from approximately 2500 B.C.; Egyptian ruins reveal evidence of decorative bead use as well. The netting technique, or gourd stitch, was developed around 500 B.C. and was used in ritual practices and royal adornment. Drawn glass beads, developed around 200 B.C., were of uniform size and shape and, due to their limited availability, came to be used as currency. Explorers and traders bargained with native tribes, exchanging beads for various goods or services. As the bead-making process was streamlined, supplies went up and the trading value declined (Benson, 2001). Today, intricate beadwork is still an important cultural craft in many Native American societies.

Beads can be strung or woven, or sewn or glued on clothing or objects. Beads can be made of any hard material, including glass, plastic, metal, wood, or natural materials such as pearls or shells. Occupational therapists have commonly used bead stringing as a repetitive task to improve bilateral fine motor coordination, employing it more as an enabling activity than as a purposeful or occupational one. Beading activities in therapy have been associated mostly with children, but with the surge in popularity of beaded jewelry over the last several years, beadwork may now be a more acceptable adult craft intervention. Wirework and macramé are also included in this chapter since they are commonly used in combination with beads in making jewelry or other decorative objects, and their manipulation requires many of the same skills.

Tools and supplies essential to beadwork and wirework include wire/cord, fasteners, pliers, cutters, needles, and glues. Cord comes in a range of materials and thicknesses, from nylon to hemp, leather to elastic. Needles must be those specially designed for use with beading; the type will depend on the project and the style of beads used. Wire may be steel, copper, or other metal and comes in different gauges or thicknesses (see Metal Craft Chapter 8); it is most commonly round, half round, or square. Pliers with

Tubbs, C., & Drake, M. *Crafts and Creative Media in Therapy, Fourth Edition (pp. 201-210).*

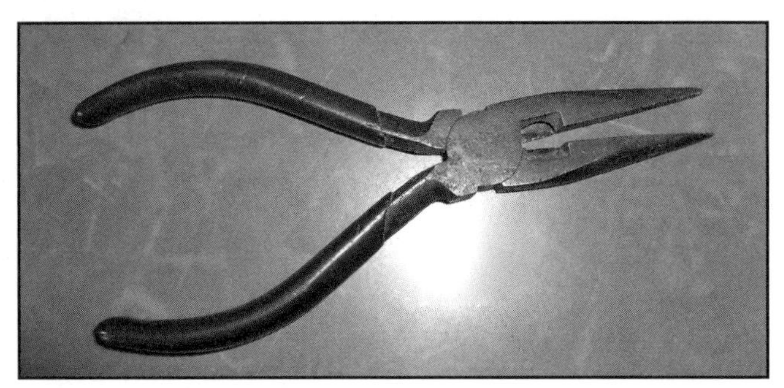

Figure 16-1. Needle nose pliers.

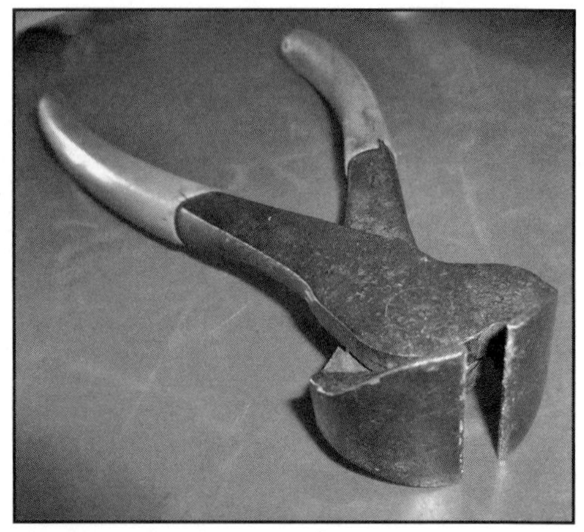

Figure 16-2. Side cutters for wire.

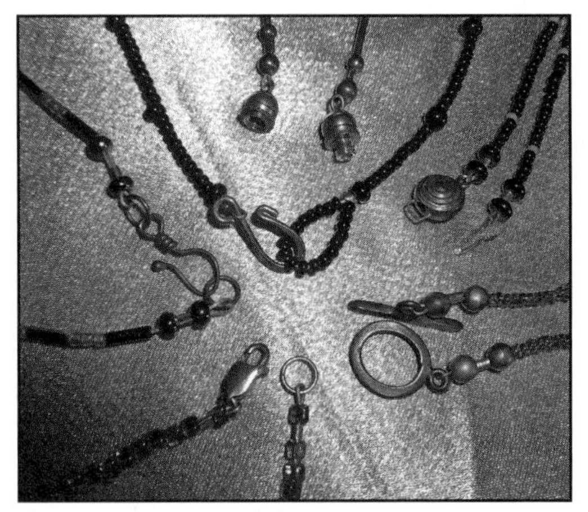

Figure 16-3. Assorted clamps.

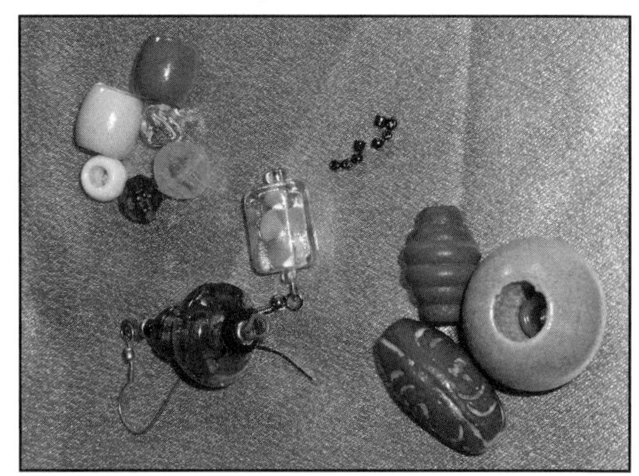

Figure 16-4. Assorted bead styles: wooden, glass, and plastic.

different ends have different functions, including chain nose for wrapping and crimping, round nose for making loops, and needle nose (Figure 16-1) for gripping in small spaces. Wire cutters are generally side- or flush cutters (Figure 16-2), with flush cutters leaving the smoothest edge. Sharp cord and thread cutters are also needed for clean cuts with no fraying. Several types of glues are satisfactory for beadwork, but they must be clear, permanent, quick-drying, and nonrunning. Other basic supplies needed are clasps (Figure 16-3) and assorted other small parts called "findings" that include bead tips, joining rings, crimp beads, ear wires (for earrings), and head pins (Kanan, 2001). Other items that may prove useful in beadwork or wirework are tweezers, bead boards, bead looms, vises or clamps, magnifiers, and small cordless rotary grinders. The therapist who decides to include beadwork in the craft repertoire should be familiar with these tools and supplies before purchasing and should be competent in their use before attempting this craft with clients. Many of the tools are relatively inexpensive but beads and findings can become quite costly. Ideal for children's activities, plastic beads are naturally the least expensive but also the least attractive. Bead styles include but are not limited to seed beads, bugle beads, fancy glass beads of all sizes, and beads of semiprecious stones (Figure 16-4; Benson, 2001). Beads and cords should be purchased together to ensure that they are compatible with each other. Kits are available that contain all supplies needed for one or multiple projects; these also vary considerably in cost. Hemp cord—popular in jewelry for children and adolescents—is available in assorted colors. This same cord, in thicker ply, is used to make macramé hangers and decorative wall hangings. Fishing line is an inexpensive cord option, but it is usually not intended to be visible in the finished project, so using it will require more beads overall. Clasps and other findings vary in price, so the therapist is advised to shop around.

Macramé

This ancient craft of knotting was used by the pharaohic Egyptians, Chinese, Maoris, and Peruvians. The word *macramé* has an Arabic origin meaning a veil of protection, or ornamental fringe. Because sailors used novel combinations of square knots to make nets, hammocks, and other articles, it is probable that the art of macramé migrated around the world through seafaring (Moseley, Johnson, & Koenig, 1962; *Reader's Digest*, 1979).

Macramé can be accomplished with almost no tools except scissors and a measuring device, therefore simple projects can be done with tools already on hand in the clinic. Some individuals use special macramé boards and pins but these are not necessary. Macramé cord is available in natural jute, acrylic, or cotton and varies in ply or thickness. Large macramé projects are not only dated, but also time consuming and consequently not appropriate for most inpatient therapy applications. The macramé process is generally done with four basic knots, with several variations for each (Octopus Books, 1973), but more than 30 complicated knots can be incorporated if more complexity is desired (Abraham, 1964). This craft is easily graded up or down, and examples of projects include key chains, belts, purses, bags, jewelry, wall hangings, and potted plant hangers (*Reader's Digest*, 1979). In current craft applications, macramé knotting is most commonly used with smaller cord to make belts and jewelry.

Special Considerations and Precautions

Regarding beadwork, expense is probably the primary disadvantage of its use in therapy. The cost of cord, findings, and beads can add up quickly. As with any craft, however, the persistent therapist can find a way to minimize the expense if the client is truly interested and would benefit from this occupation. For example, the client could provide all the supplies and the therapist could then grade or adapt the process as appropriate. Plastic beads may be satisfactory for some clients, especially children, and they are certainly available in a wide range of colors and styles. Small projects using wirework or macramé can be done economically, possibly even with scrap materials.

The wire and cord cutters are sharp and pointed, as is the metal wire itself, so care should be used in their handling. Some authors recommend protective eyewear and gloves when working with wire (Hall, 2001; Hill, 2008). Considering the crafts in this chapter, wirework poses the most consistent hazards, macramé the least. Some forms of beadwork require precision handling and repetition, so the client must be somewhat frustration tolerant. In working with adults, the therapist should try to choose projects that will not appear childish.

There are a few general tips for beadwork: use a work surface that will minimize rolling/loss of beads, for example, an inverted box lid with a nappy fabric lining; make sure the cord, when doubled, is narrow enough to fit through all bead holes; and, if using costly beads, knot between each one to avoid loss in the event of cord breakage (*Reader's Digest*, 1979). It is advisable to plan and lay out the design before stringing to assure you will achieve the desired look.

Project—Nylon Cord Choker Necklace

Plan It

As written, this project calls for reasonably good fine motor and visual skills, although the number of repetitive steps is minimized (Figure 16-5). A beaded bracelet or necklace can be an extremely simple craft, or a highly complex one that requires precise manipulation, good visual acuity, and patience. It is also a craft that can be done inexpensively or can require quite an investment. The therapist should take these factors into account and stock the supplies that are appropriate across a range of the typical client population in their facility. Primary disadvantages of this craft are that it may not interest males and the less expensive materials may not appeal to adults.

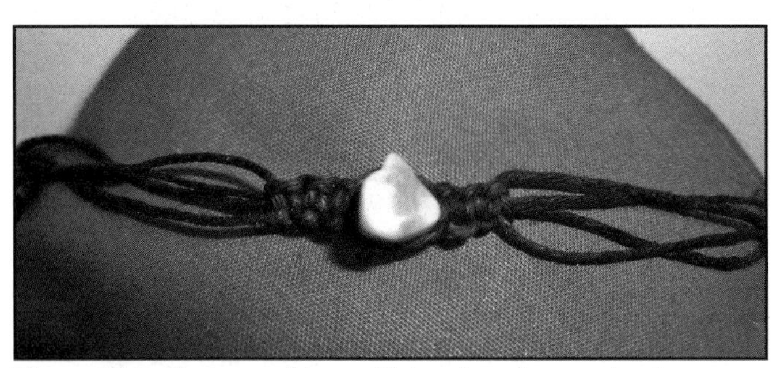
Figure 16-5. Choker necklace with beads and square knots.

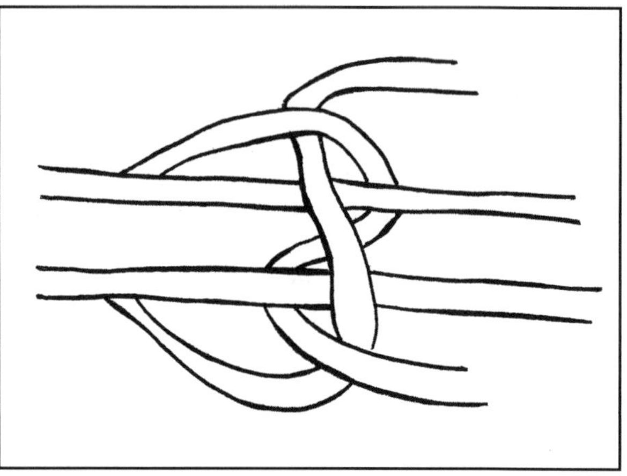
Figure 16-6. The half square knot. One working cord in front of center cords; one working cord behind center cords.

Get Ready

Supplies

- 2 yards waxed nylon (or other) cord
- Clear-drying glue
- Beads of complementary color and style. Make sure 2 strands of the cord will fit through the bead holes
- Necklace hook or clasp

Tools

- Measuring tool
- Scissors
- Small dowel or eye hook

Time required: 30 minutes

Approximate cost: $1 to $2, depending on beads selected

Do It

Process

1. Cut cord into two 1-yard lengths.
2. Fold cords evenly in half around a small dowel or eye hook that has been secured in a vise or clamp (or by some other means). You will have four cords—two outside (working) and two inside (center) cords.
3. About 3 inches from the dowel, tie three square knots (Figure 16-6), add a bead, then tie three more square knots (Figure 16-7). Tighten knots by alternating pulling outward on side cords, then pulling down on center cords to avoid puckering.
4. Skip about 2 inches of cord, then repeat step 3, but this time, switch inner and outer cords. Keep consistent tension on successive knots for a neat look.
5. Continue as above until the desired length is reached, ending with three square knots. Be sure to leave enough loose cord on the end to tie it to the clasp hook.
6. To finish off, tie a hook clasp at the end, again making sure the length is what you want. Trim raw ends of cord and secure with a drop or two of glue.

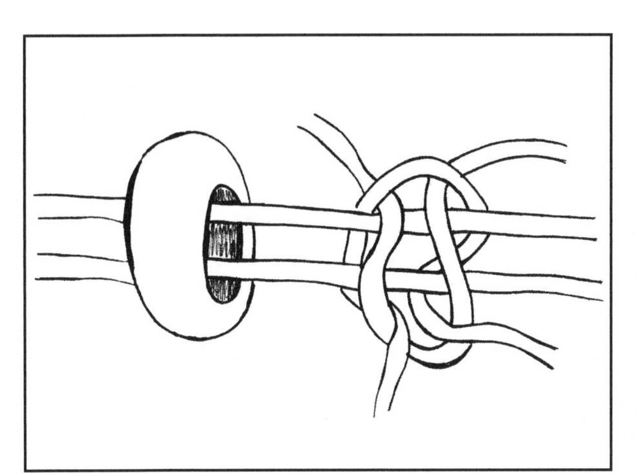

Figure 16-7. Full square knot with bead on center cords.

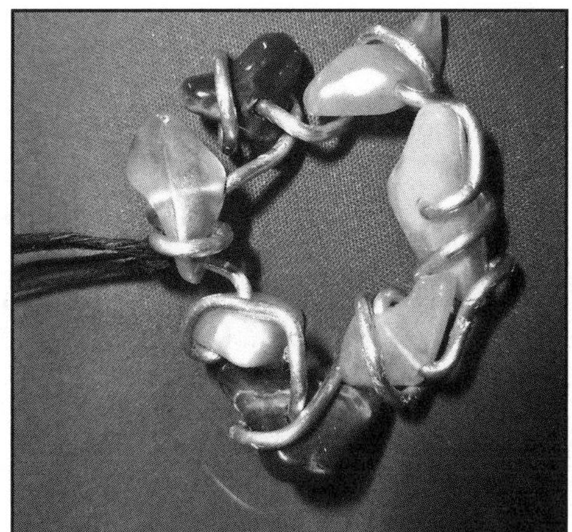

Figure 16-8. Bead and wire ornament or pendant.

Change It

For an easy variation, use only half square knots, which will result in a spiral effect instead of the flat surface of full square knots. Or instead of stringing beads on the necklace cord, add beads to a short length of wire, one at a time, adding twists around or in between as desired using needle nose pliers (Figure 16-8), then hang it as a pendant on the cord. To grade the project up, use more knots and beads, or vary their arrangement in a pattern that has to be followed. To grade the project down, use a single length of thicker cording and simply add the number of beads desired, with or without granny knots in between (Figure 16-9). As a rule, thinner cord is harder to manipulate, thicker is easier.

Document It

Below are a few examples of ways to report the therapeutic application of this activity:

- "The client was able to use both hands in a coordinated fashion to tie a square knot using a thin nylon cord."
- "The client was able to utilize learned stress management techniques when the activity became frustrating. Client reported feeling relaxed at the end of the session."
- "The client was able to attend to a jewelry making activity for 15 minutes without redirection to task."

Other Ideas and Grading

Items incorporating beadwork and wire sculpting need not be limited to jewelry. Multiple combinations of bead and cord types, wire, and other materials are possible, and other articles to consider making include ceiling fan or lamp pulls; wine goblet markers; bookmarks; and decorative tassels to embellish bookmarks, zipper pulls, or curtain tiebacks. Beads can be sewn onto clothing, threaded together into strands and glued onto box tops, or woven into wire and wrapped around objects such as candlestick holders or vases. For a more complex process, beads can be woven on a small loom to make bracelets, barrettes, chokers, or even small bags. Beads threaded onto wire and alternated with wire coils and loops make festive napkin rings or hanging ornaments. Seed beads can be strung and sewn on as edging for coasters or placemats. Make inexpensive beads with paper (see Chapter 15, Figure 15-9) and string as any other bead. Wire can be twisted to form interesting effects: hold the ends of several wires in a vise, grab the other ends together with a vise grip or rotary hand drill, and twist. Wire can be shaped and joined to form baskets around dishes or candleholders (Hill, 2008; Wood, 2002). Shaped wire inserted into various bases can become photo holders. Make whimsical creatures or people by combining bent wire with beads. See References and Resources at the end of this chapter for more comprehensive design ideas and instructions.

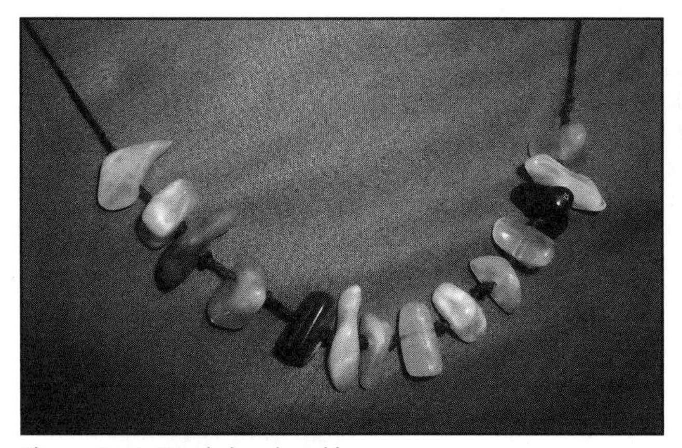

Figure 16-9. Simple bead necklace.

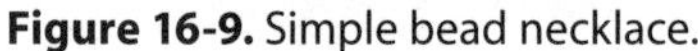

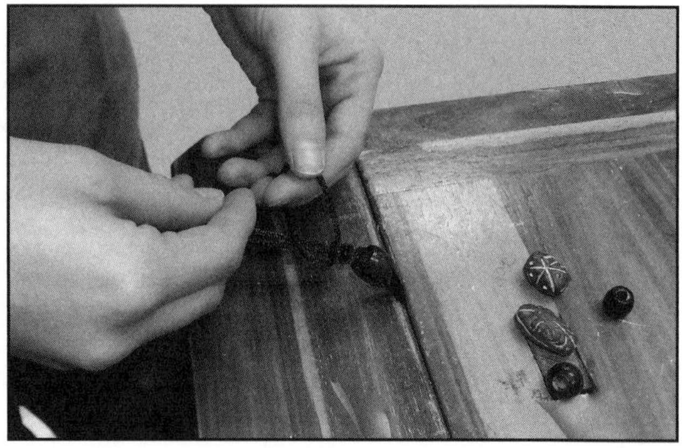

Figure 16-10. Tying a square knot requires bilateral and hand-eye coordination.

Beading projects can be simplified by increasing the size of the beads and cording, and/or by decreasing the complexity of the design. Random patterns are easier because they require less planning and the client does not have to adhere to a particular color or sequence, however, following a pattern may be an element of the therapeutic objective. Consecutive stringing is simpler than stringing using interspersed knots or filler beads. In wirework, free-form bending is much easier than trying to create a specific shape. Although thicker wire requires more force to bend, it is easier to control. Re-bending wire repeatedly may cause it to become brittle and break. Using a tool to stabilize the stationary end of the wire usually results in a more successful bend but requires two hands to accomplish. Offering pictures, samples, and demonstrations are also ways of simplifying the activity.

Main Therapeutic Applications

Physical Dysfunction

Beadwork, wirework, and macramé knotting all have relatively high fine motor demands. Most activities normally require the use of two hands, but a stabilizing device may be used in some instances. These would make excellent activities for clients with hand injuries or other orthopedic problems who need to work on manipulation skills (Figure 16-10). Many forms of this craft offer little or no resistance so they would be appropriate for clients with weak or fragile joints, such as in rheumatoid arthritis (Deshaies, 2006) or for clients with low endurance. Some projects can be positioned to require reaching, providing a way to work on range of motion or endurance for more proximal joints. Some beadwork requires intact visual acuity and perception, so it may not be suitable for the visually impaired or individuals with neurological deficits that result in visual field or depth perception problems. Other projects, however, can be structured such that they can capitalize on and develop tactile skills as compensation for vision loss. Clients with ataxia or apraxia may find some of these activities too difficult. Bear in mind that beads on the floor could present a fall hazard and the therapist may want to place beads in a concave dish or on a towel to prevent them from dropping or spilling easily.

Mental Health

Beading activities can be graded to allow participation of individuals functioning at different cognitive levels. Beadwork is a component of one craft in the Allen Diagnostic Module and it is suggested that clients functioning at cognitive level 4-5 can complete it (Earhart, Allen, & Blue, 1993). Clients experiencing depression or the negative symptoms of a psychotic disorder can follow simple, repetitive patterns (Early, 2009). Clients can be offered choices in terms of color or style and thus achieve some feelings of control and self-determination. Personalized bead creations that can be worn may improve self-concept, body awareness, and self-esteem. Beadwork also offers opportunities to make gifts for others, which also increases feelings of self-worth and societal contribution. One mentally retarded participant at an adult day program was able to help make jewelry that was sold as part of a family business, allowing her both vocational and family engagement and facilitating a transition to a more independent lifestyle (Winkle & Cobb, 2010). Clients with poor tolerance for precise or tedious work will have difficulty with this craft. Those with a short attention span can be successful, however, because most projects can be stopped and restarted at any point. Clients with aggressive tendencies should be supervised when using sharp items such as needles, pliers, and cutters. The therapist may want to use wire with caution, as it could also be used as a weapon and is difficult to inventory before and after sessions. Some clients with psychiatric diagnoses also exhibit deficits in motor planning/manipulation, so this should be considered in choosing this media.

Pediatrics

Most children love beads. The bright colors are visually interesting and the varying shapes and textures offer diverse tactile stimulation, as well as opportunity to practice manipulation skills (Henderson & Pehoski, 2006). Even fairly small children can string beads and may enjoy making elastic bracelets and anklets for themselves or for friends. Elastic cord and assorted plastic beads can be purchased cheaply in bulk and assembly requires no tools or other materials. Beadwork presents children with simple decision making and design opportunities with a high likelihood of success. Simple projects can be completed quickly, thus keeping the child's attention. Older children may enjoy making macramé key rings or chokers, or decorating clothing with beaded edging. As with needlework, this craft may be more suitable for girls than for boys; the therapist should be attuned to current trends and fashions. Wirework is not recommended for children. Wire lengths can be awkward to manage and may pose a danger to self or others. Children may also have difficulty envisioning the finished product, reducing their interest in the activity. A plastic-coated wire, such as Twisteez (available from www.twisteezwire.com) could be a safer substitute material to use with children.

Adolescents

Beading, wirework, and macramé are all appropriate crafts for the adolescent client. Given the ability to meet motor, sensory, and cognitive skill demands mentioned in previous sections, many adolescents will enjoy making jewelry for themselves or others. This craft offers an avenue for self-expression, helping to establish a sense of identity and display of personal taste. The popularity of "retro" fashion fluctuates over time, but some type of knotting such as macramé is usually in vogue in the form of jewelry or other accessories. These crafts offer a means to work on attention, sequencing, following directions, and fine motor skill, and adolescent girls in particular may find them rewarding. Given the current popularity of beadwork and ready availability of supplies, this could develop into a productive hobby from which the individual will continue to benefit.

Older Adults

Typical impairments in elderly clients, including decreased visual acuity and discrimination, peripheral sensation, and manipulation skills secondary to musculoskeletal changes, may affect the ability or desire to participate in beading projects. A client who has previously engaged in (and enjoyed) similar activities is likely to have the most interest in this type craft. They may derive satisfaction from being able to make simple beaded jewelry for grandchildren or friends. As previously noted, this craft requires minimal physical strength, but coordination and manipulation skills are necessary. The therapist should also consider that this is traditionally more consistent with women's occupations.

Groups

Beadwork is not typically utilized as a group activity, but simple projects could be completed in a group setting. Participants could share bead containers and assist one another in design decisions. Any complex bead or wirework activity would be difficult in a group due to the need for one-on-one assistance and/or supervision with tool and material use.

Case Study

Arlita, age 30, had just become established as a successful realtor when she was diagnosed with multiple sclerosis. She had noticed her increasing fatigue and clumsiness, but had attributed it to her long work hours. Finally, after falling one afternoon at a client's home, she decided to consult her physician. He started her on a medication trial, and referred her to a local outpatient therapy clinic for evaluation and education. Arlita was reluctant to take time off work to go, but the physician emphasized that overwork would only exacerbate her condition.

The occupational therapist evaluated Arlita using the Occupational History Interview and the facility's generalized musculoskeletal assessment, which included goniometry, strength, and sensory testing. Her theoretical approach combined aspects of the Model of Human Occupation and the Biomechanical Model. The therapist learned that Arlita had been divorced for 7 years and had no children. She was an only child who had been raised by her aunt and uncle, and a drive for vocational success and financial security had turned her into a self-described "workaholic." She had received her realtors' license not long after her divorce and had since built a thriving business. The physical assessments revealed that Arlita had mild to moderate weakness throughout her extremities with some peripheral sensory loss, particularly in her feet. Her endurance for physical exercise was about 10 minutes, although she could tolerate sedentary activities (e.g., driving and computer work, for much longer periods of time). Reinforcing the physician's recommendations, the occupational therapist explained to the client that allowing herself to become fatigued was detrimental to her condition.

Together, the therapist and Arlita decided that she needed to work on learning energy conservation/work simplification techniques, developing an overall wellness program, and exploring leisure activities that would foster relaxation while still fulfilling her need to feel busy. They set the following goals: to consistently incorporate work simplification and energy conservation techniques into daily activities, documenting accomplishments and problems in a diary as possible; to participate in a range-of-motion exercise program at least one time daily; to learn and utilize a variety of stress management strategies; and to consistently participate in a leisure activity/relaxation technique/hobby.

Arlita was very motivated to maintain or improve her health, so she was receptive to learning and practicing the techniques presented by the therapist. The therapist also offered her several crafts activities; she chose to try a simple beaded bracelet. She found it challenging to handle the small beads, but was very pleased with the end result. She started a necklace project and took it with her to complete at home. She reported to the occupational therapist that she found the activity relaxing and felt like it was also helping her maintain her range of motion and manipulation skills. She had also quickly learned to use vision when necessary to compensate for sensory deficits. Arlita also stated that having a pleasurable activity to do at home was some consolation for having to reduce her hours at work. She said she planned to visit the local craft store and possibly invest in some basic tools and instruction books.

Discussion Questions

1. Due to the nature of multiple sclerosis, this client may one day develop visual problems. How might you adapt her new found hobby so she can continue it?
2. Would you recommend wirework or macramé for this client? Why or why not?
3. Arlita may eventually lose income because of her illness. How might she use her new jewelry-making skill to help compensate for this? What therapy activities might be of benefit in planning for this eventuality?

Resources

The Illustrated Guide to Crafting With Tin, Wire, and Foil
By Simona Hill
Southwater/Anness Publishing, 2008

Teach Yourself Visually: Jewelry Making and Beading
By Chris Franchetti Michaels
Visual, 2007
Step-by-step instructions with photographs for many techniques.

Bead Simple: 150 Designs for Earrings, Necklaces, Bracelets, Embellishments and More
By Susan Beal
Taunton Press, 2008
Projects designed with improvisation in mind.

The Bead Jewelry Maker: Stylish Handcrafted Jewelry to Make at Home
By Cheryl Owen
Barrons Educational Series, 2005

Easy Beading, Vol. 4: The Best Projects From the Fourth Year of BeadStyle Magazine
By Beadstyle (Books and Magazines)
Kalmbach Publishing, 2008

Creating Wire and Beaded Jewelry: Over 35 Beautiful Projects Using Wire and Beads
By Linda Jones
North Light Books, 2004

Making Beaded Jewelry
By Barbara Case
David and Charles Publishers, 2003

References

Abraham, R. M. (1964). *Diversions and pastimes with coins, cards, string, paper and matches.* New York, NY: Dover Publications.
Benson, A. (2001). *Beading for the first time.* Ogden, UT: Chapelle Ltd.
Deshaies, L. (2006) Arthritis. In H. M. Pendleton, & W. Schultz-Krohn (Eds.), *Pedretti's occupational therapy: Practice skills for physical dysfunction* (6th ed.). St. Louis, MO: Mosby Elsevier.
Earhart, C. A., Allen, C. K., & Blue, T. (1993). *Allen diagnostic module.* Colchester, CT: S & S Worldwide.
Early, M. B. (2009). *Mental health concepts and techniques for the occupational therapy assistant.* Philadelphia, PA: Lippincott Williams & Wilkins.
Hall, M. A., Wrobel, J., & Salamony, S. (2001). *Decorative crafts sourcebook.* San Diego, CA: Thunder Bay Press.
Henderson, A., & Pehoski, C. (2006). *Hand function in the child: Foundations for remediation* (2nd ed.). St. Louis, MO: Mosby/Elsevier.
Hill, S. (2008). *The illustrated guide to crafting with tin, wire, and foil.* London, UK: Anness Publishing/Southwater.
Kanan, D. (2001). *The basics of bead stringing.* Santa Monica, CA: Borjay Press.
Moseley, S., Johnson, P., & Koenig, H. (1962). *Crafts design.* Belmont, CA: Wadsworth.
Octopus Books. (1973). *The basic book of macramé and tatting.* Hong Kong, China: Mandarin Publishers.
Pendleton, H. M., & Schultz-Krohn, W. (Eds.). (2006). *Pedretti's occupational therapy: Practice skills for physical dysfunction* (6th ed.). Philadelphia, PA: Elsevier.
Reader's Digest. (1979). *Crafts and hobbies.* Pleasantville, NY: Reader's Digest Association, Inc.
Winkle, M. Y., & Cobb, A. L. (2010). Plotting next steps: Transitions for adults with developmental disabilities, *OT Practice, 15*(21), 13-16.
Wood, D. (2002). *Creative glass.* San Diego, CA: Laurel Glen Publishing.

Section IV

Miscellaneous Crafts

17

Electronic Media

Charla Renée Bullard, MA, ATR-BC, LPAT and Lori Dawn Lockhart, MAEd;
Fourth Edition updated by Carol Crellin Tubbs, MA, OTR/L

Objectives

The student should be able to:

- Understand basic computer terminology and list commonly used equipment
- Describe advantages and limitations of using electronic media for creative activities in therapy
- List current software programs that incorporate artwork
- List ways to grade computer art activities
- List assessments used to determine a client's ability to utilize various software programs and/or need for adaptive devices
- Explain ways of applying creative electronic media with various client populations

This chapter explores computer use for engaging in creative activities in the therapeutic setting. Special emphasis will be placed on considerations necessary for success in the physical, cognitive, and emotional realms of therapy and rehabilitation when using computers with clients. Assistive technology and the use of expressive arts software as a component of rehabilitation will be the focus.

The computer, as we know it, started around the early 1940s with the invention of the IBM Automatic Sequence Controlled Calculator (IBMASCC). This computer was created by Howard H. Aiken and was 8 feet tall by 51 feet long (IBM Corporation, 2005). In the span of about 70 years, the technology has advanced from a computer that took up a whole room to computers that are not only portable, but can fit in the palm of your hand and connect with almost any place in the world via the Internet. With this portability has come unlimited opportunity for development of hardware and software for use in a therapeutic setting.

When first introduced, computers held a new fascination for individuals of all ages. People were accustomed to watching a magic show, for example, with its spectacular process, but when working with computers, most people saw only the spectacular output. A few years ago, this seemingly "magic" technology was only available to the wealthy, able-bodied person. However, thanks to the decreasing costs of computers and the development of advanced assistive devices, computers are currently used by people of all ages, cognitive levels, and physical abilities. There are now Web sites that provide efficient and effective health-related services and information. According to Rogers (2005), the future (and in some instances, the present) in health care entails computerized scheduling of doctor's appointments, sharing of digital (only) medical records, and relaying diagnostic information from home via the internet. Prescriptions will be transmitted

Tubbs, C., & Drake, M. *Crafts and Creative Media in Therapy, Fourth Edition (pp. 213-224).*

to the pharmacy via computer and hospital medical bracelets will contain radio chips to assure accurate administration of medication. Computer technology permeates our everyday lives.

Hardware

In order to use computers within the realm of therapy, certain hardware is necessary. The first necessary piece of hardware is the computer itself. There are many types of computers on the market. When using a computer for therapy, the brand of computer does not matter, nor does the particular operating system. The only thing to take into consideration when choosing an operating system is compatibility with the software that will be used. When using computers in therapy sessions, input devices (e.g., keyboards, mice, touch-screens, switches, scanners, and digital cameras) and output devices (e.g., CD burners, 3½-inch disk drives, and printers) are needed. Those devices, too, must be compatible with the computer in use.

Many different computers input devices are available, thanks to the advance of *assistive technology*. The Assistive Technology Act of 1998 (Tech Act), which is an Amendment to IDEA (Individuals with Disabilities Education Act), defines an assistive technology device as "Any item, piece of equipment, or product system, whether acquired commercially, off-the-shelf, modified or customized, that is used to increase, maintain or improve functional capabilities of individuals with disabilities" (U.S. Government Printing Office, 2005).

There are several types of assistive input devices for the computer that help individuals with disabilities gain access. Some typical assistive technology devices that are used with expressive arts software are alternative mice, joysticks, alternative keyboards, touchscreens, switches, head pointers, stylus and pad, and microphones. The client should be carefully evaluated before choosing an input device.

Computer mice come in all shapes and sizes. There are typical mice that are about the size of an average adult's palm. Mice may have buttons on both the right and left sides. If an individual is left-handed or if he or she has had an accident/disabling condition that has made it impossible for him or her to use his or her dominant right hand, mouse button controls can be reversed in the Control Panel Settings of most computers. There are smaller mice that are wonderful to use with children. In some cases, these smaller mice are designed to look like mice, frogs, and other objects like cars and airplanes. These themed mice make it fun for children to use and they are the perfect size for little hands. There are also trackball mice that work by moving either a small or large ball with a finger or hand. Trackballs and trackball mice are extremely beneficial for individuals who have had a stroke or problems with fine- or gross-motor control. Joysticks were originally created for use with video games; however, after their invention, it was found that they had wonderful capabilities as an alternate mouse-like device for individuals with difficulty grasping or difficulty with fine motor control. Joysticks consist of a pivoting stick, usually mounted to a square base. The cursor is moved on the screen by the individual moving the joystick from side to side or front to back. Joysticks also have a button or buttons that can be pressed to make a selection. Touch pads are typically found on laptop computers; however, they have made their way onto various condensed keyboards. A touch pad allows movement of the cursor by moving a finger across a touch-sensitive pad.

A typical QWERTY keyboard is an effective input device; however, sometimes individuals need alternative keyboards to gain computer access. There are many types of alternative keyboards such as Big Keys, ABC Keyboard, IntelliKeys, and various condensed keyboards. The Big Keys keyboard has large, colorful letters that are laid out in alphabetical order. This keyboard is very beneficial to younger children, who have not learned the QWERTY layout and have problems hitting small keys. The ABC Keyboard looks like a regular keyboard but the keys are laid out in an alphabetical rather than QWERTY layout. The IntelliKeys keyboard has overlays that can be made to match various IntelliTools software. The overlays are put on top of a touchboard-like input device and generally have pictures to represent selections. Condensed keyboards are excellent options for individuals who, for whatever reason, have lost the use of one hand. The various types of condensed keyboards are useful for one-handed typists because the keys are closer together and the hand does not have to move very far to go from one side of the keyboard to the other. Some condensed keyboards even come with a built-in touch pad so the keyboard and mouse are within easy reach of one hand.

Touch screens come either as a complete monitor or as a screen that can be mounted to the front of a regular computer monitor. Touch screens typically are activated by either the breaking of a light beam or the detection of an electrical charge on someone's finger (Cook & Hussey, 2002). There are switches for just about every moveable body part. The most typical switches are head switches, foot switches, and hand switches. Switches require switch hoppers or a switch interface box in order for them to be connected to a computer. Please note that in order to use switches, switch accessible/scanning software must be installed. Infrared head pointers are becoming more frequently used. Infrared head pointers work by placing a dot on someone's forehead. An infrared mechanism is attached to the computer and it reads the movements of the dot. As someone moves his or her head, the cursor will move on the screen. Infrared head pointers and head switches are especially helpful when working with individuals with cerebral palsy or quadriplegia. A stylus and pad can be effectively used when working with younger children or when working with individuals who feel more comfortable using a more familiar and traditional tool to access the computer. A stylus and pad resemble a pencil and a writing pad. The touch pad is connected to the computer and reads whatever movements the stylus makes on it. Microphones provide an excellent way for visually-impaired individuals to interact with a computer. When using microphones to access the computer, specific software such as Dragon Naturally Speaking, Jaws, and Jawbone is essential.

Just as assistive equipment is important for input into the computer, output devices are also essential to the therapeutic session. Regardless of how much or how little work is done on the computer, the ability to provide a copy of the work gives a feeling of accomplishment and may also provide some sense of control over the environment. Output devices allow individuals to have hard copies (paper) of their work and also to have digital copies (disk) that they can edit at a later time. The most common output devices are CD burners, 3½-inch disk drives, and printers. The user can also save the image to a flash drive, or email it, to be viewed or printed at another location. Printers output hard copies of work completed during the session, which can be shared with others after the therapy session to further benefit the individual. Magnetic printer paper is available and would allow the artwork to be posted on a metal surface, such as the ubiquitous "refrigerator art" seen in many households. An individual's work can be burned onto a CD for the individual to have a digital copy. Please be aware when burning CDs that there are two different types: 1) CD Recordables (CD-Rs) where you can only burn a file to the disk one time and 2) CD Recordable-Writables (CD-RWs) where the individual is able to edit the work at a later date and burn over the first draft file.

Special Considerations

There are certain factors to take into account when using computers in therapy. The first consideration should always be for the safety of the individual using the computer. Computers and televisions have been known to cause seizures in some individuals with seizure disorder. It is highly important when working with an individual who has seizure disorder or a history of having seizures to consult the individual's medical doctor before using a computer with the individual. Another consideration that should be thoroughly contemplated when using computers in therapy is cost. Computers, assistive technology, and software programs range from inexpensive and readily available to highly expensive. Computers typically are priced from several hundred dollars to several thousand dollars, although costs have continued to decline in recent years. Naturally, adding special features to the basic package will increase the final cost as well. The new iPad and iPad II offer both portability and exceptional flexibility in use, including the capability to run art applications, but they are typically just as costly as a full-sized computer with monitor. A final consideration is the therapist's previous computer knowledge and experience. The therapist should experiment and become familiar with the computer, assistive technology, and software before using it in a session. If a therapist has no previous computer knowledge, there are classes at various colleges/university and online to help build the necessary skills. The Internet for Classrooms Web site at www.internet4classrooms.com has some excellent training modules on things like the Windows and Macintosh Operating Systems, Internet Explorer, Microsoft Word, Microsoft PowerPoint, Microsoft Excel, Hyperstudio, Inspiration, and Kidspiration (Brooks & Byles, 2000).

Assessments

Before implementing computerized art activities with a client, medical, physical, and emotional needs and abilities should all be considered, and a variety of assessment tools may be utilized. There are multiple assessment tools available to help determine the type of assistive device needed to access the computer, many of which were designed for a specific diagnosis. In 2002, a French standardized assessment was translated to English, titled "Assessment of Computer Task Performance," and was adapted to aid therapists in selecting assistive technology for a broad range of diagnoses (Dumont, Claude, & Mazer, 2002). Other assessments to consider are the Allen Sementic Differential Scale for response to interventions through Web pages, the Assistive Technology Evaluation for assistive devices necessary for increased independence, the Computer Attitude Scale to rate the individual's motivation toward using the computer, and the Computer System Usability Questionnaire for grading software/user compatibility (Boop, 2003).

After evaluating an individual and providing them with appropriate adaptive devices, choosing appropriate software is the next consideration. As with all interventions, the individual's age, cognition, and physical abilities should be considered when choosing software.

Art-Based Software Programs

Both occupational therapists and art therapists have used art-based software programs in therapy for many years (Collie & Čubranić, 1999; Cromwel, 1986; Drake, 1992; Malchiodi, 2000; McLeod, 1999; Parker-Bell, 1999). Following are descriptions of art-based software programs with examples of interventions to address physical, cognitive, and emotional goals in therapy.

Kid Pix Deluxe 4 is an educational and creative software program designed for use with children from kindergarten through eighth grade and can easily be adapted for use in individual or group therapy settings. Features of the program include the ability to limit certain options and printing capabilities for use with young children, the ability to add customized templates, and to switch between English and Spanish computer speech and text.

Because this software program provides not only visual but also auditory stimulation each time a selection is made and the curser is moved, it gives additional motivation to the child to work on physical skills such as extending, reaching, pointing, and grasping input devices such as the joystick, mouse, touch screen, or stylus. As with traditional art materials, the process of creating on the computer can likewise encourage fine-motor function and training in various visual and perceptual skills. Interventions using computer-based art can address visual focus, attention, and eye-limb/hand-eye coordination, depending on how input device is controlled. For those who access the computer using the laser-sensor or mouthstick, the process of making artwork may better motivate the patient to actively control head position and subsequently strengthen neck muscles.

Children experiencing low energy due to physical or medical issues may find using traditional art materials very frustrating and difficult. However, a sense of success may be experienced when filling the screen with color, images, and sounds of personal choice using the fill and stamp tools. The success is realized by placing a hand (hand, finger, side of hand, or thumb) on the touch screen or by moving a finger up-and-down to click the mouse.

Children who are resistant to communicate verbally, who have minimal or no fine-motor functioning, or who have become ventilator-dependent and need to work on coordinating speaking with ventilator breathing may benefit from using a microphone input device. The microphone in combination with the microphone paint tool could prove to be a positive intervention in motivating the child to self-expression through actualizing an abstract image on the monitor by varying voice tone and pitch.

To address cognitive issues, a child may utilize the draw, paint, fill, background, mixer, stickers, text, stamp, music, and animation tools, which are most efficient to actualize an idea. The child can be encouraged to verbally communicate ideas before creating them to enhance cognitive functioning. Additionally, the therapist may demonstrate single- or multi-stepped tasks on the monitor for the individual to retain and then execute, helping to enhance memory skills. The slideshow is another function in which problem solving, sequencing, and planning skills can be addressed when used in combination with previously created and saved images.

Sound evoked from the various modes of access coupled with brightly colored images addresses cognitive functioning related to cause-and-effect. Each art tool has its own realistic sound (e.g., the marker squeaks as if applying heavy pressure and the scissors sound as if cutting thick paper). Additionally, there is also a music tool in the program that allows a child with low vision or blindness to "create" a picture of sounds.

The 83-color pallet, images, music, and comments surrounding the process of art making may provide an avenue for addressing feelings and issues surrounding the child's diagnosis. The editing capability to move, copy, paste, rotate, flip, scale, and delete images promotes individual autonomy and increases sense of self.

One intervention that may be beneficial to the child on an emotional level is to use the slideshow to review images in chronological order throughout therapy. This may help the child symbolically "see" progressive improvement in therapy. The child with low energy or initiation skills can utilize the pre-drawn images such as rubber stamp, stickers, background, and animation tools to receive immediate gratification and increase sense of self. As with freehand drawn images, pre-drawn images selected by the individual may convey personal ideas and stimulate conversation that relate to issues that need to be addressed in therapy.

For children who are resistant to speaking due to emotional issues or those who are struggling with speaking after becoming ventilator-dependent, the novelty of hearing one's voice coming from the computer may be therapeutic. Using the microphone icon in the paint toolbox, the child selects a pattern of choice, then talks or sings into the microphone. Depending upon the child's pitch and tone of voice, colorful images explode on the screen to create an abstract picture. The child can also make brief recordings using the music tool and microphone. Those created images and chosen sounds can be incorporated into a graphic image or slideshow presentation. Furthermore, the child does not have to speak but rather can convey thoughts and ideas through typed words using the text tool. When the text box is highlighted and read text icon selected, typed words are read by the computer. This function may prompt conversation or motivate the child to respond by repeating the words. An important note to add is that the program has an editing feature that allows accurate pronunciation of words (Tools for Learning, 2000-2004).

If the therapist is unable to acquire Kid Pix Deluxe 4, but has a computer with a draw/paint program, the book *Kids Computer Creations* is a task resource for children ages 4 through 10. It provides 52 graded tasks organized by theme and grade-level of difficulty. In addition, a brief history of computers is included, providing helpful computer tips, answers to common questions, and definitions of computer terminology interspersed throughout the book (Sabbeth, 1995).

Flying Colors 2 Paint is an art-based software program developed for children, adolescents, and adults. The program provides three different working levels that each limit tool options according to age and/or skill level. Tools included in the program are text, draw, paint, stamp, stencil, symmetry, background, borders, and patterns. The tools give access to thousands of detailed theme-based images, colorful patterns, animated gradient colors, and percussion sound effects that correlate with placing images, patterns, and colors on the screen (Magic Mouse Productions, 2006).

This program's draw/paint tools can be used for interventions similarly to other art-based programs. However, there are two features unique to this program worth highlighting: the symmetry tool, which rotates drawn images around a pre-selected point; and the playback tool, which records all cursor movements during the process of creating artwork. Creating a "Name Kaleidoscope" (G. Wright, personal communication, March 14, 2005) is an intervention that can be used during the initial part of therapy to help maintain the session's focus on the individual as when establishing rapport, acquiring past history, and setting therapeutic goals. The nature of the task is open-ended, encourages spontaneity, and is not intimidating or overwhelming to the inexperienced computer-user or individual being introduced to an art-based program for the first time. The task is also appropriate for use with individuals of all ages and with a range of diagnoses.

To create a Name Kaleidoscope using Flying Colors 2 Paint, access the symmetry tool in the advanced level of the program. Determine the origin point and choose the number of segments (or copies) based on paper size and printer specifications. Then, using the paintbrush tool with tight spacing, write a name in one segment ensuring that letters extend between the height and width of the segment. Lines, shapes, and colors may be added in the negative space around letters. As soon as an image is placed on the computer screen, the program instantaneously duplicates it around a central point to create the kaleidoscope effect. If using the stamp tool, images do not pivot around the point of origin but instead rotate vertically around the point. Artwork created can be simple and realized in a matter of seconds, or elaborate and require a majority of the session to complete. After completion of the Name Kaleidoscope, the individual can "watch" an animated version of the process of creating the artwork from start to finish by selecting the playback tool in the advanced level (Flying Colors 2 User Manual, 2003).

Adobe Photoshop Elements 9.0 is a photo-enhancing software program that provides creating, organizing, editing, printing, and slideshow capabilities for digital images. Images used can come from files created directly from the software program, as well as a variety of input devices such as scanners, digital cameras, card readers, and camera phones. The latest software versions have simplified the object-selection process for editing purposes with simply clicking and dragging the cursor on the desired object, instead of what used to be a tedious and labor-intensive process of "tracing" an object (Adobe Photoshop, 2005). It is recommended that adolescents and adults who have a high level of cognitive functioning, excellent visual acuity, and outstanding fine-motor functioning would benefit from this program because of necessary attention to detail required for a multi-level, multi-step process required to effect a single change. However, just as the therapist makes modifications using traditional art materials for a particular task or diagnosis, the therapist can modify tasks or adapt files to best meet an individual's needs. Each new edition of this program has some modification of features, although newer is not necessarily better in terms of usefulness in therapy. Therapists are advised to compare features of each version and decide which are most useful for their particular client population.

This software program allows individuals who may be experiencing physical discomfort to use the art-making process as a positive distraction through experimentation with the effects of different filters using provided sample images. By downloading personal graphics and editing selected images using transformation tools or the color palette, the individual may create original graphics using the painting and drawing tools. In addition, individuals who are visually impaired may use the program to create a musical slideshow composed of music selections combined with the client's recorded voice.

Specific uses for Photoshop Elements are practically unlimited. For example, using the program to create a calendar from the template provided in the program might be an appropriate intervention for an individual with memory deficits. Images of personal choice, such as familiar people and places, with typed daily reminders, may be included in the calendar. The therapist may also encourage the individual to verbally communicate ideas and the steps necessary before executing them, also facilitating memory skills. At the close of the session, the client may again review, or "teach" the steps taken to complete the task to the therapist, a peer, or family member, thus combining the cognitive and creative aspects to reinforce new skills learned. iPhoto, a software program that is included on Macintosh computers at an extra cost, is similar to Photoshop and relatively simple to use.

Individuals in need of an emotional or expressive outlet can manipulate photos that best convey their thoughts and ideas through a photo collage, using the various edit tools to change colors or to cut-and-paste. The slideshow feature may be used to record the client's images chronologically and combine them with the client's recorded personal thoughts and feelings related to the image. This may prove beneficial for the client to "see" and "hear" progress in therapy. The slideshow can then be burned to a CD or DVD for the client to take upon discharge. This software is a powerful photo-editing tool limited only by the individual's imagination and motivation.

Print Magic includes many step-by-step art tasks using Photoshop Elements, or similar photo manipulation program, to make personalized decals, window clings, and fabric transfers for various projects that can be tailored to address individual goals in therapy (Bradley, 2005). Several other art-based software programs are also available and each has both advantages and disadvantages. For all those listed below, the therapist should ensure that it is compatible with the computers being used.

Crayola Art Studio, available from several retailers, including www.crayolastore.com, is designed for children age 4 and up. It has 12 art "tools" and over 1,000 images that can be added to user-created artwork. It is basic enough for clients with little or no computer or artistic skills and its progressive undo and redo features encourage experimentation. The program includes a "Begin to Draw" level and the simplified screen is easy for children to operate. One advantage that it has over some other programs is that it can be installed on more than one computer, although only used on one at a time. Reviewers give it high marks for ease in use.

The Art Explosion Greeting Card Factory Deluxe 6.0 and Hallmark Card Studio 2011 are both programs that allow the user to create custom greeting cards and other items such as calendars, stationery, labels, and gift tags. The user can incorporate program images/clipart, text effects, and greetings, but also personal photos. The Greeting Card Factory has photo editing and photo effect capabilities and can capture photos directly from the user's camera if desired. In addition, its text effects and clipart can be loaded directly onto the computer so the creator does not have to go and forth to the menu for those items. This program works well with both inkjet and laser printers. The Hallmark Card Studio allows the user to print, email, or create a file of their work for sharing with others.

The Scrapbook Factory Deluxe 4.0 software allows users to make digital scrapbooks using the program's thousands of designs and images in combination with their personal photos. It has a built-in photo editor and is capable of creating CD photo scrapbooks that can be watched on TV. The program can also make photo calendars in numerous formats, such as weekly, monthly, or yearly. Pages can be saved as a .jpg or .pdf file for printing or emailing. One disadvantage of this software is that the entire program has to be loaded onto the hard drive and it requires 3 GB of memory. It also works best with a wide format printer.

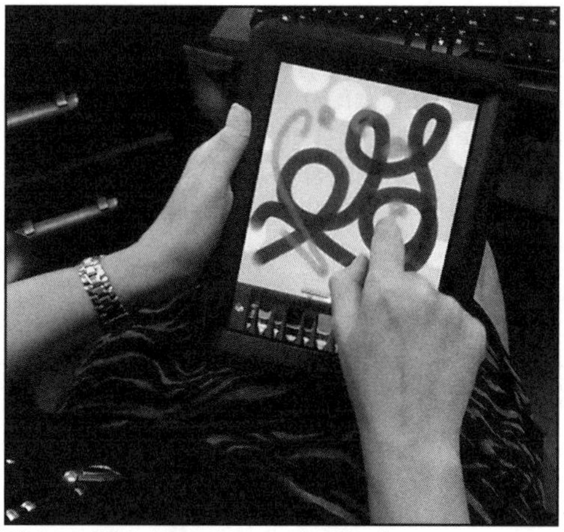

Figure 17-1. Drawing on the iPad.

The greeting card and scrapbook software are somewhat unique in that they allow the client to create something more functional than works of art. They are able to make items for gifts or to send personal greetings to friends or loved ones that they may not be able to produce without the aid of a computer. The program images and messages can provide a sort of compensation for limited physical or cognitive ability and the end product can look just as attractive as one created by an able-bodied individual.

Arts- and Crafts-Based Video Games

One interesting twist on art software is the creativity-based video game. Nintendo (www.nintendo.com) produces both Crafting Mama and Art Academy, games that require the player to create something as he or she moves through the levels. To play Crafting Mama, one of a series of "Mama" games, the gamer uses a stylus to fold, sew, glue, paint, and perform other actions used in crafting. The game has 40 different projects to choose from and the user can select colors, fabrics, and so on to make unique items each time it is played. Once made, the creations can be used to play mini-games or to accessorize the Mama character. The game projects are diverse: candles, jewelry, needle felt, pressed flowers, floral garland, and more. The "Mama" series also includes Cooking Mama and Gardening Mama, which, like Crafting Mama, may offer the user a virtual experience of common leisure activities in which they may be more independent.

Art Academy, which also requires a Nintendo DS, allows the gamer to create virtual artwork, and it will even frame and save artwork so that it can be displayed as a slideshow or viewed individually. The works created are somewhat impressionistic, which is good for the beginner, and there are quiet music and sound effects during the game that may enhance relaxation. Virtual tools include different types of pencils and brushes, and colors can be easily mixed or diluted. The game has an in-game tutor that teaches "real world" art techniques and includes demonstrations, examples, and tips. The user can get ideas from included stock images or personal photos. One disadvantage is that there is no way to move images to a PC or to print them, and this may be unsatisfactory for a client who wants to create art to use or give away.

Art Applications for the iPad

The iPad offers several unique features over the standard computer, including the ability to easily and inexpensively load many diverse applications (Figure 17-1). Among those are three art programs: ArtStudio, Brushes, and Sketchbook Pro. All have features in common (e.g., undo and zoom) and individually they have unique abilities and advantages/disadvantages.

ArtStudio has the ability to both import and export, and it has multiple brush choices and a sophisticated color palette. One helpful feature is the in-app art lessons, which use animated steps and figures that can be drawn over. The lessons also have a shake-for-menu feature, but it requires two hands to use. The user can send artwork via email or upload it into the program's online Flickr gallery. One disadvantage of this application is that it does not have an autosave, so the user must remember to save work frequently to protect it.

Brushes has a nice gallery view feature that frames your work and hangs it on a virtual wall, where each piece is labeled with title, artist name, and date. This application also has a playback feature for created works so that user can watch as his or her work is re-created, stroke by stroke. The toolbars are accessed by tapping the screen but it does not have a quick tool access function or in-app assistance.

Sketchbook Pro has the most brush choices and also the most complex user interface. Advantages are the in-app assistance and the top-only toolbar, which minimizes the chance that the user will accidently hit it and disrupt the work in progress. This application allows the user to export art for use in Photoshop. Although certain functions are opened/operated with simple finger swipes, the toolbar does not stay visible and the user has to tap each time it is needed again. All three applications allow the user to operate the program with either a finger or with a stylus. One compatible and lightweight stylus is the Pogo Sketch (Pigott, 2010).

Miscellaneous Technology-Assisted Art

One last idea for technology-assisted creativity is the PicoCricket Kit from Playful Invention Company (PICO). The company was founded by an assistant professor from MIT but children helped in the development of the craft projects in this kit. The kit comes with various Lego craft materials but also includes technological additions such as sensors for sound, light, and touch; USB to serial cable; a beamer; motorboard; soundbox with display; and software for programming the creations made with the materials. The kit goes "back to the future to bring arts and crafts into the 21st century." By using the software program, in which program sequences are depicted as puzzle pieces, children can create commands for their creations and have them react to their environment. The PicoCricket combines kinetics with sensory experiences. Examples of items made include a magic lantern, a mechanical puppet, kinetic sculptures, interactive jewelry, a birthday cake that sings when you blow out its candles, and various musical instruments made with unusual household items. The creative aspect of these projects teaches problem-solving strategies that can be generalized to common daily activities. The overall mission of the product is to expand the ways that people can create and learn (Brown, 2007).

As discussed, the process of "creating" with art-based software or other technological means proves beneficial on many different physical, cognitive, and emotional levels in the therapeutic setting. Another rapidly expanding dimension of computer technology where image and sound are combined for therapeutic use is in virtual reality. Just as the magician creates an illusion to transport the viewer's imagination and stimulate the mind with wonder and curiosity, likewise does the visual image—real or imagined. According to Riccio, Nelson, and Bush (1990), the therapeutic benefits of visual imagery, guided imagery, role play, and simulated environments have been known for years to be beneficial in therapy. The imagery helps to draw from the individual emotions and memories that bring purpose, meaning, and success to therapy.

> *Virtual reality* is defined as an immersive and interactive three-dimensional (3D) computer experience occurring in real time (Pimental & Teixeira, 1995). Virtual reality applications use 3D computer graphics, which respond to the users movements, thereby giving the user the sense of being immersed in the virtual environment (Reid, 2004, p. 133).

There have been several studies examining the benefits of virtual reality. For example, cognitive function in children diagnosed with traumatic brain injury increased when a virtual environment was combined with physical activity (Grealy & Heffernan, 2001). Upper-limb function was improved in those experiencing the effects of a stroke by having them reaching and grab for objects that change colors, move, and disappear on the screen (Rydemark & Broeren, 2002). In children diagnosed with cerebral palsy, playfulness can be assessed using virtual activities such as painting, playing soccer, and driving a car (Reid, 2004). Fall risk can be reduced in a geriatric population through increased standing tolerance and balance gained by reaching for balls that transform into colorful particles or flying birds (Cunningham & Krishack, 1999). Virtual reality has the capability "to improve life skills, mobility and cognitive abilities, quality of life, and social opportunities" (Reid, 2004, p. 134).

Regardless of mode of intervention, the ultimate goal of therapy is for newly acquired skills to generalize into other areas of the client's life. The prestige associated with computer use may provide a sense of empowerment in feeling "connected" to society (Swenson Miller, Bunch-Harrison, Brumbaugh, Kutty, & FitzGerald, 2005). In addition, utilizing basic key commands to navigate the art-based software is a skill that may increase competence in using other software programs or in surfing the Internet. Because new technology is constantly being developed, some of the programs or devices in this chapter may be outdated or upgraded even by the time of publication. Therefore, the therapist who decides to employ computer or other technology-assisted arts and craftwork in therapy is advised to take steps to stay current with the latest programs and devices. The Internet makes this relatively easy with a small investment of time. With the use of technology, both children and adults with severe physical disabilities have a vast potential for engaging in and enjoying the benefits of creative expression that others take for granted.

The following clinical vignette (Drake, 1999) is just one of many that reflect how the use of computer technology, adaptive equipment, and art-based software enhances lives. In this study, a 10-year-old female was helped to realize her potential and, in some respects, accomplish the unbelievable.

Case Study

Emily is a 10-year-old client with severe motor control impairment due to cerebral palsy. Until she was 8 years old, it was unknown that she had an IQ of 110. Because she was so physically handicapped and her language was limited, and because there was no one trained to test her IQ by non-pencil-and-paper methods before, it was thought that she was mentally retarded as well as physically limited. Emily was born in New York City but at age 2 1/2 she and her mother moved back to her mother's home in the South. Shortly thereafter, her mother, who had been a drug addict, died of an overdose and Emily was taken to live with her grandmother in a rural community. She had no schooling except what she saw on television. When Emily was 8, her grandmother died and no one else in the family was willing or able to care for her, as she required total personal care, including feeding, diapering, and bathing.

The state department of human services made a decision to place her in an intermediate care facility for the developmentally disabled. She was finally evaluated and measured for a custom wheelchair and was enrolled in a special education class. All the members of the treatment team evaluated her, and at that time, her IQ was discovered to be 110. A concerted effort was made by all the professionals involved to help her make up for the time she was without schooling. They were assisted by the state assistive technology reference guide (Thompson, Bethea, Rizer, & Hutto, 1998). The occupational therapist used a combination of theories, including Learning/Cognitive Disabilities and the Model of Human Occupation. Emily's upper extremity athetosis made most occupational activities difficult for her, so the therapist planned to use compensatory physical methods combined with remedial cognitive/academic ones. Emily's occupational therapy goals were to increase self-care such as self-feeding, learning to sit on the toilet, and control the timing of toileting; develop/enhance visual, perceptual, and motor performance skills; enhance and stimulate visual attention; improve upper extremity fine motor coordination and dexterity; utilize her motivation to learn to overcome performance deficits; develop a feeling of independence and autonomy.

She was evaluated for appropriateness of computer use. The therapist found that Emily could begin to control the screen by using a joy stick on her wheelchair lap board. The schoolteacher working with Emily began a program to teach her to read. She had taught herself some words by simply watching television. While attending occupational therapy, she worked with the computer graphics as a reward for feeding herself and waiting to sit on the toilet to urinate and defecate. She started out with a simple program of lines and shapes that she could color in and move around the screen. But, she rapidly advanced to a more sophisticated program involving assembling designs on the screen. The therapist worked with her on visually scanning her work, developing figure ground perception by seeing shapes within shapes and figures, on color discrimination and sequencing her actions to get the effects she wanted, and from there to drawing and painting on more sophisticated software. The occupational therapy clinic did not have a color printer so the therapist attached her work to an email and sent it to the curriculum center at the board of education building to have the graphics printed out from Emily's drawings. Soon Emily was skilled enough to draw her own cartoons, which she used on greeting cards.

The school staff used her enlarged cartoons for signs and warnings around the school building. Emily was seen as a good candidate for a new group home for the disabled that was about to be funded by a grant. The occupational therapist worked with the grant writers to see that money was included to buy computers for each resident's room.

Discussion Questions

1. How could the possibility of increasing Emily's social isolation be avoided as she became more involved with the computer?
2. Could any of the movements she learned to make with the joystick be transferred over to help her in increasing her independence in self-care?

Resources

Books

Creative Computer Crafts: 50 Fun and Useful Products You Can Make With Any Inkjet Printer
By Marcelle Costanza
No Starch Press, 2006

Digital Expressions: Creating Digital Art With Adobe Photoshop Elements
By Susan Tuttle
North Light Books, 2010
Clear step-by-step instructions, excellent blending of art and technology.

Digital Scrapbooking for Dummies
By Jeanne Wines-Reed and Joan Wines
Wiley Publishing, 2005

Photocraft: Cool Things to Do With the Pictures You Love
By Caroline Herter, Laurie Frankel (photos), and Laura Lovett (illustrations)
Bulfinch Press 2005

Photoshop Elements 4: One-on-One
By Deke McClelland with Galen Fott
Deke Press with O'Reilly Media, Inc., 2005
A compact disc is included with this book. Many books for newer versions of Photoshop Elements are also available.

The Arts and Crafts Computer: Using Your Computer as an Artist's Tool
By Janet Ashford
Peachpit Press, 2002

Microsoft Image Composer for Dummies
By Brian Johnson
IDG Books Worldwide, Inc., 1998
This guide starts with the most basic images and advances to web page design.

Painter 11 Wow!
By Cher Threinen-Pendarvis
Peachpit Press; 2010
For beginners to the most sophisticated artists.

Scrapbooking Digitally
By Kerry Arquette, Darlene D'Agostino, Susha Roberts, Andrea Zocchi
Taunton Press, 2008

Web sites

PC Magazine—Online magazine that provides information on the latest PC computer hardware and software products.
http://www.pcmag.com/

Computing With Kids—A weekly online magazine that reviews children's products, such as software, Web sites, video games, and smart toys.
http://www.computingwithkids.com/

Art Educational Web site—For children and adults.
http://www.doodlestudio.com

Magic Mouse Productions—Developer of Flying Colors 2 Paint.
http://www.magicmouse.com/

Mind Play: Educational Software—For children and adults.
http://www.mindplay.com/

Riverdeep: The Learning Company—Developer of educational and creative software Kid Pix Deluxe 4.
http://www.riverdeep.net/index.jhtml

Brighter Child: Publishers of Children's Educational Products
http://www.brighterchild.com/

Crayola—Creator of art and educational software product Crayola Dream Makers.
http://www.crayola.com/index.cfm?mt=topbar_home

Bright Minds: The Critical Thinking Company
http://www.brightminds.us/home/index.jsp

References

Adobe Photoshop Elements 4.0 Users Guide for Windows [Software manual]. (2005). San Jose, CA: Adobe Systems.

Boop, C. (2003). Assessments: Listed alphabetically by title. In E. B. Crepeau, E. S. Cohen, & B. A. B Schell (Eds.), *Willard and Spackman's occupational therapy* (10th ed., pp. 981-1004). Philadelphia, PA: Lippincott Williams & Wilkins.

Bradley, H. (2005). *Print magic: Creating crafts using digital photos and art.* Upper Saddle River, NJ: Creative Homeowner.

Brooks, S., & Byles, B. (2000). *On-line practice modules. Internet for classrooms* [On-line]. Retrieved from www.internet4classrooms.com/on-line.htm.

Brown, E. J. (2007). Digi-handcrafting: Have you discovered the digital arts revolution? *Advance for Occupational Therapy Practitioners, 23*(15), 42.

Collie, K., & Čubranić, D. (1999). An art therapy solution to a telehealth problem. *Art Therapy: Journal of the American Art Therapy Association, 16*(4) 186-193.

Cook, A. M., & Hussey, S. M. (2002). *Assistive technologies: Principles and practices* (2nd ed., p. 24). St. Louis, MO: Mosby.

Cromwel, F. S. (1986). *Computer applications in occupational therapy.* New York, NY: Howarth Press.

Cunningham, D., & Krishack, M. (1999). Virtual reality: A wholistic approach to rehabilitation. *Studies in Health Technology and Informatics, 62*, 90-93.
Drake, M. (1992). *Crafts in therapy and rehabilitation*. New York, NY: McGraw Hill
Drake, M. (1999). *Crafts in therapy and rehabilitation* (2nd ed.). Thorofare, NJ: SLACK Incorporated.
Dumont, C., Claude, V., & Mazer, B. (2002). Development of a standardized instrument to assess computer task performance. *American Journal of Occupational Therapy, 56*, 60-68.
Flying Colors 2 Users Manual [Software manual]. (2003). Inverness, CA: Magic Mouse Productions.
Grealy, M. A., & Heffernan, D. (2001). The rehabilitation of brain injured children: The case for including physical exercise and virtual reality. *Pediatric Rehabilitation, 4*(2), 41-49.
IBM Corporation (2005). *IBM's ASCC introduction*. IBM [On-line]. Retrieved from www-03.ibm.com/ibm/history/exhibits/markI/markI_intro.html.
Magic Mouse Productions (2006). *Flying colors 2 example compositions* [On-line]. Retrieved from www.magicmouse.com/.
Malichiodi, C. A. (2000). *Art therapy & computer technology: A virtual studio of possibilities*. London, UK: Jessica Kingsley.
McLeod, C. (1999). Empowering creativity with computer-assisted art therapy: An introduction to available programs and techniques. *Art Therapy: Journal of the American Art Therapy Association, 16*(4) 201-205.
Parker-Bell, B. (1999). Embracing a future with computers and art therapy. *Art Therapy: Journal of the American Art Therapy Association, 16*(4), 180-185.
Pigott, S. (2010). *Three amazing art apps for the iPad: A review and comparison*. Retrieved from www.macgasm.net/2010/05/18/amazing-art-apps-ipad-review-comparison.
Reid, D. (2004). The influence of virtual reality on playfulness in children with cerebral palsy: A pilot study. *Occupational Therapy International, 11*(3), 131-144.
Riccio, C. M., Nelson, D. L., & Bush, M. A. (1990). Adding purpose to the repetitive exercise of elderly women through imagery. *American Journal of Occupational Therapy, 44*, 714-719.
Rogers, M. (2005). *Physician, wire thyself: Health care system needs major dose of technology* [On-line]. Retrieved from www.msnbc.msn.com/id/9274039/.
Rydmark, M., Broeren, J., & Pascher, R. (2002). Stroke rehabilitation at home using virtual reality, haptics, and telemedicine. *Studies in Health Technology and Informatics, 85*, 434-437.
Sabbeth, C. (1995). *Kids computer creations: Using your computer for art and craft fun*. Charlotte, VT: Williamson Publishing.
Swenson Miller, K., Bunch-Harrison, S., Brumbaugh, B., Kutty, R. S., & FitzGerald, K. (2005). The meaning of computers to a group of men who are homeless. *American Journal of Occupational Therapy, 59*, 191-197.
Thompson, A. R., Bethea, L. L., Rizer, H. F., & Hutto, M. D. (1998). *Students with disabilities and assistive technology: A desk reference guide*. Jackson, MS: Mississippi Department of Rehabilitation Services/Project START.
Tools for Learning (Kid Pix Deluxe 4 for Schools) [Software manual]. (2000-2004). Navato, CA: Riverdeep.
U. S. Government Printing Office (2005). *Public Law 105-394. GPO* [On-line]. Retrieved from www.frwebgate.acess.gpo.gov/cgi-bin/getdoc.cgi?dbname=105_cong_public_laws&docid=f:publ394.105.

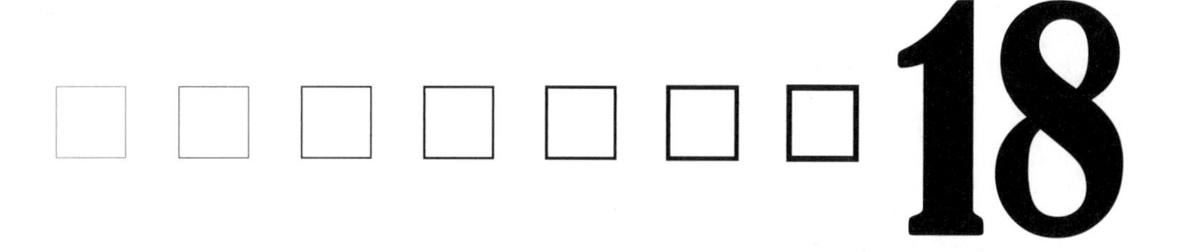

Expressive Media

Objectives

The student should be able to:

- Describe historical/cultural examples of the use of various expressive media
- List basic supplies, materials, and methods for making puppets, doing face painting, and doing simple magic tricks as for a performance
- Discuss advantages and limitations of expressive activities in therapy
- List precautions of using various expressive media
- Articulate the use of various expressive activities with different client populations

While we may not think of performance activities as crafts, many of those components that accompany a performance, such as set design and creation of props and costumes, would most certainly be considered crafts, "activity that is done with artistic skill, or to produce with ingenuity" (Merriam Webster's Collegiate Dictionary, 10th ed., 1994).

The media in this chapter are somewhat different than most of the others in this book in that they are principally expressive in nature, that is, their purpose is to tell a story or portray an emotion and not to fulfill a function or be an object of beauty. Many crafts have self-expression as a by-product; here, it is the primary objective. These media are used most often with children and adolescents, but in some situations may be beneficial for adults as well. This chapter describes therapeutic applications, adaptations, and considerations for several activities that could become part of a performance, including puppets, masks, face painting, magic, and body decoration. Pantomime and drama are also discussed briefly to illustrate how these elements may be combined and used therapeutically. One suggestion for using the techniques described below is to plan a production that could incorporate both crafting and performing, customized to meet the needs of individual group members.

Puppets

Puppets have been used for thousands of years in dramatic presentations; artifacts have been found in Greece, Rome, Egypt, India, and China (May, 1989; Philpott, 1966). In civilizations where writing was rare or

Tubbs, C., & Drake, M. *Crafts and Creative Media in Therapy, Fourth Edition (pp. 225-238).*

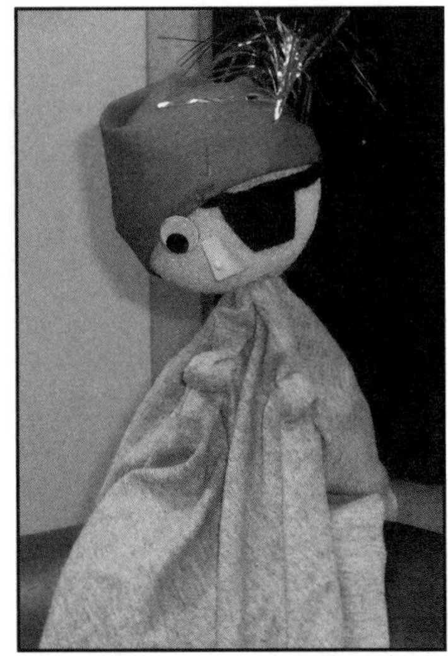

Figure 18-1. A simple hand puppet.

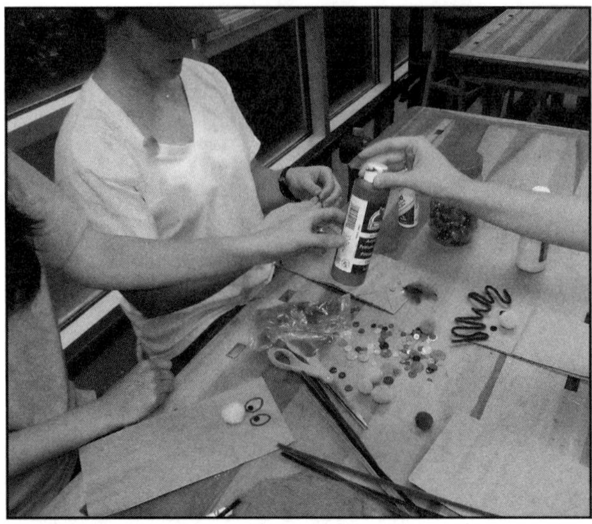

Figure 18-2. Group members make puppets for a production, sharing supplies and ideas.

nonexistent, puppets played an important role in storytelling, the primary means of passing down historical information (Philpott, 1966). Puppets really provide two crafts in one: first is the fabrication of the puppet; second is its employment in a dramatic presentation. Methods used in fabrication may fall under a number of other craft categories, including needlework, paper crafts, and even woodwork. Puppets are generally one of four basic types: marionettes, hand puppets, rod puppets, or shadow puppets. Marionettes are controlled by strings or wires from overhead. Hand puppets may be of many styles, but all are made such that the fingers and thumb operate—or are—the moving parts. Rod puppets are moved from below via one or more attached rods. Shadow puppets are intricately cut, two-dimensional forms whose shadows are projected onto a screen (May, 1989). Modern puppets may be quite sophisticated but retain the basic characteristic of requiring human movement to bring them to life. Hand puppets are the type most commonly made and used in therapy applications (Figure 18-1).

Puppets are especially suitable for children, but may also be used with adults in some situations. Children or adults can use puppets to express disagreeable feelings or ideas more freely. Groups of children can also use puppets to do serial storytelling, providing an outlet for their fertile imaginations and an opportunity to practice taking turns. This method may also be useful for letting adolescents compare their ideas and worldview with those of their peers. Puppets can be employed in mutual storytelling—child and therapist—which gives the therapist a chance to voice alternative solutions/scenarios for problem behaviors (Parham & Fazio, 1997). Fabrication of the puppet can require a range of motor, cognitive, and sensory skills, depending on construction type. Controlling the puppets is primarily a motor operation, but incorporating them into a production—with a storyline or dialogue—will add cognitive and possibly interactional demands as well. Puppet shows can be done as solo presentations or by a group of performers. In putting on a puppet show for entertainment purposes, the following pointers may help. Start with a written script; ad-lib is difficult for amateurs. Remember that puppets should move around when talking, and only the one talking should move. Lastly, have someone able to provide feedback during rehearsal, since it is hard to critique yourself (Wright, 1989). Puppets can also be part of a conversational dialogue; again, this may be a more comfortable communication approach for children or adults who experience distress in interpersonal situations.

Puppets can be made with very inexpensive, even castoff materials. Suggested bases for puppets include paper plates, socks, gloves, paper bags or boxes, and papier-mâché forms; even a painted hand can be a puppet. One author suggests making puppets—made with basic household materials—that go along with popular children's songs. (Ross, 2002). A simple puppet can easily be completed in one treatment session, and of course, the therapist can grade the project according to construction design and details. Used as a group activity, puppet making can provide a venue for participants to share materials, and the therapist can facilitate discussion and interaction as they work (Figure 18-2).

Project—Spoon Puppet

Plan It

This puppet can be made with mostly scraps and a few basic craft supplies. The therapist could also choose a theme and have fabric that corresponds to it, for example use shiny or filmy fabric for fairy tale characters, or furry fabric for animals. It may be a good idea to have some samples and limit supply choices if doing this activity with young children. Having fabric pieces pre-cut will eliminate the need to use scissors. This activity might be a good opportunity to work on sharing materials and supplies and/or to talk about different emotions and how their puppet face might look in order to express them.

Get Ready

Supplies

- A large wooden spoon
- Yarn and fabric scraps
- Glue
- Markers or paint
- Rubber band
- Beads, sequins, etc. (optional)
- Foam scraps

Tools

- Scissors
- Paint brushes

Time required: 30 minutes or less

Approximate cost: Less than $1

Do It

1. Paint the spoon bowl and upper part of the handle the desired skin tone color (optional). Allow to dry.
2. Cut a rectangle of fabric large enough to easily cover the hand plus a little extra.
3. Bunch one long edge of fabric around the "neck" of the spoon and secure with a rubber band.
4. Hold spoon handle under fabric and judging position of thumb and index finger, cut a hole for each. When you operate the puppet, your pinky and thumb will be the arms (Figure 18-3).
5. Cover the rubber band with yarn or a strip of fabric, glued or tied in the back
6. Cut a 2-inch wide strip of foam and wrap and tape it around the spoon handle 1 to 2 inches below the rubber band (under the fabric). This will give the puppeteer something to hold onto while operating the puppet.
7. Decorate the head/face as desired (e.g., glue on yarn for hair, paint or glue on eyes, mouth, etc.).
8. Decorate fabric with buttons, bows, and so on, as desired (Figure 18-4).

(Adapted from Buetter, 1996)

Change It

The spoon puppet can be varied in many ways depending on the materials available or the preference of the creator. Different fabrics and materials can be used for the clothing and hair and the face can be painted or not. One way of grading the activity down is to simplify any embellishment, or paint a face on the spoon

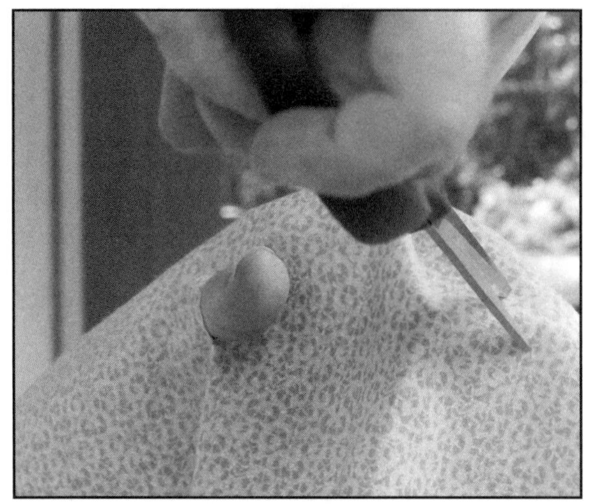

Figure 18-3. Holes cut for the thumb and finger.

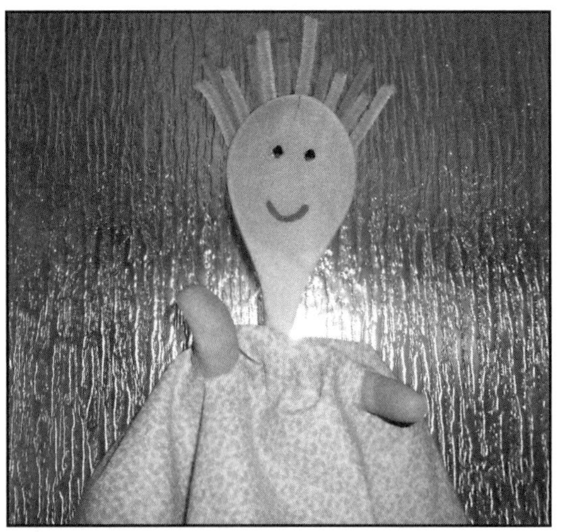

Figure 18-4. "Ms. Spoonhead."

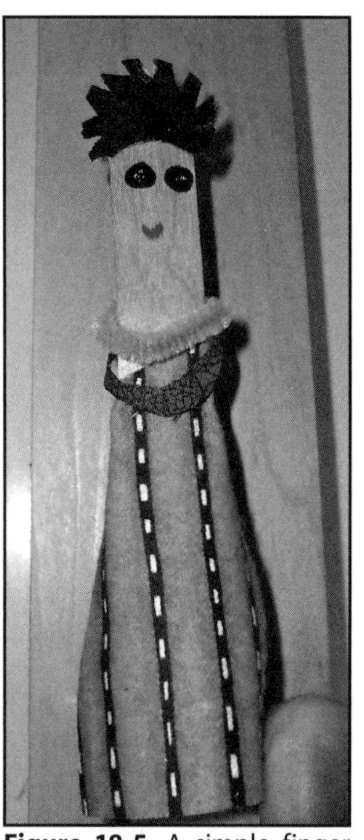

Figure 18-5. A simple finger puppet.

ahead of time and just have the client add the clothing. Another simple variation is to make a finger puppet as described next. Grade the activity up by adding extra items to the clothing such as buttons, bows, pockets and so on. To make a finger puppet, use a tongue depressor instead of a spoon, and attach a 2-inch piece of hook Velcro to one side. With glue, add facial features, hair, and clothing as desired, then use a piece of pile Velcro to strap around the finger (Figure 18-5).

Document It

Below are some suggestions for documenting various therapeutic applications this project.

- "The children were able to share glue and one container of sequins without an altercation."

- "The client was able to use adapted to scissor for cutting fabric and stayed within 1 inch of the marked lines."
- "While using her puppet in 'dialogue' the client expressed fears about her classmates and her schoolwork."

There are many sources of inspiration for puppet making. Libraries, bookstores and Internet retailers will have books with puppet making and puppet show ideas, especially in the kids or juvenile crafts section. Designs may be based on a particular story or theme, or just the product of an active imagination. In therapy, clients should be encouraged to experiment; success is ensured since there is no standard right or wrong.

Masks

Masks, like puppets, can be made from varied materials and may incorporate crafts methods discussed elsewhere in this book. Masks have been used for thousands of years in dances, plays, ceremonies, and celebrations (Schwarz, 2002). Masks are often part of full costumes and they allow the wearer to portray an emotion, engage in fantasy, or entertain other people. Wearing a mask is also a way of symbolically becoming someone else, and may enable expression of ideas and feelings that the wearer would otherwise conceal. Aside from the psychological implications, making masks is simply a fun craft that will provide the participant enjoyment while addressing a variety of motor and process skills.

Using common household products makes construction of a mask an economical craft limited only by imagination. Mask bases may be paper plates, cardboard sheets or boxes, papier-mâché forms, caps, large plastic jugs, or plain white plastic mask forms (Green, 1992; Lamĕrand, 2003; Schwarz, 2002). Masks can be decorated with yarn, raffia, or ribbon for hair; with paint, construction paper, felt, glitter, or feathers for facial features or added details; with straw as antennae, pipe insulation as long noses, or pudding cups as "bug-eyes" (Lamĕrand, 2003; Schwarz, 2002).

Project—Basic Mask

Plan It

In preparing for the project, be sure that the jug to be used is clean and dry and free of any odors. Some clients may not be able to cut the plastic material, so the therapist may need to do this beforehand. If the client is to cut the plastic independently, be aware that even the plastic edges can be sharp. It is a good idea to have some samples since this an imagination-based activity and some individuals, especially children, may require more structure. This activity may not be appropriate for someone who has tactile sensitivity or is uncomfortable having something on the head or over the face.

Get Ready

Supplies

- Empty 1-gallon bleach bottle or milk jug
- Colored raffia or yarn
- Glue
- Tape
- Paint
- Glitter
- White foam coffee cup
- Elastic band

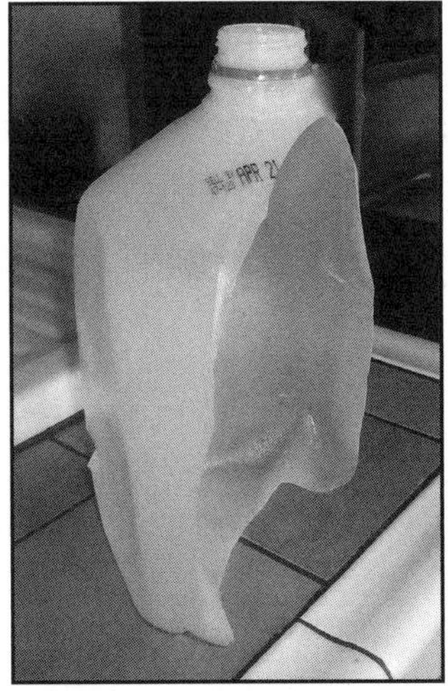

Figure 18-6. Handle side of jug cut away.

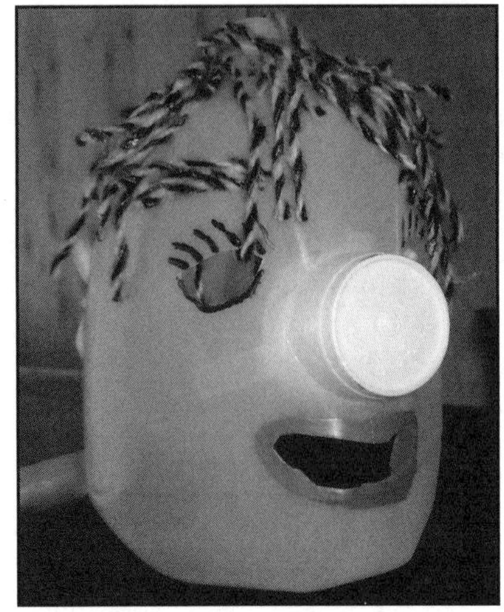

Figure 18-7. Completed jug mask.

Tools

- Scissors
- Craft knife
- Paint brushes
- Hole punch or awl
- Pen/pencil

Time required: 45 minutes

Approximate cost: Less than $1

Do It

Process

1. Cut away the handle side of the jug, but leave the narrow end intact, to create an opening for the head. Some or all of the bottom of large end of the jug may need to be cut away and adjusted for fit (Figure 18-6).
2. Use a punching tool to punch holes on either side of the head opening for insertion of the elastic head strap.
3. Punch more holes all around the top for insertion of the hair.
4. Mark and cut two holes in the appropriate place for eyes.
5. Mark and cut a hole for the nose, larger than the bottom of the foam cup, but smaller than the top of the cup.
6. Twist together a few strands of raffia or yarn and tie a knot in one end. Push the free ends through a hole, pull up to the knot, then tie snugly just on the other side of the hole.
7. Repeat to fill all holes with "hair."
8. Insert cup through nose-hole, bottom end out. You may have to trim the top of the cup, depending on how much you want the nose to protrude. Add tape on the inside to hold.
9. Add decoration as desired using paint, glitter, etc.
10. Insert elastic band through the strap holes on each side and knot; length will depend on head size (Figure 18-7).

Change It

For a variation, add ears to top or sides; use a different object, such as a paper towel tube, to make a nose; paint the entire jug before decorating; or punch holes in other places to insert whiskers, antennae, or other appendages. To grade the activity down, cut the plastic and punch the holes ahead of time. Or glue on hair instead of tying it through punched holes. To grade the activity up, have the client use more hair or add extra features as described above. Or have the client try to recreate an animal or creature from a two-dimensional drawing.

Document It

The therapist can document different aspects of the activity, as shown in the examples below.

- "The client demonstrated increased hand strength in ability to cut through plastic material with scissors."
- "The therapist instructed the client to copy the sample exactly, using the same colors and shapes, in order to increase visual attention and color and shape discrimination."

Masks are ideal in working with children with psychological or physical problems, or both. Children love to pretend and are not intimidated by fantasy or silliness. In fact, fantasy can help a child explore feelings or resolve conflict (Parham & Fazio, 1997). One author suggests the use of popular children's books to create themes for play and dress-up, as a way of engaging a child's interest and attention (Sladyk, Berry, Brenner, Hengeveld, & Moisan, 2002). Some adult clients may also take pleasure in making masks, especially around the time of Mardi Gras or Halloween, when it may seem more socially appropriate. The type and complexity of masks can be easily graded to suit the client's skill level and the therapeutic challenge desired.

Face Painting

Face painting, a direct descendent of clown make-up, has been used for centuries by actors, clowns, and mime artists, but has more recently become a common sight at craft fairs, festivals, and carnivals and is a great attraction for children. Face painting done with grease paint or theatrical make-up is more durable and gives a professional look. Although it can be done with common ordinary cosmetic make-up or acrylic paints, it is more likely to run and smear. Face painting supplies are widely available around Halloween but can be purchased at hobby stores or from catalogs year round. Face painting can be used to portray a character, express an emotion, or simply as a part of play.

Supplies

- Paper and pencil
- Grease paint
- Baby oil
- Cold cream (optional)
- Talcum powder
- Facial tissue

Tools

- Make-up brushes
- Mirror

Process

1. On paper, draw a face depicting the make-up plan.
2. Use brushes to apply face paint or grease paint to the skin, using the paper template as a guide. If using grease paint, apply cold cream first. Apply colors in this order: white, pastels, primary colors, then black.

3. Powder each color after applying it. Brush excess powder away with a powder brush.
4. Clean grease paint brushes with baby oil and wipe them dry.
5. Disinfect the brushes between clients.

Variations: Add fine glitter to discrete areas for highlighting. Rather than doing traditional make-up, simply paint pictures on the skin in the fashion of tattoos.

It is probably a good idea to use hair clips or tie-backs during paint application, and to cover the client with a smock or old T-shirt to protect clothing (Silver, 2000).

The main precautions for using face paint are to be aware of allergies to make-up and to avoid breathing the talcum powder. Be sure to keep paint and glitter away from eyes as well. For clients with dermatitis, acne, or respiratory ailments, face painting should be avoided.

Children and teenagers especially enjoy face painting. It may be a component of a play or other dramatic presentation, or it may be done simply for fun or to lighten the mood during a therapy session. Face painting is usually an indispensible part of clowning and mime; in these crafts, most of the face is painted. For children and teens, however, a simple design such as a flower, butterfly, or lone teardrop is often sufficient (Baygan, 1982; Buchman, 1975; Harris, 1985; Stolzenberg, 1981).

Face painting is safe and allows the participant to see more clearly than when wearing a mask (Silver, 2000). Children will have fun becoming their favorite characters and can act out or express themselves in situations in which they might otherwise be uncomfortable. Children might enjoy painting each other's faces but may have difficulty doing their own.

Magic

Magic as entertainment has been around for over 4,000 years. Some early magic employed natural scientific phenomena; others used sleight-of-hand (Klingel & Noyed, 2002). Some people may think magic always refers to the supernatural (e.g., casting a spell or conjuring a spirit, for example) but in occupational therapy it is neither supernatural nor scary. Occupational therapists have been using magic as a medium of treatment for almost three decades. Project Magic, a program developed in 1982 by magician David Copperfield and occupational therapist Julie DeJean, seeks to link therapists and magicians to work together in teaching magic tricks to clients ("David Copperfield Works Magic," 2002). The program, endorsed by the American Occupational Therapy Association ("The King of Magic," 2004) provided a trick manual along with lists of local magicians with an interest in working with rehab clients. Tricks are used with one-handed clients, head trauma clients, or anyone who needs to improve manual dexterity (Krinsky, 1998). It is useful for individuals with physical, psychosocial, or developmental disabilities; it improves motivation and self-confidence while simultaneously working on motor and cognitive skills (Civichino, 2003). While an original Project Magic manual may be difficult to locate, magic tricks are still a useful therapy activity.

Magic is a novelty for clients who have become bored with other types of treatment, such as repetitive exercise, and is an appropriate therapeutic tool for both children and adults. Simple magic tricks commonly involve the use of cups, balls, coins, or cards (Klingel & Noyed, 2002). Numerous books on magic are available in the juvenile section of the library (Gibson, 1980; Lopshire, 1969; Milner, 1987b; Severn, 1964, 1965, 1977; Waters, 1985) and of course from online retailers. Tricks can be simple and silly or sophisticated and difficult (Gibson, 1980). The therapist should select tricks based on client interest, deficit areas to be addressed, and reasonable chance of a successful outcome. All tricks require practice to be performed smoothly and the skilled performer will develop the skill of "patter," or talking and moving to distract the audience (Civichino, 2003; Milner, 1987b). Practice of processes and movements is integral to improvement of the client's motor control and cognitive/process skills such as attention, memory, and sequencing. Clients may enjoy demonstrating their newly learned skills in front of an "audience" of fellow clients or magic can be included as a portion of a longer performance with multiple "cast" members. Since the magician should be able to perform the trick almost automatically, this craft may be too difficult for clients with severe motor planning or coordination deficits. It is also not recommended for clients who are delusional or for children under the age of 5 (Civichino, 2003).

Project—Pick-a-Card Magic Trick

Supplies:

- One deck of standard playing cards

Process:

1. Shuffle the cards.
2. Holding them face down, fan them out and ask the subject to pick a card and remember it without showing it to you.
3. Meanwhile, put the rest of the deck behind your back and turn the bottom card over.
4. Present the deck to your subject, bottom up (he or she should still see the top of the card) and ask him or her to insert his or her card back in the deck.
5. Once again, put your hands behind your back and turn the bottom card back over.
6. You should now have all the cards facing the same way except the card that your subject picked.
7. Proudly announce your subject's card!

Body Decoration

Although tattooing and other forms of permanent body art are certainly beyond the realm of occupational therapy, some other types of body decoration may prove appropriate and beneficial as therapeutic media. Decoration of the human body has been done for centuries across many cultures. For example, in India, hands—and sometimes feet—are painted in lines, dots, and blocks of henna color in an art form called mehndi (MacLeod-Brudenell, 1994).

In current American culture, especially among female adolescents and young adults, nail and hair adornment is perennially popular and the temporary nature of this art makes it safe to experiment and express oneself. Nail polishes are easy to find and some can be purchased with kits that include design ideas. They are relatively inexpensive and can be used with multiple clients. Nail polishing is an excellent paired activity; it could facilitate interpersonal interaction while allowing participants to work on fine motor skills at the same time. Unless incorporated into a manicure, painting nails requires only nail polish and possibly a cuticle stick. Removing nail polish will additionally require polish remover and cotton balls or paper towels. The therapist should be aware of any adverse response to the fumes of the polish or polish remover.

Hair braiding, twisting, plaiting, and corn-rowing are practiced cross-culturally. Many people choose hairstyles that they think display their personality or membership in a group. Rastafarians, for example, wear dreadlocks as a part of their religion; in western Africa, hair plaiting is considered an art form (MacLeod-Brudenell, 1994). While the therapist may or may not be able to teach these skills, clients already familiar with them may enjoy using them as a novel way to work on upper extremity function and new hairstyles sometimes provide a boost to self-esteem. Another related activity is doing hair wraps. Heavy cotton thread of different colors is wrapped tightly around a small gathering of hair strands; the wrapping can extend for just a few inches, or for the full length of the hair. Books, magazines, and Internet sites can provide ideas in keeping with the most current fashions. See Resources section at the end of the chapter for other sources of information and ideas. Many hair design activities would require only combs/brushes, assorted hair accessories, and a willing "customer." Hair design projects are excellent for use as paired activities. They can boost the self-esteem of both participants, in addition to fostering communication and possibly even friendship. In the appropriate setting, the occupational therapist might even set up an ongoing "beauty shop," stocked with general supplies, where clients could act as customers and/or beauticians. All tools would need to be sanitized after each use, or be inexpensive enough to either give to the client or discard.

Pantomime and Drama

Pantomime, sometimes abbreviated as mime, is the art of gesture and pose. It is essentially a means of storytelling through bodily movements and facial expression. Some attribute its origin to the Greeks who so richly developed drama and its associated techniques. Others say the earliest humans mimicked animal movements as part of storytelling and worship rituals. Tribal dances of Native Americans, Arabs, and Africans are indeed pantomime dances, sometimes done in preparation or celebration of particular cultural practices such as the hunt. In a more modern iteration, silent movie actors used a form of mime—incorporating props and sets—to communicate the plot in early movies.

Although described here as a dramatic art form, the use of gesture is a universal means of communication. For example, when communicating with someone who speaks a foreign language, we automatically augment speech with gestures to emphasize the message. Nonverbal communication comes naturally to humans and precedes use of language in the same way drawing comes before writing. Because of its utility in both facilitating self-expression and in teaching specific communication skills, occupational therapists have been using drama in therapy for decades (Keysell, 1975; Pardoe, 1931; Phillips, 1996).

One purpose of using mime with clients is to help them learn to communicate more effectively, both as sender and recipient of information. Mime is a fun, nonthreatening way to express oneself and to work on understanding the body language and social cues of others. Pantomime is particularly good for children who have difficulty sharing thoughts and feelings with verbal communication, or who are overly reliant on verbal communication (Parham & Fazio, 1997). It may be used to re-enact a client's problem situation, or as part of role playing. Each mime session should start with a warm-up in which clients can stretch and explore their body movements. For a more structured exercise, the therapist may instruct the clients to move only one particular body part, or to focus on keeping one part fixed, or to mimic demonstrated motions or actions (Phillips, 1996). Musical or percussion instruments can be added to stimulate movement rhythms. An example of an appropriate warm-up for children ages 3 to 8 years is pretending to be a wind-up toy. The therapist would demonstrate with a real wind-up toy, then pretend to "wind up" the children and allow them to move. Other warm-ups for children could be pantomimes of playing with different kinds of balls, or imitating animals or vehicles. Warm-ups for children ages 8 to 12 years could be occupational or sports related, such as making a bed or swinging a baseball bat. Adolescents may relate more to interpersonal dramatization or putting on make-up and clothes. Adults can be asked to do movements that simulate abstract concepts such as extroversion or introversion, closeness or distance. Since adults are more likely than children to be self-conscious about acting, they may be more comfortable portraying emotions or ideas, which can be accomplished with less body movement. Older adults may also enjoy pantomiming famous people or scenes from well-known movies or books in an activity similar to charades.

Miming can be made even more challenging by having clients suggest scenarios for role play. The therapist may have to provide prompting to help clients visualize situations in which they would have to utilize newly learned behaviors such as assertiveness. For example, an individual in a chemical dependency unit might role play the appropriate reaction/response to being offered drugs or a drink. During the miming of problem scenarios, the therapist can intervene with alternative suggestions, or other group members can offer interpretations or critiques of their peer's performance. By paying attention to the details of communication, clients are often able to learn how their behavior may unintentionally affect other people. Pantomime is a safe way to use the trial-and-error method of improving communication skills; scenes can be replayed until the client, therapist, or audience is satisfied. In closing a mime session, clients may enact various common goodbye rituals—waving, hugging, or shaking hands (Alberts, 1971; Aubert, 1976; Blatner, 1973; Buchan, 1972; Corsini & Cardone, 1966; Gray & Percival, 1962; Straub & Straub, 1984; Weisberg & Wilder, 1985) which will serve to provide a symbolic boundary between acting and reality. In day-to-day therapy sessions, time will likely not permit face painting or other make-up for a mime session; however, if a group wants to elaborate on its ideas and plan a performance, this may be an occasion to experiment with make-up or grease paint. For some clients, the experience of miming in therapy may lead them to pursue acting avocationally in other venues such as community centers or local playhouses (Wetherd, 1973).

Drama, in its many forms, has been a therapeutic tool in multiple disciplines, including occupational therapy, for many years. It can be utilized in many forms, including individual or group, competitive or cooperative (Fidler & Velde, 1999) and, in the past, was found to be especially beneficial with psychiatric clients with extended lengths of stay (Phillips, 1996). The benefits of group performance can occur in multiple formats. For example, a group of elderly subjects participated for 12 months in a chorus with regular rehearsals. At the conclusion of the year, those who participated had higher overall self-ratings of health, increased overall activity participation, and decreased falls (Cohen et al., 2006). More recently, one group of mental health clients found that aspects of theatrical activity were relevant to their problems. The participants reported the flexible nature of the activity was valuable and that the audience augmented their enjoyment and sense of competence (Fleury, Marazzani, & Saucier, 2004). Dramatic productions can also be a way of connecting clients to their cultural roots. For children in a Navajo school system, both prepartion for and re-enactment of a traditional Powwow were found by their therapist to be useful for both motor and psychosocial skill building (Crowe, 2009). Exclusive use of drama and music has developed into specialized therapy practices and will not be elaborated on in this text. It is worth mentioning, however, that a full-scale dramatic production will require sets, props, and costumes, all of which are crafts unto themselves, and create an opportunity for multidisciplinary collaboration. A Special Gifts Theater program, for example, was implemented in one community to allow children with disabilities to participate in dramatic productions and thereby work on socialization/communication skills, building self-esteem and managing sensory issues. These skills facilitated occupational performance in other areas and parents reported improvements in abilities such as coordination, attention span, and communication (Ciukaj, Suarez-Balcazar, & Field, 2009). Another program found that participation in dramatic activities improved children's reading comprehension and gave them a greater awareness of the feelings of others (Kelin, 2007). In any therapeutic use of dramatic or expressive activity, with adults or children, the therapist needs to ensure a psychologically safe environment and intervene if necessary (Diffendal, 2002; Parham & Fazio, 1997). In the appropriate setting, plays/ theatrical presentations offer a broad spectrum of creative opportunities for clients with diverse abilities and interests.

Case Study

Five-year-old Ronald, diagnosed with conduct disorder and depression, was admitted to a 10-bed children's mental health unit with an average length of stay of 3 weeks. With a few exceptions, most of the clients were diagnosed with conduct disorder and therefore the program emphasized strict behavioral limits. Children earned privileges such as television or playground time by accomplishing goals for each treatment session as well as exhibiting appropriate behavior during mealtimes and therapeutic community meetings. Since social interaction was a primary focus area, the occupational therapist performed most client evaluations and treatment in a group setting and tended to rely on developmental, behavioral, and psychoanalytic theories for activity selection. The Draw-A-Person test, the Test of Gross Motor Development (Ulrich, 1985), and the Build-a-City Assessment were all administered in a group setting. Each young child was also evaluated individually using the Stanford Pre-School Internal-External Scale (SPIES) to assess internal and external orientation to behavior and its positive or negative outcomes (Mischel, Zeiss, & Zeiss, 1974). Since Ronald was admitted on an emergency basis on a Friday afternoon, the occupational therapist decided to postpone his group evaluations until Monday, when two other children were scheduled to be admitted. Ronald's single mother, who was also responsible for caring for her two other children and her own mother, felt she could no longer assure a safe environment at home. Ronald had been verbally and physically attacking his younger siblings, as well as endangering himself by jumping off high places and riding his bike recklessly. In fact, he was just recovering from a broken arm. Results of the SPIES indicated that Ronald perceived a great deal of external control, that is, he had little responsibility for, or control over, his behavior.

On Monday morning, Tom and Paul, brothers ages 7 and 9, were admitted as scheduled. Their case worker had brought them to the hospital from their foster home. Although they had received previous psychiatric care, this was their first hospital admission. They were also both diagnosed with conduct disorder. The boys' mother had abandoned the family, and their father felt unable to care for them. His weekend visit at the foster home had precipitated an episode of disruptive and dangerous behavior on the part of the children, seemingly because he would not take them with him when he left.

The occupational therapist decided to conduct her two group assessments at their first session. The occupational therapist found that Ronald could complete gross and fine motor tasks, but his responses were somewhat delayed. She reasoned that this was likely due to slow information processing or inattention and not a true motor deficiency. He could perform tasks adequately, but only with repeated prompting to redirect his attention. Tom and Paul both scored normally on the Test of Gross Motor Development.

The therapist began the Draw-A-Person test by placing the boys as far from each other as possible at the small table. They all drew hurriedly and the two brothers made frequent aggressive comments to each other. Ronald's projective story about the two figures he drew involved stealing a cat and hurting it. While an aide took the boys for a snack, the therapist assembled the materials—empty thread spools, plasticene modeling clay, tape, glue, construction paper, colored pencils, string, blunt-end scissors, plastic table knives, wooden clay modeling tools, and foam cubes—for the Build-a-City assessment. After the boys were instructed to "build an ideal city," they all began to grab items from the table. Paul began to draw and cut out cars and Ronald began to draw a house. They worked individually for several minutes until Tom dropped his own attempt to tape sheets of construction paper together and grabbed Ronald's picture saying, "Let me show you how to make a house." He folded and taped the paper before throwing it back to Ronald saying, "Cut a door and some windows, stupid!" The therapist chose not to intervene but carefully monitored the situation. The hostile interaction soon included Paul as well, who acquiesced to his brother's orders. Tom dominated the activity and the other two boys chafed under his dictatorial manner, but neither resisted him physically.

In the follow-up discussion, the boys frequently interrupted each other as they tried to explain the importance of each object. Tom invariably won out and explained for the other boys. With guidance from the therapist, all three boys eventually helped clean up, earning privilege points and ending the session on a more positive note. In the afternoon session, the occupational therapist seated the boys at separate tables and helped them each make two paper bag puppets. These were to be used later in acting out their anger and aggression in a safe and structured way. The boys drew eyes, noses, mouths, and other features with felt pens. They pasted paper, yarn, and pieces of cloth for hats and clothes and worked more calmly than on the previous day. The next day, each boy was invited to put on a show with his two paper bag puppets. By the third puppet show, Tom allowed Ronald to help him by handling one of his puppets and helping with the dialogue. The boys were rewarded with more privilege points for this positive display of cooperation. The therapist decided to next have the boys work together on a group puppet show, with the older boys assisting Ronald as needed.

Discussion Questions

1. What other role play or dramatic activities might be beneficial for these clients? For each of your answers, describe how you could incorporate crafts, or other hands-on components. What other treatment approaches/activities might you use with these children?
2. List other treatment settings in which long-range projects, such as rehearsed puppet shows or plays, would be useful.
3. Describe a situation in which the therapist might need to intervene in a group role-play activity.

Resources

Puppet Planet: The Most Amazing Puppet Making Book in the Universe
By John Kennedy
North Light Books, 2006
Lots of patterns for colorful puppet creatures. Includes description of basic supplies and processes.

Mehndi Designs: Traditional Henna Body Art
By Marty Noble
Dover Publications, 2004

Puppet Mania: The World's Most Incredible Puppet Making Book Ever
By John E. Kennedy
North Light Books, 2004

Kids' Magic Secrets: Simple Magic Tricks and Why They Work
By Loris Bree and Marlin Bree
Marlor Press, 2003

Maskmaking
By Carol Sivin
Sterling Publishing, 1986

Macrame Hair Wraps: A Modern Folk Art
By Susan B. Frank, 2000
Susan B. Frank, publisher

Magic for Dummies
By David Pogue
IDG Books Worldwide, Inc., 1998

Hair Wraps
By Anne Akers Johnson
Klutz, 1998

Puppets and Masks: Stage Craft and Storytelling
By Nan Rump
Sterling Publishing, 1995
Good book for working with children.

The Usborne Book of Dressing Up: Costumes, Masks, and Face Painting
By Chris Caudron
E. D. C. Publishing, 1994

References

Alberts, D. (1971). *Pantomime: Elements and exercises*. Lawrence, KS: The University of Kansas Press.

Alkema, C. J. (1971). *Puppet-making*. New York, NY: Sterling Publishing Co.

Aubert, C. (1976). *The art of pantomime*. New York, NY: Arno Press.

Baygan, L. (1982). *Make-up for the theater, film, and television*. New York, NY: Drama Club Publishers.

Blatner, H. A. (1973). *Acting in: Practical applications of psychodramatic methods*. New York, NY: Springer Publishing.

Buchan, L. G. (1972). *Roleplaying and the educable mentally retarded*. Belmont, CA: Fearon Publishers.

Buchman, L. G. (1975). *Stage makeup*. New York, NY: Watson-Guptill Publications.

Buetter, B. M. (1996). *Simple puppets from everyday materials*. New York, NY: Sterling Publishing Co., Inc.

Ciukaj, M., Suarez-Balcazar, Y., & Field, S. B. (2009). Incorporating creative drama into the lives of children with disabilities: A community–based program. *OT Practice, 14*(22), 19-23.

Civichino, A. (2003). Copperfield's magic boosts rehabilitation. *Toronto Observer.* Retrieved from www.observer.thecentre.centennialcollege.ca/life/copperfield.

Cohen, G., Perlstein, S., Chapline, J., Kelly, J., Firth, K., & Simmens, S. (2006). The impact of professionally conducted culturally programs on the physical health, mental health and social functioning of older adults. *The Gerontologist, 46*(6), 726-734.

Corsini, R. J., & Cardone, S. (1966). *Roleplaying in psychotherapy.* Chicago, IL: Aldine Publishing Company.

Crowe, T. K., & Hong, N. (2009). Culturally rich, meaningful occupations. *Advance for Occupational Therapy Practitioners, 25*(10), 8.

David Copperfield Works Magic at the Program in Occupational Therapy. (2002). Washington University in St. Louis. Retrieved from http://ot.wustl.edu/ot.

Diffendal, J. (2002). Kids, through the use of their hands.... *Advance for Occupational Therapy Practitioners, 18*(22), 12.

Fidler, F., & Velde, B. (1999). *Activities: Reality and symbol.* Thorofare, NJ: SLACK Incorporated.

Fleury, F., Marazzani, M. H., & Saucier, J. F. (2004). The use of theatre in the psychosocial re-adaptation of patients with mental disorders: Participants' perspectives (English abstract). *Canadian Journal of Occupational Therapy, 71*(2), 108-115.

Gibson, W. (1980). *Big book of magic for all ages.* Garden City, NY: Doubleday.

Gray, V., & Percival, R. (1962). *Music, movement and mime for children.* Toronto, Canada: Oxford.

Green, J. (1992). *Why throw it away? Making crazy faces and masks.* New York, NY: Aladdin Books, Gloucester Press.

Harris, S. M. (1985). *This is my trunk.* New York, NY: Atheneum.

Kelin, D. A., II (2007). The perspective from within: Drama and children's literature. *Early Childhood Education Journal, 35*, 277-284.

Keysell, P. (1975). *Mime: Themes and motifs.* Boston, MA: Plays, Inc. Publishers.

Klingel, C., & Noyed, R. (2002). *Magic tricks.* Minneapolis, MN: Compass Point Books.

Krinsky, R. (1998). Have you heard the news? *Advance for Occupational Therapists, 14*(2), 12, 74.

Laměrand, V. (2003). *Making masks*. Mankato, MN: Bridgestone Books, Capstone Press.
Lopshire, R. (1969). *It's magic?* New York, NY: MacMillan Publishing.
MacLeod-Brudenell, I. (1994). *Costume crafts*. Milwaukee, WI: Gareth Stevens Publishing.
May, R. (1989). *Looking at theater.* NY: Marshall Cavendish Corp.
Merriam Webster (Ed.). (1994). *Merriam Webster's collegiate dictionary* (10th ed.). Springfield, MA: Merriam-Webster, Incorporated.
Milner, M. (1987a). Actors avoid preaching to show lighter side of living with disability. *OT Week, 1*(2), 12-14.
Milner, M. (1987b). Occupational therapist and entertainer put magic into rehabilitation program. *OT Week, 1*(50), 12-13.
Mischel, W., Zeiss, R., & Zeiss, A. (1974) Internal-external control and persistence: Validation and implications of the Stanford preschool internal-external scale. *Journal of Personality and Social Psychological, 29,* 279-287.
Pardoe, T. E. (1931). *Pantomimes for stage and study.* New York, NY: Benjamin Bloom.
Parham, L. D., & Fazio, L. (Eds.). (1997). *Play in occupational therapy for children*. St. Louis, MO: Mosby.
Phillips, M. E. (1996). The use of drama and puppetry in occupational therapy during the 1920s and 1930s. *American Journal of Occupational Therapy, 50*(3), 229-233.
Philpott, A. R. (1966). *Let's look at puppets.* Chicago, IL: Albert Whitman and Co.
Ross, K. (2002). *Crafts from your favorite children's songs*. Brookfield, CT: The Millbrook Press.
Schwarz, R. (2002). *Making masks*. Tonawanda, NY: Kids Can Press, Ltd.
Severn, B. (1964). *Magic in your pockets*. New York, NY: David McKay Company.
Severn, B. (1965). *Magic shows you can give*. New York, NY: David McKay Company.
Severn, B. (1977). *Magic with coins and bills*. New York, NY: David McKay Company.
Silver, P. (2000). *Face painting*. Niagra Falls, NY: Kids Can Press, Ltd.
Sladyk, K., Berry, C., Brenner, C., Hengeveld, T., & Moisan, M. A. (2002). Harry Potter: Occupational therapy's new magic wand. *OT Practice 7*(18), 13-18.
Stolzenberg, M. (1981). *Clown for circus and stage*. New York, NY: Sterling Publishing Co.
Straub, C., & Straub, M. (1984). *Mime: Basics for beginners*. Boston, MA: Plays, Inc.
The King of Magic. *China Daily*. Retrieved from www.chinadaily.com.cn/english.
Ulrich, D. (1985). *Test of gross motor development*. Austin, TX: Pro-Ed.
Waters, G. (1985). *Science tricks & magic*. London, UK: Usborne Publishing Ltd.
Weisberg, N., & Wilder, R. (1985). *Creative arts with older adults: A sourcebook*. New York, NY: Human Sciences Press.
Wetherd, A. G. (1973). *Movement and drama in therapy.* Boston, MA: Boston Plays, Inc.
Wright, L. (1989). *Puppets*. New York, NY: Franklin Watts, Inc.

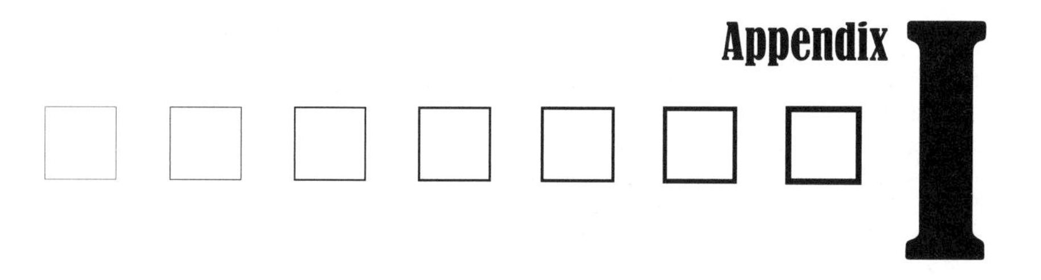

Vendors

AbleData (Technology, assistive devices)
8630 Fenton Street, Suite 930
Silver Spring, MD 20910
1-800-227-0216
1-301-608-8958 (fax)
Abledata@macrointernational.com
www.abledata.com

AMACO
6060 Guion Road
Indianapolis, IN 46254
1-800-374-1600 or 1-317-244-6871
1-317-248-9300 (fax)
salessupport@amaco.com
www.amaco.com

BJ's Craft Supplies
203 Bickford Road
Tivoli, TX 77990
1-361-286-3181
1-361-286-3719 (fax)
www.bjcraftsupplies.com

Birdsall and Company (adapted garden tools)
1540 South Broadway
Denver, CO 80210
1-303-722-2535
www.birdsallgarden.com

BitterCreek Candle Supply, Inc. (Candle supplies)
42212 County Highway East
Ashland, WI 54806
1-877-MELT-WAX (635-8929)
www.candlesupply.com

Dick Blick Art Materials
P. O. Box 1267
Galesburg, IL 61402-1267
1-800-723-2787 or 1-800-933-2542
1-800-621-8293 (fax)
www.dickblick.com

Gardening and Horticulture in Denver
(Adapted gardening tools)
888 E. Iliff Avenue
Denver, CO 80210
1-720-913-5278
denvermg@colostate.edu
www.colostate.edu/Depts/CoopExt/4DMG/Garden/special.htm
This site has other sources for adapted gardening tools as well

Healing of Magic
P. O. Box 10396
Lynchburg, VA 24506
1-434-384-4740
info@magictherapy.com
www.magictherapy.com

Tubbs, C., & Drake, M. *Crafts and Creative Media in Therapy, Fourth Edition (pp. 239-240).*

HearthSong
Madison, VA
1-800-533-4397
1-309-689-3857 (fax)
www.hearthsong.com

Mayco Colors
Ceramic products sold through local retailers
www.maycocolors.com
Mid-South Ceramic Supply Co.
1416 Lebanon Pike, Suite C
Nashville, TN 37210
1-615-242-0300
1-615-244-3191 (fax)
www.opulenceglaze.com

MisterArt
Houston, TX
1-800-721-3015
cs@misterart.com
www.misterart.com

Minnesota Clay USA
2960 Niagara Lane
Plymouth, MN 55447
1-763-432-0875
1-763-432-7675 (fax)
travis@mm.com
www.minnesotaclayusa.com

Nasco Arts and Crafts
901 Janesville Avenue
P. O. Box 901
Fort Atkinson, WI 53538
1-800-558-9595
1-800-372-1236 (fax)
custserv@nascofa.com
www.eNasco.com

National Agrability Project
www.fyi.uwex.edu/agrability/

Nature's Garden Candles
42109 State Route 18
Wellington, OH 44090
1-866-647-2368
1-440-748-0711 (fax)
info@naturesgardencandles.com
www.naturesgardencandles.com

Patterson Medical (Adaptive equipment)
1000 Remington Boulevard, Suite 210
Bolingbrook, IL 60440
1-630-378-6000
1-630-378-6010 (fax)
sp@sammonspreston.com
www.pattersonmedical.com

S & S Worldwide
(Craft supplies and educational activities)
75 Mill Street
P. O. Box 513
Colchester, CT 06415
1-860-537-3451
1-800-566-6678 (fax)
cs@snswwwide.com
www.ssww.com

School Specialty
(Formerly Sax Arts & Crafts)
1-800-513-2465
www.schoolspecialty.com

Poppy Seed Projects (Kits, group craft ideas)
(Formerly Simply Creative Crafts)
Orders@PoppySeedProjects.com
www.poppyseedprojects.com

Tandy Leather Company
1900 SE Loop 820
Fort Worth, TX 76140
1-800-433-3201
http://www.tandyleatherfactory.com
Look in a telephone book or on the web for your local Tandy store telephone number

Triarco Arts & Crafts
2600 Fernbrook Lane, Suite 100
Plymouth, MN 55447
1-800-328-3360
1-763-559-2215 (fax)
www.triarcoarts.com

Unicorn Books and Crafts, Inc.
1338 Ross Street
Petaluma, CA 94954
1-800-289-9276
1-707-762-0335
help@unicornbook.com
www.unicornbooks.com

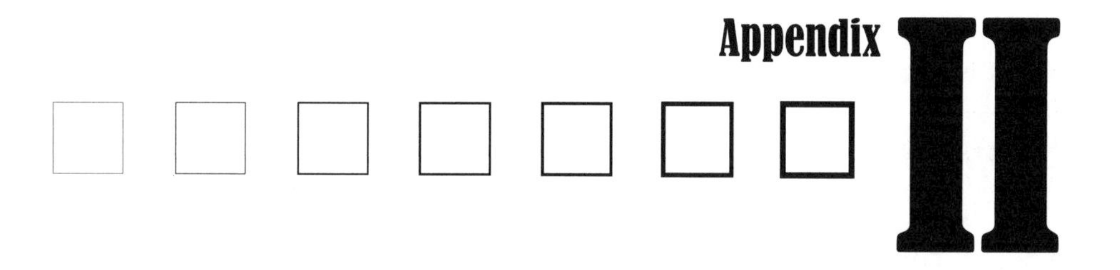

Internet Sites/Resources

Craft Ideas

- www.save-on-crafts.com
- www.homemadesimple.com
- www.createforless.com
- www.marthastewart.com/crafts
- www.craftideas.info
- www.allfreecrafts.com
- www.factorydirectcraft.com/index.php
- www.craftsfaironline.com
- www.mydailybead.blogspot.com
- www.azcentral.com/style/hfe/crafts
- www.dltk-kids.com

Videos

- www.craftvideos.co.uk
- www.craftbits.com
- www.craft-fair.co.uk
- www.diynetwork.com
- www.americanart.si.edu
- www.hgtv.com
- www.letscreate.com
- www.manataka.org
- www.craftster.org/forum/index.php?action=video
- www.youtube.com

Tubbs, C., & Drake, M. *Crafts and Creative Media in Therapy, Fourth Edition (pp. 241-242).*

- www.monkeysee.com
- www.ehow.com

Supplies

- www.kimscrane.com (origami, paper products)
- www.kyledesigns.com (switch plates, night light bases, small boxes, etc.)
- www.ssww.com/pages/?page_id=227 (S&S resource pamphlets for choosing appropriate crafts for skill level, gender, etc.)
- www.economyhandicrafts.com (economical craft kits and supplies for children)

Crafting for Charity

- www.craftbits.com/crafts/charity
- www.allfreecrafts.com/charity-crafts.shtml
- www.familycrafts.about.com/od/craftingforcharity/Crafting_for_Charity.htm
- www.craftsitedirectory.com/craft/charities
- www.marthastewart.com/article/knitting-charity

Fair Trade Craft Sites

- www.globalcrafts.org
- www.tenthousandvillages.com
- www.crsfairtrade.org/crafts
- www.ananse village.com
- www.upavimcrafts.org
- www.globalexchangestore.org
- www.fairtradequilts.com
- www.fairtradefederation.org

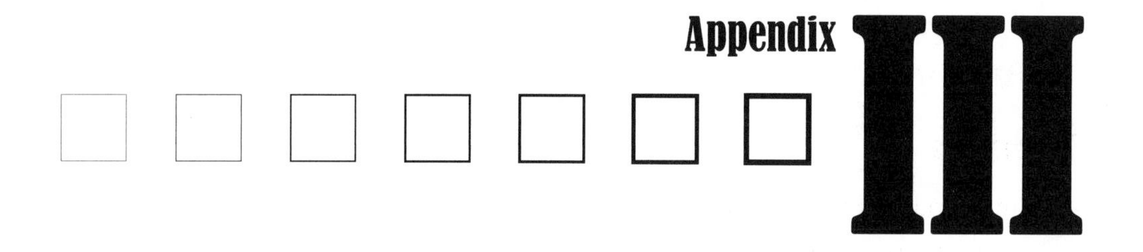

Sample Activity Analysis Form

I. **Name of activity/occupation**
   A. Brief description
   B. Major steps—Include time required for each
   C. Precautions

II. **Performance contexts and environments**
   A. Personal
      1. Age/gender
      2. Residential status
      3. Socioeconomic status
      4. Educational status
   B. Social
      1. Support system
      2. Social group membership
   C. Cultural—Cultural norms, ethnicity, customs, beliefs
   D. Physical—Treatment setting
      1. Space available, furniture arrangement
      2. Lighting, ventilation, temperature
      3. Appliances, equipment
   E. Temporal
      1. Time of day
      2. Amount of time needed, multiple sessions?
   F. Virtual—Computer use, etc.

Tubbs, C., & Drake, M. *Crafts and Creative Media in Therapy, Fourth Edition (pp. 243-247).*

III. Performance patterns

A. Habits—Does the activity utilize or reinforce useful habits?

B. Routine—Does the activity have an established sequence?

C. Roles—Is the activity consistent with customary roles of the client?

D. Rituals

IV. Therapeutic application

A. Treatment goal, relation to occupational performance

B. Appropriate population/general skills needed

1. Age range, diagnostic group
2. Motor skills
3. Process (cognitive, sensory, emotional) skills

C. Communications skills

D. Activity demands

1. Nonexpendable tools and equipment; source and cost
2. Expendable materials and supplies; source and cost
3. Space requirements
4. Sequencing and timing
5. Acceptable criteria for completion

E. Preparation

1. By whom
2. Steps and time required
3. Placement of tools and materials

F. Sensory or psychological stimulation anticipated

V. Therapeutic modification/method of instruction

A. Opportunities for grading

1. Sequence, duration, procedures
2. Working position
3. Tools (position, size, shape, texture, weight)
4. Materials (position, size, shape, texture, weight)

B. Opportunities for adapting

1. Orthotics, prosthetics
2. Assistive devices, technology
3. Preventative
   a. Energy conservation/joint protection
   b. Positioning/body mechanics
   c. Activity balance/wellness

C. Method of instruction

1. Tactile, verbal, visual cues—Type and frequency
2. Teaching-learning environment
3. Group versus individual, group member-assisted

VI. Therapeutic qualities

A. Energy patterns—Pacing, attention to task

B. Activity patterns

1. Structured versus unstructured
2. Repetitive
3. Expressive/creative
4. Tactile (equipment, materials, persons)

VII. Areas of occupation

A. IADL

B. Education

C. Work

D. Play

E. Leisure

F. Social participation

VIII. Performance skills required

A. Motor and praxis skills

1. Client position/ posture
2. Postural control
3. Position changes, ambulation
4. Trunk and limb ROM
5. Strength
6. Muscle tone
7. Endurance
8. Coordination
9. Manipulation
10. Praxis

B. Sensory-perceptual skills

1. Pacing/timing
2. Proprioception
3. Visual
4. Auditory
5. Tactile

C. Emotional regulation skills

1. Controlling emotions/frustration tolerance
2. Task persistence
3. Responding to feelings of others
4. Using coping/relaxation strategies

D. Cognitive skills

1. Judging
2. Selecting
3. Sequencing
4. Problem solving
5. Attention to task
6. Organizing

E. Communication and social skills

1. Body language and position
2. Personal space, appropriate contact
3. Exchanging information
4. Maintaining appropriate relationships

IX. Client factors—Specific skill requirements

A. Global mental functions

1. Must client be fully oriented?
2. Must client have a stable personality, behavior?
3. Must client have motivation? Impulse control?

B. Specific mental functions

1. How much attention, memory are needed?
2. Must client be able to interpret all sensory stimuli?
3. Will thought disorders interfere?
4. What language ability is required?
5. Are executive functions needed?
6. Is calculation ability required?
7. What motor planning skills are needed? (Is the task familiar or novel?)
8. Must client have intact body image, concept?

C. Sensory functions and pain

1. How much visual acuity and what types of visual perception are needed?
2. How much hearing is needed?
3. How much balance is needed?
4. Must client perceive and respond to pain?
5. Does client need to be able to discriminate other sensory stimuli?
   a. Taste, smell, touch, body movement, temperature, etc.

D. Systems function

1. What is client diagnosis/diagnoses?
2. Will the activity have an effect on respiration, blood pressure, or other cardiac function?
3. Will the activity have an effect on digestive, metabolic, endocrine, or excretory functions?
4. Will the activity have an effect of skin, hair, or nails?

E. Neuromuscular/motor function—See Motor Skills in VIII (A, B, and C)

X. Miscellaneous psychosocial considerations

A. Does the craft provide the opportunity to discover what is valuable to the client?

B. Could the craft contribute to self-esteem? How?

C. Does the craft offer opportunities for affective expression?

1. Hostility/aggression (i.e., motions such as hammering, tearing, piercing)
2. Sadness (i.e., slow movements)
3. Happiness (i.e., pride, hope, laughter)
4. Loving (i.e., stroking, holding)

D. Does the craft provide opportunities for testing reality of the client's own perceptions/beliefs?

a. Is my behavior/perception/belief normal?

E. Is there an opportunity to develop leadership skills while doing the craft?

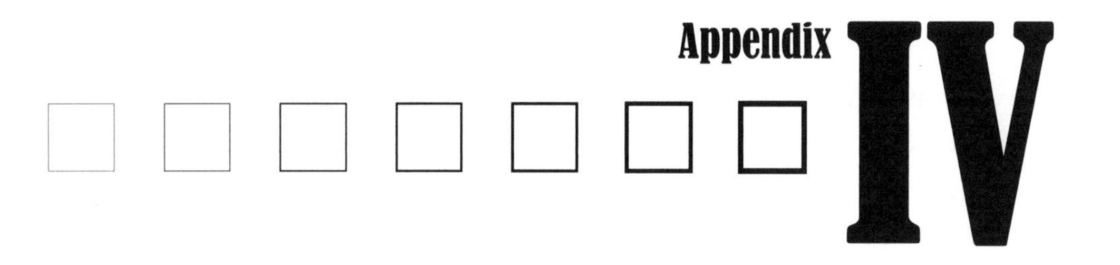

Occupational Therapy Practice Framework Summary

Collaborative Process Model

Evaluation → Intervention → Outcomes

Areas of Occupation

- ADL/self-care: All activities involving care and mobility of self
- IADL: All activities involving care of the home and others, community mobility, and community contact
- Rest and sleep
- Education: Both formal and informal, exploration and participation
- Work: Both paid and volunteer, exploration and performance; also includes retirement issues
- Play: Both exploration and participation
- Leisure: Both exploration and participation
- Social participation: At all levels

Performance Skills				
Motor and Praxis	Sensory-Perceptual	Cognitive	Emotional Regulation	Communication and Social Skills
Strength and effort, posture, mobility, coordination, manipulation, sequencing of motor acts	Receiving, discriminating, and responding to sensory input, including auditory, visual, tactile, proprioceptive, and vestibular	Attending, planning, organizing, sequencing, prioritizing; used in managing daily occupations	Identification, management, and expression of feelings, especially when interacting with others	Verbal and nonverbal behaviors used to communicate with another person

Tubbs, C., & Drake, M. *Crafts and Creative Media in Therapy, Fourth Edition (pp. 249-251).*

Performance Patterns

- Habits—Automatic behavior that is useful, underdeveloped, or overdeveloped
- Routines—Regular behavioral patterns; day-to-day structure
- Rituals—Symbolic; reinforcing of values and beliefs
- Roles—Behavioral sets

Performance Contexts

- Cultural
- Physical
- Social
- Personal
- Temporal
- Virtual

Activity Demands

- Objects and their properties—For example, tools and materials
- Space demands—For example, work area, environmental conditions
- Social demands—For example, rules, expectations
- Sequence and timing—For example, ordered steps, timing
- Required actions—For example, performance skills
- Required body functions—See Client Factors
- Required body structures—See Client Factors

Client Factors

- Values, beliefs, and spirituality:
    - Standards or principles considered worthwhile
    - Cognitive content held as true
    - Search for answers/understanding about life's ultimate questions

Body Functions

- Mental functions
    - Global mental functions such as consciousness, orientation, personality, and drive
- Specific mental function
    - Attention
    - Memory
    - Perception
    - Thought
    - Executive function
    - Motor planning
    - Emotion
    - Self-concept

- Sensory functions and pain
  - Vision
  - Hearing
  - Vestibular
  - Tactile
  - Olfactory
  - Proprioceptive
  - Pain
- Neuromusculoskeletal/movement-related functions
  - Joint mobility
  - Tone, strength, endurance
  - Reflexes, coordination;
  - Gait patterns
- Cardiovascular, hematological, immunological, respiratory
- Voice, digestive, metabolic, endocrine, genitourinary, reproductive
- Skin, hair, and nails

Body Structures

- Nervous system structures
- Peripheral sensory system structures (e.g., eyes and ears)
- Voice/speech system structures
- Internal organ system structures
- Musculoskeletal structures
- Skin and related structures

Reference

American Occupational Therapy Association. (2008). The occupational therapy practice framework: Domain and process (2nd ed.). *American Journal of Occupational Therapy, 62*(6), 625-683.

Index